Treatment of Postoperative Complications after Digestive Surgery

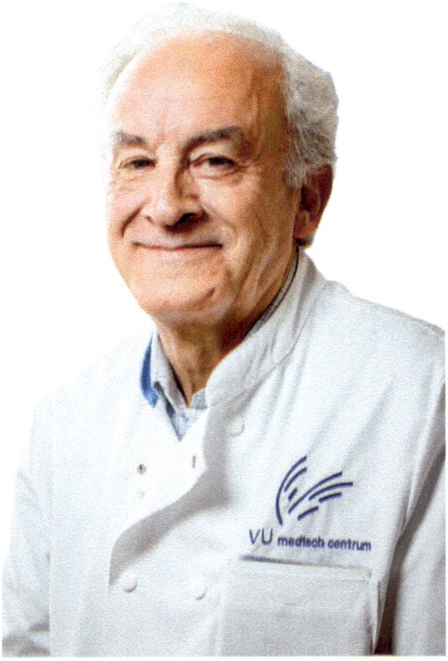

Miguel A. Cuesta

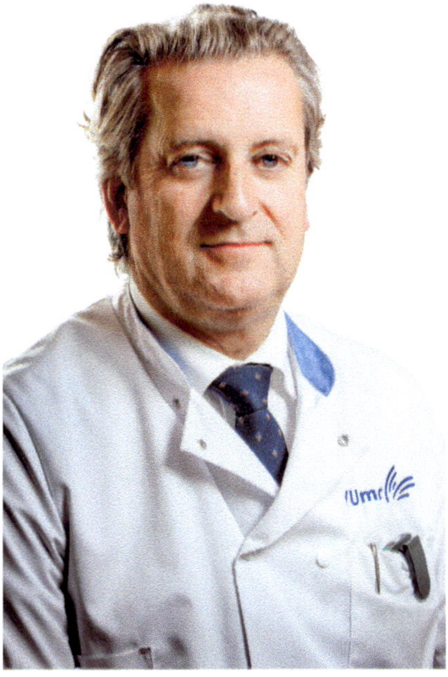

H. Jaap Bonjer

Miguel A. Cuesta • H. Jaap Bonjer
Editors

Treatment of Postoperative Complications after Digestive Surgery

Springer

Editors
Miguel A. Cuesta, MD
Department of Surgery
VU University Medical Center
Amsterdam
The Netherlands

H. Jaap Bonjer, PhD, FRCSC
Department of Surgery
VU University Medical Center
Amsterdam
The Netherlands

ISBN 978-1-4471-4353-6 ISBN 978-1-4471-4354-3 (eBook)
DOI 10.1007/978-1-4471-4354-3
Springer London Heidelberg New York Dordrecht

Library of Congress Control Number: 2013953716

Printed on acid-free paper

Springer is part of Springer Science+Business Media (www.springer.com)

We would like to dedicate this book to all patients who after a skillful and careful surgical intervention had to be treated because of a major complication. They have taught to have skills, complete dedication, compassions and humility

Contents

1 **Postoperative Consequences of Surgical Trauma** 1
Alexander A.F.A. Veenhof, Colin Sietses, and Miguel A. Cuesta

2 **Are Major Complications After Digestive Surgery Preventable?** . . . 7
Thilo Welsch and Markus W. Büchler

3 **The Clavien–Dindo Classification of Surgical Complications** 13
Daniel Dindo

4 **Diagnosis and Treatment of Major Abdominal Complications Is Multidisciplinary Work** 19
Dick J. Gouma

5 **General Principles of Recognition of Major Complications Following Surgery of the Digestive Tract** 27
Suzanne S. Gisbertz, Jennifer Straatman, and Miguel A. Cuesta

6 **Is There Less Morbidity After Laparoscopic Surgery?** 35
Antonio M. de Lacy, Salvadora Delgado, and Miguel A. Cuesta

7 **Is There Less Morbidity After Fast-Track Surgery?** 47
Christine Vermeulen, Willem A. Bemelman, and Miguel A. Cuesta

8 **Prevention and Treatment of Major Complications After Esophageal Surgery** 53
Rachel L.G.M. Blom, Donald L. van der Peet, and Mark I. van Berge Henegouwen

9 **Prevention and Treatment of Major Complications After Gastroduodenal Surgery** 75
Jose Luis Garcia Sabrido and Wenceslao Vasquez Jimenez

10 **Prevention and Treatment of Major Complications After Bariatric Surgery** 101
Frits J. Berends and Ignace M.C. Janssen

11 **Prevention and Treatment of Major Complications After Liver Surgery (and Liver Transplantation)** 123
Pascual Parrilla Paricio, Ricardo Robles Campos, and Francisco Sánchez Bueno

12 **Prevention and Treatment of Major Complications After Cholecystectomy** 143
Klaske A.C. Booij, Dirk J. Gouma, Thomas M. van Gulik, and Olivier R.C. Busch

13 **Prevention and Treatment of Major Complications After Surgery of Klatskin Tumors** 161
Geert Kazemier and Miguel A. Cuesta

14 **Prevention and Treatment of Major Complications After Duodeno-pancreatic Head Surgery** 171
Johanna A.M.G. Tol, Thomas M. van Gulik, Olivier R.C. Busch, and Dirk J. Gouma

15 **Treatment of Major Complications of Acute Pancreatitis** 191
Hein Gooszen

16 **Prevention and Treatment of Major Complications after Surgery of the Spleen, Adrenal Glands, and Distal Pancreatectomy** 199
Renske Konings, H. Jaap Bonjer, and Geert Kazemier

17 **Prevention and Treatment of Complications after Small Bowel Surgery and Appendicectomy** 209
Donald L. van der Peet and Miguel A. Cuesta

18 **Prevention and Treatment of Major Complications After Laparoscopic Ileocecal and Right Colectomy** 217
W. Jeroen Meijerink

19 **Prevention and Treatment of Major Complications After Left Colon, Sigmoid, and Rectal Surgery** 229
Cesar Reategui, Badma Bashankaev, and Steven D. Wexner

20 **Prevention and Treatment of Major Postoperative Complications After Laparoscopic Colorectal Resections** 247
Willem A. Bemelman

21 **Prevention and Treatment of Postoperative Complications After Stoma Surgery** 259
Han C. Kuijpers and Sigrun Klok

22 **Prevention and Treatment Complications in Proctology** 267
Christopher Thorn and Janindra Warusavitarne

23 Prevention and Treatment of Major Complications After Closure of Abdominal Wall and Repair of Abdominal Wall Hernias 287
Salvador Morales-Conde, María Socas, and Antonio Barranco

24 Treatment of Open Abdomen Approach 313
Miguel A. Cuesta and Jurriaan B. Tuynman

25 Establishing the Pneumoperitoneum and Closing the Trocar Sites During Laparoscopic Surgery 319
Miguel A. Cuesta and H. Jaap Bonjer

26 Final Considerations 323
Miguel A. Cuesta and H. Jaap Bonjer

Index 325

Contributors

Antonio Barranco Department of Surgery, Hospital Universitario Virgen del Rocío, Sevilla, Spain

Badma Bashankaev Department of Colorectal Surgery, Digestive Disease Center, Cleveland Clinic Florida, Weston, FL, USA

Willem A. Bemelman, MD Department of Surgery, Academic Medical Center, Amsterdam, The Netherlands

Frits J. Berends Department of Surgery, Rijnstate Hospital, Arnhem, The Netherlands

Rachel L.G.M. Blom Department of Surgery, Atrium Medical Center, Heerlen, The Netherlands

H. Jaap Bonjer, PhD, FRCSC Department of Surgery, VU University Medical Center, Amsterdam, The Netherlands

Klaske A.C. Booij Department of Surgery, Academic Medical Center, University of Amsterdam, Amsterdam, The Netherlands

Markus W. Büchler Department of General, Visceral and Transplantation Surgery, University of Heidelberg, Heidelberg, Germany

Francisco Sánchez Bueno, MD Department of Surgery and Liver Transplantation Unit, Virgen de la Arrixaca University Hospital, Murcia, Spain

Olivier R.C. Busch, MD, PhD Department of Surgery, Academic Medical Center, University of Amsterdam, Amsterdam, The Netherlands

Ricardo Robles Campos Department of Surgery and Liver Transplantation Unit, Virgen de la Arrixaca University Hospital, Murcia, Spain

Miguel A. Cuesta, MD Department of Surgery, VU University Medical Center, Amsterdam, The Netherlands

Antonio M. de Lacy Department of Gastrointestinal Surgery, Institute of Digestive Diseases, Hospital Clinic, University of Barcelona, Barcelona, Spain

Salvadora Delgado Department of Gastrointestinal Surgery, Institute of Digestive and Metabolic Diseases, Hospital Clínic of Barcelona, Barcelona, Spain

Daniel Dindo, MD Department of Visceral, Thoracic and Vascular Surgery, Triemli Hospital, Zurich, Switzerland

Suzanne S. Gisbertz Department of Surgery, Academic Medical Center, Amsterdam, The Netherlands

Hein Gooszen, MD Department of Operating Room/Evidence Based Surgery, Radboud University Nijmegen Medical Centre, Nijmegen, The Netherlands

Dick J. Gouma, MD Department of Surgery, Academic Medical Center, Amsterdam, The Netherlands

Ignace M.C. Janssen Department of Surgery, Rijnstate Hospital, Arnhem, The Netherlands

Geert Kazemier Department of Surgery, VU University Medical Center, Amsterdam, The Netherlands

Sigrun Klok Stoma Care, Gelderse Vallei Hospital, Ede, Gelderland, The Netherlands

Renske Konings Department of Surgery, VU University Medical Center, Amsterdam, The Netherlands

Han C. Kuijpers, MD, PhD Department of Gastrointestinal Surgery, Gelderse Vallei Hospital, Ede, Gelderland, The Netherlands

W. Jeroen Meijerink, MD Department of Surgery, VU University Medical Center, Amsterdam, The Netherlands

Salvador Morales-Conde Department of Surgery, Hospital Universitario Virgen del Rocio, Sevilla, Spain

Pascual Parrilla Paricio Department of Surgery and Liver Transplantation Unit, Virgen de la Arrixaca University Hospital, Murcia, Spain

Cesar Reategui Department of Colorectal Surgery, Digestive Disease Center, Cleveland Clinic Florida, Weston, FL, USA

Jose Luis Garcia Sabrido Department of General Surgery III and Liver Transplant Unit, Hospital General Universitario Gregorio Marañón, Madrid, Spain

Colin Sietses Department of Surgery, Gelderse Vallei Hospital, Ede, The Netherlands

María Socas Department of Surgery, Hospital Universitario Virgen del Rocio, Sevilla, Spain

Jennifer Straatman Department of Surgery, VU University Medical Center, Amsterdam, The Netherlands

Johanna A.M.G. Tol Department of Surgery, Academic Medical Center, University of Amsterdam, Amsterdam, The Netherlands

Christopher Thorn Department of Colorectal Surgery, St Mark's Hospital Harrow, London, UK

Jurriaan Tuynman Department of Surgery, VU University Medical Center, Amsterdam, The Netherlands

Mark I. van Berge Henegouwen, MD, PhD Department of Surgery, Academic Medical Center, Amsterdam, The Netherlands

Thomas M. van Gulik Department of Surgery, Academic Medical Center, University of Amsterdam, Amsterdam, The Netherlands

Donald L. van der Peet, MD Department of Surgery, VU University Medical Center, Amsterdam, The Netherlands

Wenceslao Vasquez Jimenez, MD, PhD Department of Surgery III, Gregorio Marañon Hospital, Madrid, Spain

Alexander A.F.A. Veenhof Department of Surgery, VU University Medical Center, Amsterdam, The Netherlands

Christine Vermeulen Department of Surgery, VU University Medical Center, Amsterdam, The Netherlands

Janindra Warusavitarne Department of Colorectal Surgery, St Mark's Hospital Harrow, London, UK

Thilo Welsch Department of General, Visceral and Transplantation Surgery, University of Heidelberg, Heidelberg, Germany

Steven D. Wexner, MD, PhD(Hon), FRCS, FRCS(Ed) Department of Colorectal Surgery, Digestive Disease Center, Cleveland Clinic Florida, Academic Affairs Florida Atlantic University College of Medicine, Clinical Education Florida International University College of Medicine, Weston, FL, USA

Introduction

Surgeons continually strive to provide the best care possible to their patients. Employing smaller incisions to reduce postoperative pain and lower the risk of wound infection and incisional hernia, improving technology of surgical instruments to facilitate safer dissection of tissues, and utilizing imaging techniques during surgery to perform more precise resections are some examples of the focus on enhancing quality of surgery. Major progress has been realized during the past decades; diagnostic invasive surgical procedures have been replaced by a variety of imaging techniques which provide high-resolution three-dimensional insight in the anatomical aspects of the disease allowing surgical teams to refine their surgical approach; large abdominal incisions have been replaced by stab incisions allowing patients to ambulate very early after surgery and resume their activities within days instead of long postoperative stays in the hospital, endoluminal and image-guided percutaneous placement of stents or drains to relieve obstructions or fluid collections which impede recovery of the patient.

Quality of surgery has increased greatly but many surgical interventions are still hampered by imperfect outcomes coined "complications," a term whose definition is subject to debate. Francis D. Moore described in his book *A Miracle and a Privilege* the introduction by Ernest Amory Codman of a system for classifying imperfect outcomes, as being due to errors in diagnosis, technique, or judgement. Moreover, these were sharply differentiated from a group identified as patient's disease. This classification provides an excellent platform for further improvement. Intricate knowledge of the disease the patient presents with is of paramount importance.

The natural course of the disease, the impact of the disease on other organ systems, and the expected changes after surgical intervention are front and center during assessment of the patient and determination of a plan on how to best manage the patient. This complex process requires collective intelligence of all those healthcare professionals who have profound knowledge of various aspects of the disease and participate in the care of the patient. These multidisciplinary meetings are the gold standard of surgical practice of the twenty-first century.

Preparation and anticipation are key to successful surgery. In-depth understanding of the anatomy, carefully determining the positioning of the patient, surgical approach, exposure and dissection, transection and ligation techniques, and, of great importance, discussing these with all members of the surgical and anesthesiological team are some of the elements which will determine the course of the surgery and the recovery after surgery.

Structured checklists have been implemented progressively to standardize and document the complex preoperative, intraoperative, and postoperative processes.

Management of the patient after surgery requires a team of health-care professionals that assesses the patient frequently and provides the knowledge and skills required to accelerate recovery on one hand and detect factors interfering with recovery on the other hand.

The objective of this book, *Postoperative Complications After Digestive Surgery*, presented in two volumes, is to share the expertise of more than 50 highly dedicated and experience surgeons and surgical residents to allow the reader to learn the lessons learned by their teachers and colleagues. The first volume, the main textbook, comprises 25 chapters with the focus on prevention and treatment of major complications by carefully proceeding through assessment, planning and preparation, performing surgery, and managing the patient after surgery.

In the second part, a more practical and descriptive volume comprises more than 100 case studies bringing daily surgical practice to the reader and provides a wealth of learning opportunities. Extensive imaging documentation of the different cases is provided along with drawing pictures of the pathology with great attention to anatomical detail. In this digital age, there appears to be some hesitation to choose pencil over mouse. However, translating images and anatomical experience into drawings is invaluable in preparing the surgeon's mind and that of the other members of the surgical team. Wendy Vetter, Dana Hamers, and Miguel Cuesta have illustrated selected cases which provide great insight and hopefully inspire the reader to pick up colored pencils.

We hope that this book will enrich the knowledge and understanding of surgeons and surgical residents around the world and will inspire them to contribute to improving surgery continually.

Amsterdam, The Netherlands Miguel A. Cuesta
Amsterdam, The Netherlands H. Jaap Bonjer

Chapter 1
Postoperative Consequences of Surgical Trauma

Alexander A.F.A. Veenhof, Colin Sietses, and Miguel A. Cuesta

Keywords Laparoscopic surgery • Stress response • C-reactive protein • Postoperative course • Immunosuppression • Operative trauma

Every surgical trauma is followed by unanticipated side effects such as pain and infection. A theory regarding the onset of these side effects is the surgical stress response with subsequent increased demands on the patient's reserves and immune status. A demand on organ functions is increased following surgery and is thought to be mediated by trauma-induced endocrine and metabolic changes. To circumvent this problem and reduce surgical trauma, the first minimally invasive colectomy was described by Jacobs et al. in 1991 [1]. Since, many studies have shown the clinical short-term benefits for laparoscopic colectomy over open procedures without compromising oncological outcome [2–5].

HLA-DR expression on monocytes is correlated to the competence of a patient's specific immune response. C-reactive protein levels are associated with postoperative infectious complications. Interleukin-6 levels are associated with postoperative complication rates and are a predictor of morbidity following surgical intervention. Since the introduction of laparoscopic colectomies, several studies have studied these parameters and compared the postoperative stress response between open and minimally invasive procedures. Wu et al. [6] and Harmon et al. [7] both described lower interleukin-6 levels following laparoscopic colectomy.

A.A.F.A. Veenhof • M.A. Cuesta, MD (✉)
Department of Surgery, VU University Medical Center, Amsterdam, The Netherlands
e-mail: ma.cuesta@vumc.nl

C. Sietses
Department of Surgery, Gelderse Vallei Hospital, Ede, The Netherlands

M.A. Cuesta, H.J. Bonjer (eds.), *Treatment of Postoperative Complications after Digestive Surgery*, DOI 10.1007/978-1-4471-4354-3_1,

Both interleukin-6 levels and C-reactive protein levels were found to be lower for laparoscopic colectomies by Schwenk et al. [8]. Recently, this institution published a series of 40 patients in which surgical stress response was compared between laparoscopic and open total mesorectal excision (TME) [9]. Only a significant reduction in surgical stress response regarding HLA-DR expression in monocytes and interleukin-6 levels could be found for the laparoscopic TME 2 h postoperatively. No differences regarding leukocytes, monocytes, C-reactive protein, interleukin-8, cortisol, growth hormone, and prolactin could be found at 24 and 72 h postoperatively, concluding that only a short-term benefit in surgical stress response for laparoscopic TME procedures could be proven.

Recently, the introduction of fast-track postoperative care by Kehlet [10–12] has revived the discussion regarding postoperative immune and stress response. By high thoracic epidural anesthesia, the theory is that patient's immune and stress status is reduced, therefore facilitating an enhanced postoperative recovery when compared to traditional care. Since the introduction of the fast-track multimodality postoperative care, no articles have been published to investigate the stress response and immune function between fast-track and conventional care. Therefore, two surgical departments in Amsterdam, the AMC and the VUmc, conducted a randomized trial as substudy of the LAFA trial [13] comparing open versus laparoscopic colectomy with fast-track or conventional postoperative care [14]. Patients with nonmetastasized colon cancer were randomized to laparoscopic or open colectomy with fast track or standard care. Blood samples were taken preoperatively (baseline), 1, 2, 24, and 72 h following surgery (Fig. 1.1). Systemic HLA-DR expression, C-reactive protein, IL-6, growth hormone, prolactin, and cortisol were analyzed in these blood samples. Seventy-nine patients were randomized, and patient characteristics were comparable. A significant difference in HLA-DR expression on monocytes (and therefore immune competence) was observed between the four groups (Fig. 1.2). Patient with laparoscopy and fast-track perioperative care remained the best immune competent with repeated measures of 2-way analysis of variance showing this could be attributed to type of surgery and not aftercare. Patients with open surgery and standard care were found to have higher postoperative C-reactive protein and interleukin-6 levels when compared to the other groups (Figs. 1.3 and 1.4). Once again, following repeated measures of 2-way analysis of variance, this could be attributed to type of surgery and not aftercare. Concluding, the accelerated response reported following fast-track perioperative care [10–12] could not be explained by a better preserved postoperative immune competence or reduced surgical stress response in the present study. Laparoscopy seemed to better preserve immune status and reduce postoperative surgical trauma. On the other hand, in the present study, no clinical benefits such as less postoperative complications could be found.

The discussion for a substrate as to why laparoscopy and fast-track surgery has clinical advantages remains. Up to date little evidence exists regarding a reduced postoperative surgical stress response as an explanation for enhanced patient recovery following laparoscopic colorectal surgery with or without fast-track perioperative care.

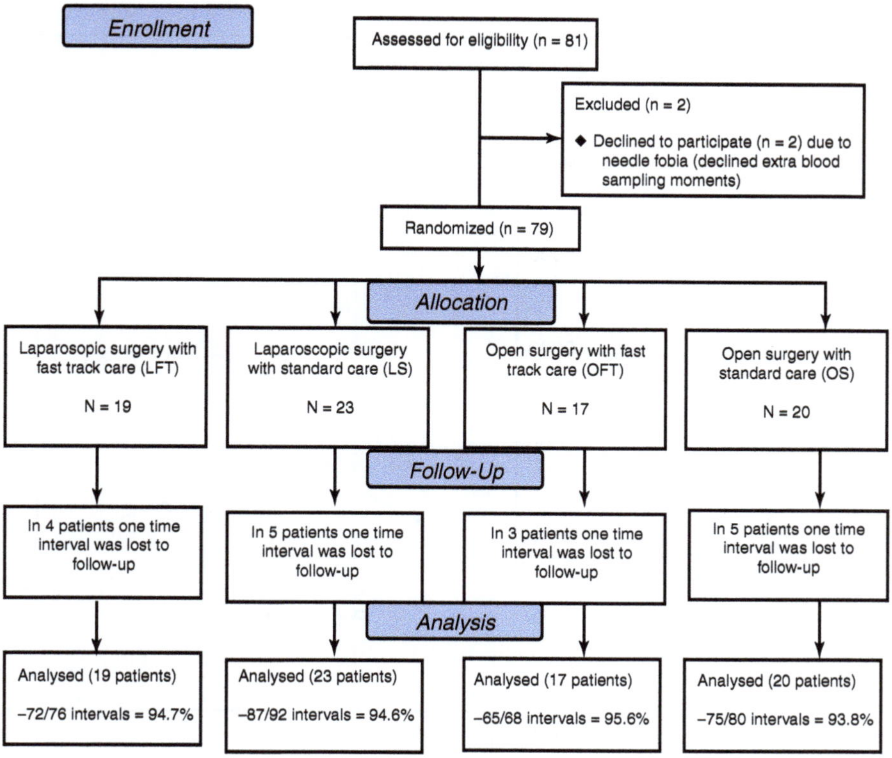

Fig. 1.1 Consort algorithm randomization

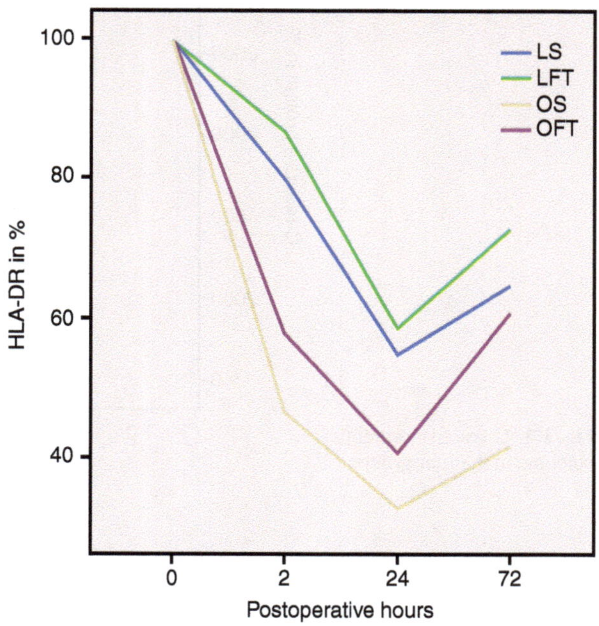

Fig. 1.2 HLA-DR outcome in the four groups

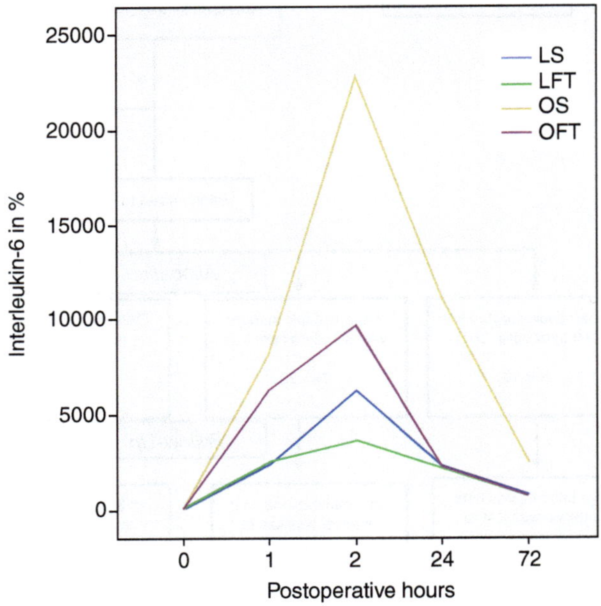

Fig. 1.3 Interleukin-6 outcome in the four groups

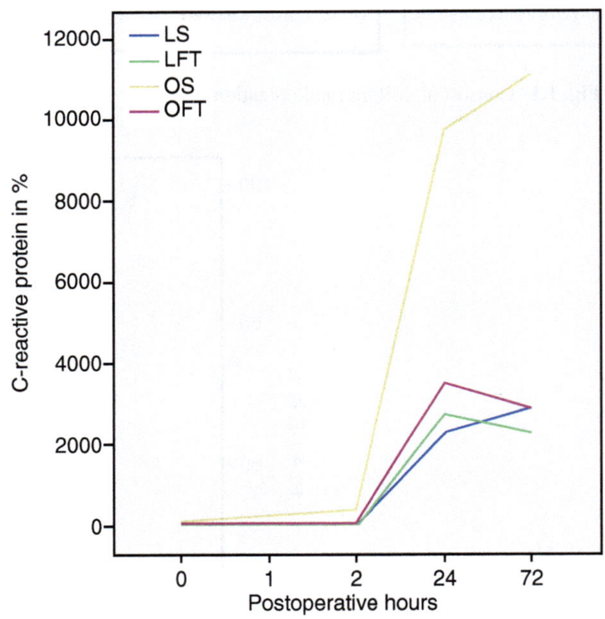

Fig. 1.4 C-reactive protein outcome in the four groups

References

1. Jacobs M, Verdeja JC, Goldstein HS. Minimally invasive colon resection (laparoscopic colectomy). Surg Laparosc Endosc. 1991;1:144–50.
2. Lacy AM, García-Valdecasas JC, Delgado S, Castells A, Taurá P, Piqué JM, Visa J. Laparoscopy-assisted colectomy versus open colectomy for treatment of non-metastatic colon cancer: a randomised trial. Lancet. 2002;359:2224–9.
3. Nelson H, Sargent DJ, Wieand S, Fleshman J, Anvari M, Stryker SJ, Beart RW, Hellinger M, Flanagan R, Peters W, Ota D. A comparison of laparoscopically assisted and open colectomy for colon cancer. N Engl J Med. 2004;350:2050–9.
4. The COlon cancer Laparoscopic or Open Resection Study Group. Laparoscopic surgery versus open surgery for colon cancer: short-term outcomes of a randomised trial. Lancet Oncol. 2005; 6:477–84.
5. Weeks JC, Nelson H, Gelber S, Sargent D, Schroeder G. Short-term quality-of-life outcomes following laparoscopic-assisted colectomy vs open colectomy for colon cancer: a randomized trial. JAMA. 2002;287:321–8.
6. Wu FPK, Sietses C, von Blomberg BME, van Leeuwen PAM, Meijer S, Cuesta MA. Systemic and peritoneal inflammatory response after laparoscopic or conventional colon resection in cancer patients: a prospective, randomized trial. Dis Colon Rectum. 2003;46:147–55.
7. Harmon GD, Senagore AJ, Kilbride MJ, Warzynski MJ. Interleukin-6 response to laparoscopic and open colectomy. Dis Colon Rectum. 1994;37:754–9.
8. Schwenk W, Jacobi C, Mansmann U, Bohm B, Muller JM. Inflammatory response after laparoscopic and conventional colorectal resections – results of a prospective randomized trial. Langenbeck's Arch Surg. 2000;385:2–9.
9. Veenhof AA, Sietses C, von Blomberg BM, Van Hoogstraten IM, vd Pas H, Meijerink WJ, vd Peet DL, vd Tol MP, Bonjer HJ, Cuesta MA. The surgical stress response and postoperative immune function after laparoscopic or conventional total mesorectal excision in rectal cancer: a randomized trial. Int J Colorectal Dis. 2011;26:53–9.
10. Wilmore DW, Kehlet H. Management of patients in fast track surgery. BMJ. 2001;322: 473–6.
11. Kehlet H. Fast-track colorectal surgery. Lancet. 2008;371:791–3.
12. Kehlet H, Wilmore DW. Evidence-based surgical care and evolution of fast-track surgery. Ann Surg. 2008;248:189–98.
13. Vlug MS, Wind J, Hollmann MW. Laparoscopy in combination with fast track multimodal management is the best perioperative strategy in patients undergoing colonic surgery: a randomized clinical trial (LAFA-study). Ann Surg. 2011;254:868–75.
14. Veenhof AA, Vlug MS, vd Pas MH, et al. Surgical stress response and postoperative immune function after laparoscopy or open surgery with fast track or standard perioperative care; a randomized trial. Ann Surg. 2012;255:216–21.

Chapter 2
Are Major Complications After Digestive Surgery Preventable?

Thilo Welsch and Markus W. Büchler

Keywords Digestive Surgery • Complications • Morbidity rates • Preoperative setting • Surgical technique • Perioperative setting • Postoperative setting • Prevention

About Morbidity Rates and Definitions

Whenever questions arise about major complications after digestive surgery, the actual morbidity rates of the respective types of surgery are warranted and important for the judgment of the clinical relevance and the continuous improvement of surgical management. There have been major advances in the reduction of postoperative complications following digestive surgery in the past years. The reasons for the improved outcome reside—beside others—in improved diagnostic tests leading to early intervention and a more precise surgical approach, better neoadjuvant treatment options, and improved peri- and postoperative care and in modified and innovative surgical techniques or devices. Surgical clinical trials have provided evidence of how to treat and prevent complications and abandoned some traditional treatment protocols that clearly had no benefit for the surgical outcome. A breakthrough in reduction of postoperative morbidity and improved surgical outcome has been provoked by the centralization of complex operations at specialized surgical high-volume centers.

Despite all medical advances, we are still lacking accurate morbidity rates of the various digestive surgical procedures when reviewing the literature. For example, anastomotic leak rates differ between 3 and 23 % after anterior rectal resection and the pancreatic fistula rates between 2 and 20 % after pancreatic resection [1, 2] depending on multiple different definitions applied in each study. This has lead to the initiation and development of internationally accepted consensus definitions for

T. Welsch • M.W. Büchler (✉)
Department of General, Visceral and Transplantation Surgery,
University of Heidelberg, Heidelberg, Germany
e-mail: markus.buechler@med.uni-heidelberg.de

M.A. Cuesta, H.J. Bonjer (eds.), *Treatment of Postoperative Complications after Digestive Surgery*, DOI 10.1007/978-1-4471-4354-3_2,

major postoperative complications that are now published for pancreatic, hepatobiliary, and rectal surgery [1–5]. Those consensus definitions also provide a discrimination of the complications into different grades, according to the clinical impact. The term "major" complication is probably best embodied by grade B and C complications based on the new consensus definitions: grade B in general implies a change in the postoperative management including interventions except re-laparotomy, and grade C complications require re-laparotomy. Grade A complications do neither necessitate a change in the clinical management nor prolong the hospital stay of the patients.

It is in the nature of every profession to strive for continuously improved outcome. All through the history of surgery, and up to now, surgeons would have positively answered the question if major complications after digestive surgery are preventable, and every surgeon would have thought about the well-known paradigma of standard surgical care that were considered lege artis, that were trained, and that were known to prevent complication rates.

The present synoptic chapter aims not to list basic surgical principles but to highlight certain fields, perioperative measures, and surgical techniques that suggest a further prospective reduction in postoperative morbidity if implemented in the broad surgical community. The following chapters of the book then provide insight into current state-of-the-art prevention and management of the various complications of digestive surgery.

Prevention of Major Complications: The Preoperative Setting

The last decade has shown that patient referral into specialized surgical high-volume centers for complex and high-risk visceral surgery is a key factor influencing postoperative outcome, i.e., morbidity, mortality, and long-term survival in case of oncologic patients [6]. Despite an observable shift of complex surgical cases to high-volume centers, there is still significant space for quality improvement through further centralization and training of surgeons from low-volume hospitals. Specialized and procedure-oriented training of low-volume medical staff by experienced high-volume surgeons has improved the quality of rectal cancer surgery in the Netherlands [7, 8] and will prospectively result in lower complication rates if this model is transferred to and practiced in other fields of visceral surgery.

Surgeons can further prevent complications through optimization of patient selection and the use of individualized treatment plans. For years, patients with necrotizing pancreatitis and infected necrosis were classically treated surgical with open necrosectomy and lavage. A Dutch trial now revealed that a minimally invasive step-up approach tailored to the individual severely ill patients with necrotizing pancreatitis results in significantly less major complications [9], exemplifying the need to evaluate the right treatment for each individual patient. Another randomized controlled landmark trial focused on patients with pancreatic head tumors and demonstrated that routine preoperative biliary stenting in jaundiced patients with pancreatic head tumors provides no benefit but increases the rate of postoperative complications [10].

Likewise, patients with impaired liver function (e.g., cirrhosis) are at increased risk to develop postoperative hepatic failure [11] and other severe, sometimes lethal, postoperative complications after hepatectomy but also after minor surgical procedures. Identification of patients at risk for postoperative liver failure is often demanding, but the ongoing development of novel diagnostic tests (e.g., based on the metabolism of methacetin [12]) suggests further progress towards the optimal indication of the type and extent of surgery or minimally invasive intervention in patients with impaired liver function.

Much is unknown about the best physical and nutritional status of the patients before undergoing visceral surgery. It sounds logic that improvement of, e.g., cardiac, pulmonary, or renal insufficiency, hepatic steatosis, extreme overweight, or physical activity prior to surgery can lower postoperative complications, but such preoperative programs are not broadly carried out and are difficult to realize and implement in daily practice. Heterogeneous results had been reported for the use of perioperative immunonutrition until a recent meta-analysis came to the conclusion that immunonutrition did positively influence gastrointestinal surgery and lowered postoperative complications [13].

Colon surgery has ever been one of the most frequently performed operations in gastrointestinal surgery, and there is still a debate about the need of preoperative mechanical bowel preparation. Randomized trials have yielded convincing evidence that preoperative mechanical bowel preparation in elective colon surgery offers no advantage with regard to postoperative complications and is no longer indicated [14]. The same results are expected for lower colorectal resections [15], but still many surgeons perform routine bowel preparation for all colorectal cases illustrating our skepticism towards advanced treatment protocols [16].

Prevention of Major Complications: Surgical Technique

The various anastomoses of the gastrointestinal tract are broadly considered as the most critical steps for a successful operation and postoperative course. Several different suture techniques, material, or devices were introduced, but none proved to be clearly superior. Besides a correct suture line, the principal factors mandatory for anastomotic healing remain a tension-free alignment of the anastomotic ends and a good blood supply and perfusion. Not long ago, we questioned elementary surgical steps that we encounter every day, i.e., if low anterior resection of the rectum necessitates the simultaneous creation of a protective stoma, if abdominal wound drains should be placed, or how to close the midline laparotomy. Randomized controlled trials have now established some degree of evidence. The rate of anastomotic leak after low anterior resection of the rectum can be significantly reduced by creation of a diverting stoma [17]. We have also learned that routine placement of abdominal wound drains is not beneficial in many elective visceral surgery cases (e.g., cholecystectomy, liver or colorectal surgery [18–20]) but that late removal of the drains increases the risk of septic complications or even pancreatic fistulas [21].

Moreover, subcutaneous drains do not prevent the development of surgical site infections.

Every day, the visceral surgeon performs the closure of the abdomen, but which technique and suture material are ideally used to prevent midline hernia? Once again, a systematic approach of randomized controlled trials and systematic analysis has provided an answer. Based on a meta-analysis, the elective midline laparotomy should be closed with a continuous, slowly absorbable suture material (evidence level 1) [22]. Most of those trials addressing the use of drains or suture material are however founded on elective procedures, and few evidence is available for treatment of emergency cases that per se have a higher postoperative morbidity.

Prevention of Major Complications: Peri- and Postoperative Setting

The successful surgical outcome is well influenced by the peri- and postoperative setting and requires a perfect interplay of the various disciplines involved in the patient's care, such as anesthesiology, radiology, the nursing staff, and physiotherapists.

For instance, the perioperative administered amount of fluids can significantly affect the postoperative outcome. Studies in colorectal surgery indicated that restrictive and goal-directed (controlled by esophageal Doppler-derived variables) fluid administration reduces the postoperative morbidity [23]. Blood transfusions probably also have a detrimental effect on the postoperative outcome. In the further postoperative course, especially after gastrointestinal surgery, patients are more and more subjected to so-called fast track or early recovery after surgery (ERAS) protocols. These protocols are a multimodal approach and combine restrictive fluid administration with optimized (epidural) analgesia, early forced mobilization, and early oral feeding beginning on the day of operation. The fast-track protocol has shown to significantly reduce postoperative complications and to shorten the length of hospital stay [24]. Patients after resection of pancreatic malignancy further benefit from prophylactic administration of somatostatin analogues that can additionally lower the overall morbidity and pancreatic fistula rate [25].

In summary, this concise update on evidence in gastrointestinal surgery substantiates that certain major complications after digestive surgery are certainly preventable and that further improvement of surgical treatment prompts the continuous generation of evidence by excellent randomized controlled trials in the future. Often, clinical trials evaluating traditional standard practice reveal surprising results and sometimes provide milestone advances in medical care. Finally, all surgeons should be encouraged to organize and participate in morbidity and mortality (M&M) conferences that immensely contribute to the continuing education of surgeons. M&M conferences should be standard integrated into every surgical center aiming to improve patient care and safety.

References

1. Rahbari NN, Weitz J, Hohenberger W, Heald RJ, Moran B, Ulrich A, et al. Definition and grading of anastomotic leakage following anterior resection of the rectum: a proposal by the International Study Group of Rectal Cancer. Surgery. 2010;147:339–51.
2. Bassi C, Dervenis C, Butturini G, Fingerhut A, Yeo C, Izbicki J, et al. Postoperative pancreatic fistula: an international study group (ISGPF) definition. Surgery. 2005;138:8–13.
3. Koch M, Garden OJ, Padbury R, Rahbari NN, Adam R, Capussotti L, et al. Bile leakage after hepatobiliary and pancreatic surgery: A definition and grading of severity by the International Study Group of Liver Surgery. Surgery. 2011;149:680–8.
4. Wente MN, Bassi C, Dervenis C, Fingerhut A, Gouma DJ, Izbicki JR, et al. Delayed gastric emptying (DGE) after pancreatic surgery: a suggested definition by the International Study Group of Pancreatic Surgery (ISGPS). Surgery. 2007;142:761–8.
5. Wente MN, Veit JA, Bassi C, Dervenis C, Fingerhut A, Gouma DJ, et al. Post-pancreatectomy hemorrhage (PPH): an International Study Group of Pancreatic Surgery (ISGPS) definition. Surgery. 2007;142:20–5.
6. Learn PA, Bach PB. A decade of mortality reductions in major oncologic surgery: the impact of centralization and quality improvement. Med Care. 2010;48:1041–9.
7. Kapiteijn E, Putter H, van de Velde CJ. Impact of the introduction and training of total mesorectal excision on recurrence and survival in rectal cancer in The Netherlands. Br J Surg. 2002;89:1142–9.
8. van Gijn W, Krijnen P, Lemmens VE, den Dulk M, Putter H, van de Velde CJ. Quality assurance in rectal cancer treatment in the Netherlands: a catch up compared to colon cancer treatment. Eur J Surg Oncol. 2010;36:340–4.
9. van Santvoort HC, Besselink MG, Bakker OJ, Hofker HS, Boermeester MA, Dejong CH, et al. A step-up approach or open necrosectomy for necrotizing pancreatitis. N Engl J Med. 2010;362:1491–502.
10. van der Gaag NA, Rauws EA, van Eijck CH, Bruno MJ, van der Harst E, Kubben FJ, et al. Preoperative biliary drainage for cancer of the head of the pancreas. N Engl J Med. 2010;362:129–37.
11. Rahbari NN, Garden OJ, Padbury R, Brooke-Smith M, Crawford M, Adam R, et al. Posthepatectomy liver failure: A definition and grading by the International Study Group of Liver Surgery (ISGLS). Surgery. 2011;149:713–24.
12. Stockmann M, Lock JF, Riecke B, Heyne K, Martus P, Fricke M, et al. Prediction of postoperative outcome after hepatectomy with a new bedside test for maximal liver function capacity. Ann Surg. 2009;250:119–25.
13. Cerantola Y, Hubner M, Grass F, Demartines N, Schafer M. Immunonutrition in gastrointestinal surgery. Br J Surg. 2011;98:37–48.
14. Slim K, Vicaut E, Launay-Savary MV, Contant C, Chipponi J. Updated systematic review and meta-analysis of randomized clinical trials on the role of mechanical bowel preparation before colorectal surgery. Ann Surg. 2009;249:203–9.
15. Van't Sant HP, Weidema WF, Hop WC, Oostvogel HJ, Contant CM. The influence of mechanical bowel preparation in elective lower colorectal surgery. Ann Surg. 2010;251:59–63.
16. Businger A, Grunder G, Guenin MO, Ackermann C, Peterli R, von Flue M. Mechanical bowel preparation and antimicrobial prophylaxis in elective colorectal surgery in Switzerland – a survey. Langenbecks Arch Surg. 2010;396:107–13.
17. Ulrich AB, Seiler C, Rahbari N, Weitz J, Buchler MW. Diverting stoma after low anterior resection: more arguments in favor. Dis Colon Rectum. 2009;52:412–8.
18. Gurusamy KS, Samraj K. Routine abdominal drainage for uncomplicated open cholecystectomy. Cochrane Database Syst Rev. 2007;CD006003.
19. Gurusamy KS, Samraj K, Davidson BR. Routine abdominal drainage for uncomplicated liver resection. Cochrane Database Syst Rev. 2007;CD006232.

20. Jesus EC, Karliczek A, Matos D, Castro AA, Atallah AN. Prophylactic anastomotic drainage for colorectal surgery. Cochrane Database Syst Rev. 2004;CD002100.
21. Bassi C, Molinari E, Malleo G, Crippa S, Butturini G, Salvia R, et al. Early versus late drain removal after standard pancreatic resections: results of a prospective randomized trial. Ann Surg. 2010;252:207–14.
22. Diener MK, Voss S, Jensen K, Buchler MW, Seiler CM. Elective midline laparotomy closure: the INLINE systematic review and meta-analysis. Ann Surg. 2010;251:843–56.
23. Rahbari NN, Zimmermann JB, Schmidt T, Koch M, Weigand MA, Weitz J. Meta-analysis of standard, restrictive and supplemental fluid administration in colorectal surgery. Br J Surg. 2009;96:331–41.
24. Muller S, Zalunardo MP, Hubner M, Clavien PA, Demartines N. A fast-track program reduces complications and length of hospital stay after open colonic surgery. Gastroenterology. 2009;136:842–7.
25. Gurusamy KS, Koti R, Fusai G, Davidson BR. Somatostatin analogues for pancreatic surgery. Cochrane Database Syst Rev. 2010;CD008370.

Chapter 3
The Clavien–Dindo Classification of Surgical Complications

Daniel Dindo

Keywords Clavien–Dindo classification • Surgical complications • Quality assurance • Morbidity • Mortality • Classifications • Medical quality

Quality assurance programs are well established in industry since decades. In the early 1950s, research in quality assessment has been first developed in Japan greatly having contributed to the success of this nation. Only many years later, the philosophy of improving quality by continuous measurement of specific outcome parameters has reached the Western industry. In medicine, however, a long time has elapsed until these principles were adopted. The lack of true competition between health-care providers has alleviated the motivation to develop quality assessment programs. Rising costs and constrained resources in health-care systems all over the world and evidence of variations in clinical practice have now triggered the interest and the development of such programs in health care. By tracking the hospitals' performances, surgical morbidity and mortality could be decreased [1]. Moreover, outcome data are starting to be publicly reported in different countries what is considered to constitute a powerful market force towards a higher standard of care at lower costs. This development is driven also by patients who are today well informed about their diseases seeking the best possible treatment. However, reliable outcome data is crucial to improve surgical performance and for benchmarking.

According to Donabedian, medical quality is determined by structure, process, and outcome [2]. In surgery, outcome is still the most frequently used indicator of surgical quality. However, there is still a lack of a precise definition of a "good" or "bad" surgical outcome. In 1992, it was proposed that "negative outcome" should be subdivided into *complication, failure to cure,* and *sequelae* [3]. Complications were defined as "any deviation from the normal postoperative course." Conditions,

D. Dindo, MD
Department of Visceral, Thoracic and Vascular Surgery,
Triemli Hospital, Zurich, Switzerland
e-mail: daniel.dindo@usz.ch

M.A. Cuesta, H.J. Bonjer (eds.), *Treatment of Postoperative Complications after Digestive Surgery*, DOI 10.1007/978-1-4471-4354-3_3,

Table 3.1 Classification of surgical complications

Grades	Definition
Grade I	Any deviation from the normal postoperative course without the need for pharmacological treatment or surgical, endoscopic, and radiological interventions Acceptable therapeutic regimens are drugs such as antiemetics, antipyretics, analgetics, diuretics, and electrolytes and physiotherapy. This grade also includes wound infections opened at the bedside
Grade II	Requiring pharmacological treatment with drugs other than such allowed for grade I complications Blood transfusions and total parenteral nutrition are also included
Grade III	Requiring surgical, endoscopic or radiological intervention
Grade III-a	Intervention not under general anesthesia
Grade III-b	Intervention under general anesthesia
Grade IV	Life-threatening complication (including CNS complications)[a] requiring IC/ICU management
Grade IV-a	Single organ dysfunction (including dialysis)
Grade IV-b	Multiorgan dysfunction
Grade V	Death of a patient
Suffix 'd'	If the patients suffers from a complication at the time of discharge, the suffix "d" (for "disability") is added to the respective grade of complication. This label indicates the need for a follow-up to fully evaluate the complication

IC intermediate care, *ICU* intensive care unit
[a]Brain hemorrhage, ischemic stroke, subarachnoidal bleeding, but excluding transient ischemic attacks (TIA)

which are inherent to the procedure and are expected to occur (such as pain or scar formation), should be discriminated from complications and be termed "sequelae." Finally, diseases that remain unchanged after surgery or reoccur (e.g., R2-resected tumor or an early recurrence of an inguinal hernia) also reflect negative outcomes, either, but constitute a failure to cure rather than a complication.

The incidence of complications is still the most often used surrogate marker for surgical quality. However, we still lack a consensus on how to define and to grade surgical complications what substantially hampers the interpretation of surgical performance. A number of attempts have been made to classify surgical complications [3–8], but none of them has gained widespread acceptance. Some surgeons advocated that intuition is an appropriate guide to define what a complication might be and for grading [9]. However, any system reporting complications must narrow the room for mistakes and subjective interpretation. Therefore, the challenge is to use a scale system, which has to be simple but must not impede accuracy or general clinical applicability.

To standardize surgical outcome reporting, we have introduced a classification of surgical complications consisting of five grades [10]. The basic principle of this classification—termed Clavien–Dindo classification—is based on the therapy needed to treat the complication (Table 3.1). The classification mainly focuses on the medical perspective, with major emphasis on the risk and invasiveness of the therapy used to correct a complication. This perspective minimizes subjective interpretation and any tendency to down-rate complications because it is based on objective data. Such an approach is especially important in retrospective studies where postoperative complications are often poorly documented, whereas the therapy to treat a complication is well recorded in both physician and nursing reports. It might be argued that policies in the management of a given surgical complication may vary among different physicians and centers or countries. As an example, an intra-abdominal abscess after bowel resection may be treated in some cases either by antibiotics, percutaneous drainage, or relaparotomy. The decision often depends on personal and somewhat subjective appraisals. Such variation is mostly due to the lack of an accepted paradigm for the "best practice" but may also depend on local determinates such as the availability of medical resources (e.g., interventional radiologist). Despite such possible variations, the use of therapeutic consequences as the basis to rank complications remains the best approach: First, this is the most readily available and objective information regarding the postoperative course. Second, the treatment for a complication may induce stress to a patient and may lead to further morbidity, which justifies inclusion in the ranking system. Third, medical resources are limited and have to be used with reluctance. The least invasive or expensive treatment that is effective should be chosen to treat a complication. The approach to use the treatment required to correct a complication is also suggested by others [11].

In 2004, our classification was validated in a large cohort of patient, and it significantly correlated with complexity of surgery as well as with the length of hospital stay [10]. Evaluated through an international survey sent to leading surgical centers, the classification demonstrated to be objective and reproducible [10]. The validity of this classification was also shown in another study [12], in which 97 % of the recorded complications were correctly graded over a 6-month study period. Five years after the first publication, we tested the general applicability of this classification [13]. For that reason, complex clinical courses with complications were collected during the weekly morbidity and mortality conferences. These clinical case scenarios were sent to different centers all over the world, which had used our classification for more than 3 years, asking them to grade each complication presented in the case scenarios. Additionally, we tested how the severity of each grade is perceived in three groups of individuals (physicians, nurses, and patients) by using predefined case presentation that had to be graded. The survey sent to the different surgical centers yielded a high and highly significant degree of agreement (> 90 %), demonstrating that the classification also withstands in complex complication scenarios, retaining its reproducibility and objectivity. Moreover, the classification significantly correlated with the subjective perception of the severity of a complication [13]. Recently, the correlation between costs and complications—as assessed by our classification—was investigated [14]. Morbidity of 1,200 consecutive patients undergoing major surgery from 2005 to 2008 was analyzed and full in-hospital costs were assessed for each patient. The overall 30-day mortality was 1.8 %, whereas the morbidity rate was 53.8 %. Patients with an uneventful course generated mean costs per case of US$ 27,946 (SD US$ 15,106). Costs increased dramatically with the severity of postoperative complications as assessed by the Clavien–Dindo classification and rose to mean costs of US$ 159,345 (SD US$

151,191) for grade IV complications. This increase in costs, up to 5 times the cost of a similar operation without complications, was observed for all types of analyzed procedures. This study demonstrates the dramatic impact of postoperative complications on full in-hospital costs per case. Furthermore, it again demonstrates the validity of the Clavien–Dindo complication classification as it considerably correlates with costs.

Classifications are mandatory to ease the interpretation of surgical performance and to assess surgical quality. However, to be valuable for clinical practice, such classifications must be reliable, objective, and easy to use. Complications are still the most often used parameter to evaluate quality in surgery. Classifications of surgical complications are therefore needed for outcome comparison. Such a classification should impede subjective interpretations of the severity of postoperative events to ensure comparability with other centers and over time. The Clavien–Dindo classification has proofed to be an objective and reproducible tool for outcome assessment. In the last few years, it gained wide acceptance not only in surgery but also in other surgical specialties (such as urology or gynecology), and it is now increasingly used in surgical literature for outcome reporting with more than 1,000 citations since 2004.

References

1. Rowell KS, Turrentine FE, Hutter MM, et al. Use of national surgical quality improvement program data as a catalyst for quality improvement. J Am Coll Surg. 2007;204(6):1293–300.
2. Donabedian A. The quality of care – how can it be assessed? JAMA. 1988;260:1743–8.
3. Clavien PA, Sanabria JR, Strasberg SM. Proposed classification of complications of surgery with examples of utility in cholecystectomy. Surgery. 1992;111(5):518–26.
4. Pomposelli JJ, Gupta SK, Zacharoulis DC, et al. Surgical complication outcome (SCOUT) score: a new method to evaluate quality of care in vascular surgery. J Vasc Surg. 1997;25(6):1007–14. discussion 1014–5.
5. Gawande AA, Thomas EJ, Zinner MJ, Brennan TA. The incidence and nature of surgical adverse events in Colorado and Utah in 1992. Surgery. 1999;126(1):66–75.
6. Veen MR, Lardenoye JW, Kastelein GW, Breslau PJ. Recording and classification of complications in a surgical practice. Eur J Surg. 1999;165(5):421–4. discussion 425.
7. Pillai SB, van Rij AM, Williams S, et al. Complexity- and risk-adjusted model for measuring surgical outcome. Br J Surg. 1999;86(12):1567–72.
8. Strasberg SM, Linehan DC, Hawkins WG. The accordion severity grading system of surgical complications. Ann Surg. 2009;250(2):177–86.
9. Woodfield JC, Pettigrew RA, Plank LD, et al. Accuracy of the surgeons' clinical prediction of perioperative complications using a visual analog scale. World J Surg. 2007;31(10):1912–20.
10. Dindo D, Demartines N, Clavien PA. Classification of surgical complications: a new proposal with evaluation in a cohort of 6336 patients and results of a survey. Ann Surg. 2004;240(2):205–13.
11. Bruce J, Krukowski ZH, Al-Khairy G, et al. Systematic review of the definition and measurement of anastomotic leak after gastrointestinal surgery. Br J Surg. 2001;88:1157–68.
12. Dindo D, Hahnloser D, Clavien PA. Quality assessment in surgery: riding a lame horse. Ann Surg. 2010;251(4):766–71.

13. Clavien PA, Barkun J, de Oliveira ML, Vauthey JN, Dindo D, Schulick RD, de Santibañes E, Pekolj J, Slankamenac K, Bassi C, Graf R, Vonlanthen R, Padbury R, Cameron JL, Makuuchi M. The Clavien-Dindo classification of surgical complications: five-year experience. Ann Surg. 2009;250(2):187–96.
14. Vonlanthen R, Slankamenac K, Breitenstein S, Puhan MA, Muller MK, Hahnloser D, Hauri D, Graf R, Clavien PA. The impact of complications on costs of major surgical procedures: a cost analysis of 1200 patients. Ann Surg. 2011;254:907–13.

Chapter 4
Diagnosis and Treatment of Major Abdominal Complications Is Multidisciplinary Work

Dick J. Gouma

Keywords Diagnosis • Treatment • Abdominal complications • Surgical treatment • Hospital volume • Surgeons volume • Mortality • Hospital resources • Process of care • Complications • Outcome • Quality assurance

Introduction

Surgical treatment of the various gastrointestinal diseases is inherently associated with risk for complications ranging from temporary disadvantage such as superficial wound infection to recovery after reoperation and even up to death.

During the diagnostic process and preoperative evaluation of patients with a GI disease eligible for surgical treatment, surgeons should always search for the balance between the potential benefits of surgery and the risk of complications of the procedure.

Several factors are important such as the general condition of the patient including age and comorbidity; the extent of the procedure; the stage of the disease, in particular for malignant tumors; and last but not least the experience of the surgeon in that particular field of GI surgery as well as the experience of the other involved disciplines in the hospital such as interventional radiology, ICU, and endoscopy to manage the complications.

Accepting these general principles of quality of care implies establishment of a multidisciplinary approach in management of these GI diseases and in particular the complications.

This chapter will recapitulate that the outcome of surgery is dependent on multidisciplinary work, facilitated by the structure of care as well as the process of care in that particular hospital because both domains will eventually determine the quality of care.

D.J. Gouma, MD
Department of Surgery, Academic Medical Center,
Amsterdam, The Netherlands
e-mail: d.j.gouma@amc.uva.nl

M.A. Cuesta, H.J. Bonjer (eds.), *Treatment of Postoperative Complications after Digestive Surgery*, DOI 10.1007/978-1-4471-4354-3_4,

Aspects of the Structure of Care

Hospital Volume/Surgeons Volume

Hospital volume and surgeon volume are the most recognized variables to be correlated with complications and in particular with hospital mortality. The majority of studies (>90 %) on high-volume versus low-volume hospitals showed a lower mortality at high-volume hospitals [1–3]. The older studies were criticized using clinical data without risk adjustment. Recent studies including a recent published meta-analysis on pancreatic resection, using risk adjustment, showed again significant lower mortality in high-volume hospitals (odds ratio 0.32; 95 % CI 0.16–0.64) [4].

The relation of surgeon volume and mortality has also been shown for several procedures with odds ratios ranging from 1.24 for lung resection to 3.6 for pancreatic resection [5]. Most studies however focused on hospital volume. One should also realize that the relative importance of surgeon's volume and hospital volume is difficult to analyze in detail because high-volume surgeons, generally after subspecialty training, are frequently working in high-volume hospitals.

A recent study evaluated hospital mortality for five different groups of hospitals assigned according to quintiles of hospital mortality varying from 3.5 to 6.9 % and analyzed rates of all complications, major complications and death in these five categories [6, 7]. They showed no significant difference in total and major complications in those hospitals, but differences in mortality of patients with major complications were found ranging from 12.5 % up to 21.4 % due to more adequate management of these complications [7]. This is another argument that besides surgeons experience the basic hospital resources are an important factor for outcome and mortality.

Nevertheless, we should realize that with more complex (laparoscopic) procedures nowadays, surgeon training and in particular subspecialty training or advanced fellow training is an important factor for outcome. It was shown recently that patients with cancer operated by board-certified surgeons had lower local recurrence rates [8].

Hospital Resources

Hospital resources are important not only for management of complications of GI surgery but also for prevention of complications.

In particular, patients undergoing high-risk surgery will need more complex perioperative care as well as complex management of severe, life-threatening complications.

The Intensive Care Unit staffing is crucial, and it has been shown that the relative risk for hospital mortality with high-intensity ICU staffing is lower 0.71 (95 % CI

0.62–0.82) compared with low-intensity ICU staffing [9]. The same has been shown for nursing staffing and up-to-date technology and equipment on ICU and surgical wards [10]. So besides the surgeon staff other hospital specialties, in particular the ICU staff, interventional radiologists, interventional endoscopists, anesthesiologists, cardiology services, pain management team, etc., are of upmost importance for treatment of postoperative complications and outcome. In some hospitals, an interdisciplinary team for the postoperative management of patients has been established to facilitate this process.

Aspects Related to Process of Care

The process of care reflects different aspects starting with patient selection and evaluation for a surgical procedure. Discussion of all patients in a multidisciplinary meeting for the indication of surgery also prevents for bias in selection due to "surgeon-related aspects."

In fact, there should be a clear general accepted (evidence-based) guideline of preoperative work-up of these patients and well-defined criteria to accept patients for a surgical procedure. All patients should have pre-assessment by the anesthesiologist before the patient is accepted for surgery, and a checklist should be used to control the completeness of the different preoperative aspects [11].

Another important factor to prevent complications is to reach a certain standard for the perioperative care and the surgical procedure. There is a wide variation of measures ranging from prophylaxis for venous thromboembolism, continuous use of cardiac medication, antibiotic prophylaxis, nutritional support, etc.

These measurements should also include other organizatorial aspects, such as preoperative control of instruments, different types of staplers, and counting gauche. Currently the checklist, including a time-out procedure, is introduced routinely in the Netherlands to facilitate this process [11].

There should also be a certain standard set of steps to be taken during the procedure. For example, the Critical View of Safety (CVS) has been included as a standard to perform before clipping the cystic duct and cystic artery during a laparoscopic cholecystectomy.

The next step for prevention of complications is adequate care on the ward and control by an experienced nursing and surgical staff. The multidisciplinary approach is also useful in terms of pain management together with anesthesiologists and interaction with general medicine staff for medication of cardiopulmonary disorders during the ward rounds.

One of the advantages of fast-track surgery or early recovering programs is that most postoperative measurements are standardized and by that more adequately managed/controlled by the nursing staff [12].

The last but probably most important step in this process is early recognition of a complication and by that early intervention, for example, before hemodynamic instability due to persistent sepsis after leakage of an anastomosis. The enormous development of radiology during the past decades improved diagnostic accuracy for intra-abdominal complications such as leakage, fluid collections, and abscess formation considerably.

Despite the progress of diagnostic tools, clinical observation and continuity of care to facilitate the observation of changes in the clinical condition are of upmost importance.

The "classical paper" of M. Trede on management of complication after pancreatic resection is still of inestimable value, and he already summarized nicely that changes in clinical finding are crucial for early diagnosis [13]. The simple clinical findings suspect for leakage of the anastomosis are beginning of abdominal tenderness, in particular if none before; tongue slightly drier; a rise in temperature and pulse; respiratory rate is higher; oliguria; and barely perceptible agitation.

Laboratory tests will endorse infection/sepsis, and abdominal CT will facilitate to confirm the diagnosis within hours and probably identify the intra-abdominal cause and subsequently lead to early intervention.

Generally intervention of complication can be performed by local staff (surgeons/radiologists) in the particular hospital of initial surgery.

For some complications, for example, a bile duct injury after laparoscopic cholecystectomy, it has been shown that treatment by the initial surgeon, who performed the procedure, will lead to higher mortality compared with referral to centers [14].

In the earlier years, abdominal complications were generally managed by relaparotomy and subsequent drainage of collections or management of postoperative bleeding. Nowadays, most interventions are done nonsurgically by interventional radiologists or endoscopists [15]. The 7 x 24 h availability of intervention radiology is however not available in each hospital. The strategy is therefore highly dependent on local expertise and, for example, patients with a bile duct injury still undergo relaparotomy in 20–30 % without further preoperative evaluation of the type of injury.

Referral to centers should be performed depending on the clinical situation of the patient combined with hospital resources (local expertise). The complications and management of complications of most GI surgery procedures will be discussed in detail in the next chapters.

Birkmeyer already reported extensively about the conceptual model of the relationship between the structure, process of care in hospitals, and outcome of surgery [6, 7] (Fig. 4.1).

Monitoring System for Complications and Outcome

Quality assessment and continuous monitoring of specific aspects of outcome, for example, complications, is an important factor in stimulating improvement of quality of care. Therefore, surgical performance is now monitored in most countries and connected directly with quality improvement programs.

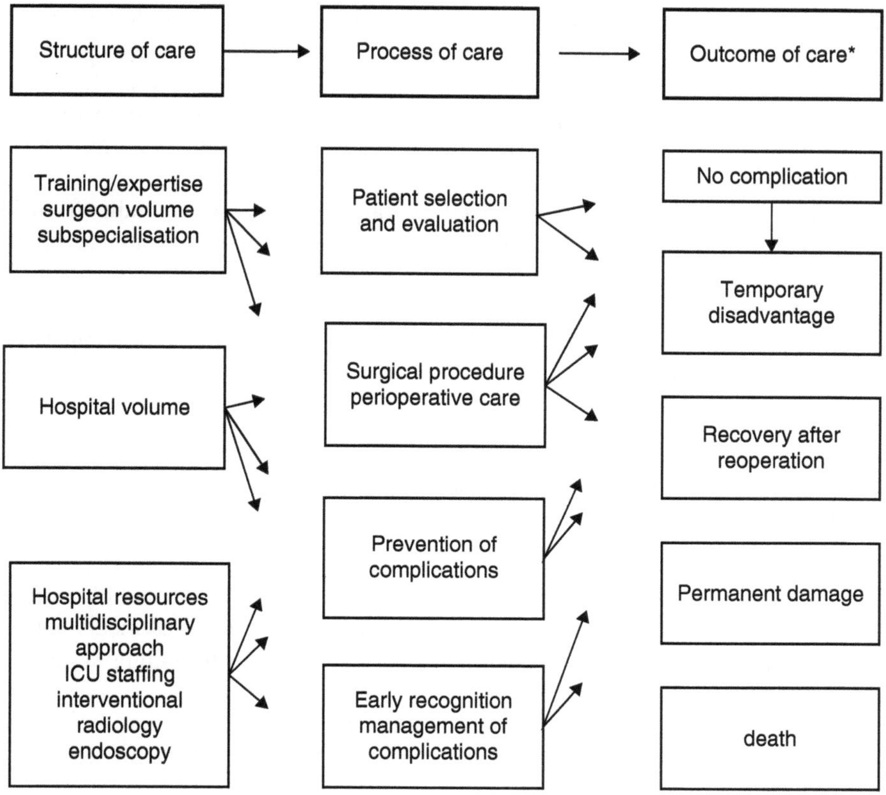

Fig. 4.1 Relation between structure and process of care and outcome in terms of complications and mortality. *Complication scale according to the National Surgical Complication Registry in The Netherlands (Adapted from the conceptual model from Birkmeyer and Dimick [6])

The definition of surgical complications is however not well defined, and many different definitions have been used [16]. The development of these definitions is a challenging task, and Sokol already discussed that the more the definition is specified, the more restrictive it will be. In the Netherlands, there has been a plea to be more inclusive rather than exclusive, and a broad definition is used in the Dutch National Surgical Complication Registry (LHRC), for uniform registration of surgical complications [17]. A complication is an unintended and undesirable event or condition following medical treatment, that is, harmful for the patient and necessitates adjustment of medical treatment or that leads to permanent harm.

The complication registry includes all patients that are admitted under responsibility of the Department of Surgery, and the complication must have occurred during the treatment or in a period of 4 weeks after discharge. The severity of every complication is graded as follows: zero: no harm; 1: temporary disadvantage, no [re]operation; 2: recovery after reoperation; 3: probably permanent damage/disability; 4: death; and 5: unclear due to untimely death. These data are linked to admission and discharge data, operative procedure details, and epidemiological data (i.e., age, sex, American Society of Anesthesiologists [ASA] classification). These systems allow analysis of a wide variety of complications and give valuable tools for quality improvement. This includes surgical and technical aspects as well as other aspects of care. Currently the system is modified to allow comparison of hospitals in the Netherlands, but sofar this is still impossible without correction for risk adjustment of patients.

A study from the USA already showed that ranking of hospital mortality from 44 hospitals might change enormously by using unadjusted versus risk-adjusted mortality with a maximum change from 7 up to number 39 [18].

The National Surgical Quality Improvement Program (NSQIP) in the USA even incorporated five critical elements necessary to ensure validity for comparison between different hospitals:

1. Standardization of endpoints
2. Standardization of definitions and terms
3. System for data collection and prospective collection
4. Data collectors themselves grading and training
5. Validated system for risk adjustment

So accepting the ongoing attempts for transparency about outcome of surgical procedures and quality assessment, the abovementioned critical elements and in particular risk adjustment is mandatory before a general open grading system of quality of care can be accepted.

The abovementioned aspects of the structure and progress of care as well as the monitoring systems of complication and mortality should be taken into account in the following chapters on specific complications in GI surgery.

References

1. Birkmeyer JD, Siewers AE, Finlayson EV, Stukel TA, Lucas FL, Batista I, Welch HG, Wennberg DE. Hospital volume and surgical mortality in the United States. N Engl J Med. 2002;346(15):1128–37.
2. Gouma DJ, van Geenen RC, van Gulik TM, de Haan RJ, de Wit LT, Busch OR, Obertop H. Rates of complications and death after pancreaticoduodenectomy: risk factors and the impact of hospital volume. Ann Surg. 2000;232(6):786–95.
3. van Heek NT, Kuhlmann KF, Scholten RJ, de Castro SM, Busch OR, van Gulik TM, Obertop H, Gouma DJ. Hospital volume and mortality after pancreatic resection: a systematic review and an evaluation of intervention in the Netherlands. Ann Surg. 2005;242(6):781–8. discussion 788–90.
4. Gooiker GA, van Gijn W, Wouters MW, Post PN, van de Velde CJ, Tollenaar RA, On behalf of the Signalling Committee Cancer of the Dutch Cancer Society. Systematic review and meta-analysis of the volume-outcome relationship in pancreatic surgery. Br J Surg. 2011;98(4): 485–94.
5. Birkmeyer JD, Siewers AE, Finlayson EVA. Surgeon volume and operative mortality in the United states. N Engl J Med. 2003;349:2117–27.
6. Birkmeyer JD, Dimick JB. Understanding and reducing variation in surgical mortality. Annu Rev Med. 2009;60:405–15.

7. Ghaferi AA, Birkmeyer JD, Dimick JB. Variation in hospital mortality associated with inpatient surgery. N Engl J Med. 2009;361(14):1368–75.
8. Bilimoria KY, Phillips JD, Rock CE, Hayman A, Prystowsky JB, Bentrem DJ. Effect of surgeon training, specialization, and experience on outcome for cancer surgery: a systematic review of the literature. Ann Surg Oncol. 2009;16:1799–808.
9. Pronovost PJ, Angus DC, Dorman T, Robinson KA, Dremsizov TT, Young TL. Physician staffing patterns and clinical outcomes in critically ill patients: a systematic review. JAMA. 2002;288(17):2151–62.
10. Bottger TC, Hermeneit S, Muller M, et al. Modifiable surgical and anesthesiologic risk factors for the development of cardiac and pulmonary complications after laparoscopic colorectal surgery. Surg Endosc. 2009;23(90):2016–25.
11. de Vries EN, Prins HA, Crolla RM, den Outer AJ, van Andel G, van Helden SH, Schlack WS, van Putten MA, Gouma DJ, Dijkgraaf MG, Smorenburg SM, Boermeester MA, SURPASS Collaborative Group. Effect of a comprehensive surgical safety system on patient outcomes. N Engl J Med. 2010;363(20):1928–37.
12. Vlug MS, Wind J, Hollman MW, et al. Laparoscopy in combination with fast track multimodal management is the best perioperative strategy in patients undergoing colonic Surgery: a randomized clinical trial (LAFA-study). Ann Surg. 2011;254:868–75.
13. Trede M, Schwall G. The complications of pancreatectomy. Ann Surg. 1988;207(1):39–44.
14. Flum DR, Cheadle A, Prela C, Dellinger EP, Chan L. Bile duct injury during cholecystectomy and survival in medicare beneficiaries. JAMA. 2003;290(16):2168–73.
15. de Castro SM, Kuhlmann KF, Busch OR, et al. Delayed massive hemorrhage after pancreatic and biliary surgery: embolization or surgery. Ann Surg. 2005;241:85–91.
16. Sokol DK, Wilson J. What is a surgical complication? World J Surg. 2008;32:942–4.
17. Goslings JC, Gouma DJ. What is a surgical complication. World J Surg. 2008;32:952.
18. Khuri S, Daley J, Henderson W, et al. The Department of Veterans Affairs NSQIP: the first National Validated, Outcome–Based, Risk-Adjusted and Peer-Controlled Program for the measurement and enhancement of the quality of surgical care. Ann Surg. 1998;224:491–550.

Chapter 5
General Principles of Recognition of Major Complications Following Surgery of the Digestive Tract

Suzanne S. Gisbertz, Jennifer Straatman, and Miguel A. Cuesta

Keywords Postoperative complications • Surgery • Digestive tract • Morbidity • Mortality • C-reactive protein (CRP) • Imaging techniques • CT scanning

Introduction

Major complications following surgery of the digestive tract are associated with increased morbidity, prolonged intensive care and hospital stay, and even mortality [1–10]. Infectious complications are frequent; an infectious complication rate of 21 % has recently been described following colorectal surgery [11]. Among the most severe infectious complications are anastomotic failures. Reported leakage rates range from 0.6 to 23 % [1–10]. The reconstruction following resections, and not so much dissection and resection itself, causes most surgical adverse events. The frequency and consequences vary according to the target organ and the executed operation. A postoperative mortality of 12–39 % following anastomotic leakage has been reported, compared to 2–5 % without leakage [1, 2, 12, 13]. On the opposite, incidence of clinical anastomotic leakage was 42 % among patients who died and 11 % in the uneventful group in a large population-based trial [3].

Even if an anastomosis can be preserved, late complications are observed frequently, such as anastomotic strictures leading to obstruction or continence problems. Furthermore, anastomotic leakages may result in permanent stomata. Conflicting results persist whether anastomotic leakage is associated with an increased local recurrence rate and a worse oncologic outcome [4, 12, 14].

S.S. Gisbertz
Department of Surgery, Academic Medical Center, Amsterdam, The Netherlands
e-mail: ma.cuesta@vumc.nl

J. Straatman • M.A. Cuesta, MD (✉)
Department of Surgery, VU University Medical Center, Amsterdam, The Netherlands
e-mail: ma.cuesta@vumc.nl

M.A. Cuesta, H.J. Bonjer (eds.), *Treatment of Postoperative Complications after Digestive Surgery*, DOI 10.1007/978-1-4471-4354-3_5,

Early recognition and intervention can prevent severe consequences of major complications, such as systemic inflammatory response syndrome (SIRS), sepsis, multiple organ failure, and death [1–3, 5]. Early diagnosis and repair within 5 days following initial surgery was not associated with mortality in a retrospective analysis of 655 patients, whereas repair in a later postoperative course was associated with a mortality rate of 18 % [5].

Sepsis can be difficult to distinguish from the systemic inflammatory response related to surgical trauma. Since clinical features of complications can be nonspecific and interpretation of diagnostic tests can be incorrect, early diagnosis remains a challenge, even in the era of the widespread availability of imaging techniques. A median time to clinical diagnosis of a complicated postoperative course was 8 days in recent studies [15].

These results emphasize the importance of early recognition of complications. The question remains when anastomotic dehiscence occurs after a standard operative procedure. The daily assessment of patients' clinical condition is the most important guidance for the surgeon. A patient has to clinically improve every day during a normal postoperative course, and every decline should prompt evaluation of the possible problem.

This chapter focuses on clinical features and diagnostics contributing to early recognition of major complications following abdominal surgery.

Clinical Principles

Clinical parameters such as pain, ileus, fever, tachycardia, hypotension, oliguria, and hypoxemia may raise the suspicion of postoperative complications. Most signs, however, are nonspecific. The occurrence of a combination of clinical signs yields a higher positive predictive value for anastomotic leakage [5]. Recently, a standardized postoperative surveillance protocol has been developed, consisting of the following clinical parameters: fever, heart rate, respiratory rate, urinary production, mental status, clinical condition, ileus, gastric retention, fascial dehiscence, abdominal pain (other than wound pain), leukocytes and CRP, urea and creatinine, and nutritional status [2]. This "leakage-score" is linked to a decision tree indicating diagnostic and treatment actions. Introduction of this standardized surveillance has resulted in a decrease in median time to the diagnosis of anastomotic leakage and a diminished delay in diagnosis of anastomotic leakage compared to a historical cohort [2]. Furthermore, a decrease in mortality following anastomotic leakage was observed, although this was statistically not significant [2]. These results show that although clinical signs are often nonspecific, a standardized approach increases the awareness to the occurrence of possible complications. Additionally, this awareness should be increased in patients at risk. Established risk factors for postoperative morbidity are older age, male gender, comorbidity, smoking, steroid use, higher American Society of Anesthesiologists (ASA) classification, perioperative blood transfusion, intraoperative septic conditions, the distance of the anastomosis to the anal verge in rectal surgery, malnutrition, weight loss, hypoalbuminemia, and longer operation or anesthesia time [5, 16–19].

Laboratory Principles: The Value of CRP

C-reactive protein (CRP), an acute-phase reactant in peripheral blood, has been shown to be of predictive value for infectious complications [11, 15]. In contrast with other laboratory tests, such as determination of interleukins, CRP is widely available, clinically applicable, and not expensive. CRP is stimulated by interleukin 6 (IL-6) and tumor necrosis factor α (TNF-α) in response to inflammation. CRP acts as an early defense against infection in the innate immunity system by assisting complement binding to foreign and damaged cells and enhancing phagocytosis by macrophages [20]. In a recent study, CRP was determined daily until discharge in 160 patients undergoing elective colorectal resection for cancer. Overall infectious complication rate in this study was 21 %; 3 % of complications consisted of anastomotic leakage. CRP value was significantly higher in the infectious complication group from the 2nd postoperative day onwards. The point at which CRP achieved the highest combined sensitivity and specificity for infectious complications was on postoperative day 4, with an optimum cut-off value of 145 mg/l. The negative predictive value of CRP < 145 mg/l for an infectious complication on postoperative day 4 was 96 %; the corresponding positive predictive value was 61 % [11]. These results are in concordance with the results by Welsch et al., who reported an optimal cut-off value of 140 mg/ml and a predictive value of 50.5 % on day 4 in their series of 380 patients undergoing resection for rectal cancer [15].

Other studies describe a persistent elevation of CRP levels when complications occur, and not so much the rise in CRP levels, observed in all postoperative patients [13].

Radiology Principles: The Value of CT Scanning

CT scanning is currently the most readily available diagnostic in the work-up of major complications [10, 21, 22]. Interpretation, however, can be difficult, since CT features and criteria for diagnosis of anastomotic leakage are not well established. Additionally, there can be overlap in signs on CT images between patients with and without complications. Furthermore, signs of leakage may be confused with signs of local recurrence [10].

Recent literature analyzes predictors of anastomotic leakage on CT scanning. A case–control study compared postoperative CT findings in 73 patients with a small or large bowel anastomosis with 26 patients following partial hepatectomy (control group) [21]. A CT scan was performed in both groups for suspicion of septic complications. A peri-anastomotic fluid collection containing air was the only finding that was statistically significantly in the anastomotic leakage group compared to the group without leakage, 30.4 % versus 10 %, odds ratio 3.9 [confidence interval (CI) 1.1–14.1; $p=0.04$] [21].

A retrospective series described CT scan findings for leakage following rectal surgery for cancer. Features included fluid collections in the pelvis, thickening in the presacral region, and an extraluminal contrast collection. Only the last is specific for an anastomotic leakage; there is an overlap for the other two findings between patients with and without leakage [10].

Own Study Results

We have reviewed 196 consecutive patients who were operated in our institution between January 2010 and December 2010. All patients underwent colorectal (122 patients), upper gastrointestinal (43 patients), or hepato-pancreatico-biliary (31 patients) surgery. The aim of the study was to analyze the value of CRP and CT scanning in the detection of complications following major abdominal surgery. We analyzed clinical parameters and complications in relation to perioperative CRP values and possible performed CT scans. Fifty-five patients (28 %) clinically deteriorated. Seven (3.5 %) were reoperated without a preceding CT scan (two anastomotic failures, one postoperative hemorrhage, one necrotic colostomy, one fascial dehiscence, one empyema following transthoracic esophageal resection, one small bowel perforation). In 48 patients (24.5 %), one or more CT scans were performed during the postoperative course, after a median of 7 days (SD ± 11) postoperatively. Eleven (35 %) CT scans were performed following hepato-pancreatico-biliary, 13 (30 %) following upper gastrointestinal, and 24 (20 %) following colorectal surgery. The diagnosis of a major complication was made after a median of 8 days (SD ± 9) postoperatively. Twenty-one of 48 (44 %) scanned patients were diagnosed with a major complication (14 anastomotic failures, 6 abscesses, 1 diaphragmatic hernia following transhiatal esophageal resection). Reinterventions in these patients included 13 reoperations (5 colostomies) and 7 percutaneous drainages. In one patient, a drain was already in situ from the initial operation. In 26 patients (56 %), no reintervention was carried out following the results of the CT scan; in 14 patients, there were no abnormal findings, 5 patients were diagnosed with an ileus, and in 5 patients, a pulmonary complication was identified. There was one false-positive CT result: a CT scan performed on the fourth postoperative day showing free air was interpreted by the radiologist as an anastomotic failure. This patient was managed successfully conservatively despite the CT scan results. One patient was reoperated despite a negative CT scan. Besides some ascites, no major complications were identified during relaparotomy. In this small retrospective trial, the sensitivity of a postoperative CT scan is 96 %, the specificity 100 %, the positive predictive value 100 %, and the negative predictive value 96 %. These results confirm the accuracy of CT scanning in the detection of major complications in the postoperative course following major abdominal surgery. Additionally, we have analyzed perioperative CRP values in relation to a complicated postoperative course and CT scan results. CRP values were significantly higher in patients in whom a CT scan was performed on postoperative days 4, 6–8, and 10–12. Subsequently, CRP values were significantly higher in patients with complications compared to patients with an uneventful postoperative course on days 2, 4, and 7–13 and in patients with major complications compared to patients with no or minor (no reinterventions) complications on days 4, 6, 7, and 11. The largest observed difference between minor/no and major complications was present on the fourth postoperative day, with a cut-off value of 217 mg/l ($p = .027$). However, with a CRP value of > 217 mg/l, the positive predictive value and the negative predictive value were only 69 %, the sensitivity 52 %, and the specificity 82 %. Finally, the median CRP in patients with major complications was 248 mg/l (range 125–539 mg/l) and in patients with minor/no complications 167 mg/l (range 51–325 mg/l). These results endorse the value of perioperative CRP determination as additive in postoperative decision making, with the remark that the positive predictive value and the negative predictive value are only 69 %.

Discussion

Early detection and solution of postoperative surgical complications, especially anastomotic leakages, is imperative to reduce morbidity, preserve anastomoses, and reduce mortality. The opposite is related to delay in diagnosis and treatment of the problem.

There are two methods to detect complications: clinical assessment and the combination of CRP and CT scanning. Clinical parameters are in our opinion essential in order to signalize problems; clinical interruption in the recovery phase of a patient, fever and abdominal pain are important signs. These factors will link with the performance of a CT scan without delay. In this way, the surgeon can adopt a treatment policy, which will constitute sometimes of a wait-and-see policy and other times warrant interventions, such as antibiotic treatment, percutaneous drainages, or reoperations. Currently, the policy to wait without progression of a patient to recovery is unacceptable and outdated. In our study, CT scanning has shown to be of value in the detection of postoperative complications with high positive and negative predictive values and the possibility to immediately treat certain complications by percutaneous means. Furthermore, this implies adoption for processes of quality control after surgery of any kind, but especially after major abdominal surgery. Quality control is a normal aspect in every industrial process, as in the car industry. In surgery, quality control is mostly based on the experience of the surgeon. In addition, most of this control is subjective, such as the color of the bowel as a representative for perfusion, the avoidance of tension at an anastomotic site, patency control of the anastomosis using our fingers, control of correctness of the anastomosis by inspection, completeness of doughnuts, methylene blue dye, saline, or air control. Quality control does not exist as a routine. Therefore, one should consider whether to perform a standard postoperative CT scan following major abdominal surgery and define its results as possible discharge or reintervention criteria. Before this strategy can be implemented, more research is needed. We are currently investigating this in a large prospective trial.

References

1. Isbister WH. Anastomotic leak in colorectal surgery: a single surgeon's experience. Aust N Z J Surg. 2001;71:516–20.
2. den Dulk M, Marijnen CA, Collette L, Putter H, Påhlman L, Folkesson J, Bosset JF, Rödel C, Bujko K, van de Velde CJ. Multicentre analysis of oncological and survival outcomes following anastomotic leakage after rectal cancer surgery. Br J Surg. 2009 Sep;96(9):1066–75.
3. Matthiessen P, Hallböök O, Rutegård J, Sjödahl R. Population-based study of risk factors for postoperative death after anterior resection of the rectum. Br J Surg. 2006 Apr;93(4): 498–503.
4. Park IJ. Influence of anastomotic leakage on oncological outcome in patients with rectal cancer. J Gastrointest Surg. 2010 Jul;14(7):1190–6.
5. Alves A, Panis Y, Pocard M, et al. Management of anastomotic leakage after nondiverted large bowel resection. J Am Coll Surg. 1999;189:554–9.
6. www.clinicalaudit.nl
7. Rahbari NN, Weitz J, Hohenberger W, Heald RJ, Moran B, Ulrich A, Holm T, Wong WD, Tiret E, Moriya Y, Laurberg S, den Dulk M, van de Velde C, Büchler MW. Definition and grading of anastomotic leakage following anterior resection of the rectum: a proposal by the International Study Group of Rectal Cancer. Surgery. 2010 Mar;147(3):339–51.
8. Bertelsen CA, Andreasen AH, Jørgensen T, Harling H, Danish Colorectal Cancer Group. Anastomotic leakage after curative anterior resection for rectal cancer: short and long-term outcome. Colorectal Dis. 2010 Jul;12(7 Online):e76–81.
9. Bruce J, Krukowski ZH, Al-Khairy G, Russell EM, Park KG. Systematic review of the definition and measurement of anastomotic leak after gastrointestinal surgery. Br J Surg. 2001;88:1157–68.
10. DuBrow RA, David CL, Curley SA. Anastomotic leaks after low anterior resection for rectal carcinoma: evaluation with CT and barium enema. AJR Am J Roentgenol. 1995;165:567–71.
11. MacKay GJ, Molloy RG, O'Dwyer PJ. C-reactive protein as a predictor of postoperative infectious complications following elective colorectal resection. Colorectal Dis. 2011 May;13(5):583–7.
12. Kube R, Mroczkowski P, Granowski D, Benedix F, Sahm M, Schmidt U, Gastinger I, Lippert H, Study group Qualitätssicherung Kolon/Rektum-Karzinome (Primärtumor) (Quality assurance in primary colorectal carcinoma). Anastomotic leakage after colon cancer surgery: a predictor of significant morbidity and hospital mortality, and diminished tumour-free survival. Eur J Surg Oncol. 2010 Feb;36(2):120–4.
13. Woeste G, Müller C, Bechstein WO, Wullstein C. Increased serum levels of C-reactive protein precede anastomotic leakage in colorectal surgery. World J Surg. 2010 Jan;34(1):140–6.
14. den Dulk M, Noter SL, Hendriks ER, Brouwers MA, van der Vlies CH, Oostenbroek RJ, Menon AG, Steup WH, van de Velde CJ. Improved diagnosis and treatment of anastomotic leakage after colorectal surgery. Eur J Surg Oncol. 2009 Apr;35(4):420–6.
15. Welsch T, Muller SA, Ulrich A, et al. C-reactive protein as early predictor for infectious complications in rectal surgery. Int J Colorectal Dis. 2007;22:1499–507.

16. Mäkelä JT, Kiviniemi H, Laitinen S. Risk factors for anastomotic leakage after left-sided colorectal resection with rectal anastomosis. Dis Colon Rectum. 2003 May;46(5):653–60.
17. Konishi T, Watanabe T, Kishimoto J, Nagawa H. Risk factors for anastomotic leakage after surgery for colorectal cancer: results of prospective surveillance. J Am Coll Surg. 2006 Mar;202(3):439–44.
18. van Sandick JW, Gisbertz SS, ten Berge IJ, Boermeester MA, van der Pouw Kraan TC, Out TA, Obertop H, van Lanschot JJ. Immune responses and prediction of major infection in patients undergoing transhiatal or transthoracic esophagectomy for cancer. Ann Surg. 2003 Jan;237(1):35–43.
19. Bertelsen CA, Andreasen AH, Jørgensen T, Harling H, Danish Colorectal Cancer Group. Anastomotic leakage after anterior resection for rectal cancer: risk factors. Colorectal Dis. 2010 Jan;12(1):37–43.
20. Gabay C, Kushner I. Acute-phase proteins and other systemic responses to inflammation. N Engl J Med. 1999;340:448–54.
21. Power N, Atri M, Ryan S, Haddad R, Smith A. CT assessment of anastomotic bowel leak. Clin Radiol. 2007 Jan;62(1):37–42.
22. Khoury W, Ben-Yehuda A, Ben-Haim M, Klausner JM, Szold O. Abdominal computed tomography for diagnosing postoperative lower gastrointestinal tract leaks. J Gastrointest Surg. 2009 Aug;13(8):1454–8.

Chapter 6
Is There Less Morbidity After Laparoscopic Surgery?

Antonio M. de Lacy, Salvadora Delgado, and Miguel A. Cuesta

Keywords Morbidity • Laparoscopic surgery • Minimally invasive surgery (MIS) • Esophageal surgery • Gastric surgery • Rectal cancer surgery • Cancer survival • Quality of life-short term results

Since the systematic introduction of minimally invasive surgery (MIS) beginning 1990, questions continue to arise whether MIS compares to conventional surgery in terms of efficacy and safety. Two special triggers for this quest were first the appearance of the port-site metastases after laparoscopic colon resection for cancer and second the progressive imperative to make surgical practice an objective science. Since then evidence-based surgery (EBS) has known a tremendous advancement.

The first publications regarding the port-site metastasis have notably stimulated the performance of randomized control trials, mostly done multicentric, by which conventional surgery for cancer has been compared with its corresponding laparoscopic approach.

The reasons to think that the complication rate after a MIS-procedure could be lower than following its conventional counterpart are multiple: (a) a careful dissection technique, (b) less blood loss, (c) avoidance of huge-approach wounds such as with laparotomy or thoracotomy, and (d) systematic dissection by planes.

A.M. de Lacy
Department of Gastrointestinal Surgery, Institute of Digestive Diseases,
Hospital Clinic, University of Barcelona, Barcelona, Spain

S. Delgado
Department of Gastrointestinal Surgery, Institute of Digestive and Metabolic Diseases,
Hospital Clínic of Barcelona, Barcelona, Spain

M.A. Cuesta, MD (✉)
Department of Surgery, VU University Medical Center,
Amsterdam, The Netherlands
e-mail: ma.cuesta@vumc.nl

M.A. Cuesta, H.J. Bonjer (eds.), *Treatment of Postoperative Complications after Digestive Surgery*, DOI 10.1007/978-1-4471-4354-3_6,

In this chapter we will try to answer the question if a laparoscopic approach causes a change in complication patterns of certain operative techniques by using primarily studies classified at the level of evidence I, randomized studies, and meta-analysis in which randomized studies have been included.

Esophageal Surgery

Single series and systematic reviews have been published regarding different MIS approaches for esophageal cancer.

With respect to morbidity and cancer survival, Smithers et al. have compared patient outcomes from esophageal resection holding for three procedures: (a) open thoracotomy and laparotomy, (b) a thoracoscopic/laparotomy approach (thoracoscopic-assisted), and (c) a total thoracoscopic/laparoscopic approach (total minimally invasive esophagectomy, MIO) [1].

Drawing from a prospective database of all patients managed with cancer of the esophagus or esophagogastric junction, Smithers et al. designed a database for assessing certain postoperative variables, the adequacy of cancer clearance, and survival.

The number of patients selected for each procedure was as follows: (a) open esophagectomy, 114; (b) thoracoscopic-assisted, 309; and (c) total MIO, 23. The three groups were comparable with respect to preoperative variables. The differences in the postoperative variables were found to be the following: less median blood loss in the thoracoscopic-assisted (400 mL) and total MIO (300 mL) groups versus open (600 mL), longer time for total MIO (330 min) versus thoracoscopic-assisted (285 min) and open (300 min), longer median time in hospital for open (14 days) versus thoracoscopic-assisted (13 days) and total MIO (11 days), and less stricture formation in the open (6.1 %) versus thoracoscopic-assisted (21.6 %) and total MIO (36 %). There were no differences in lymph node retrieval for each of the approaches. The open group had more stage III patients (65.8 %) versus the thoracoscopic-assisted (34.4 %) and total MIO (52.1 %) groups. There was no difference in survival rate when the groups were compared stage for stage for an overall median of 3-year survival span.

Hence, minimally invasive techniques to resect the esophagus in patients with cancer were confirmed to be safe and comparable to an open approach with respect to postoperative recovery and cancer survival.

Recently, Butler et al. published a review about MIO current status and future direction [2]. They reviewed 31 articles at level III; they included single-center cohort studies and comparative series. Concerning morbidity and mortality, they analyzed data for anastomotic leakage, respiratory morbidity, and mortality. Regarding the first point, they concluded that the MIO leakage rate ranged between 2.2 % and 52.9 %. This is at least comparable to those leakage rates reported following the open esophageal resections. Moreover, there is no apparent difference between leakage rates in thoracic or cervical anastomosis following MIE. Concerning respiratory morbidity, 12 series on MIO provide a weighted median respiratory complication rate of 31.7 % which is somewhat lower than the rates of the open transthoracic approach as found in the randomized study by Hulscher et al., who compared the transhiatal to the transthoracic esophageal resection—postoperative respiratory infections being in the transthoracic approach 57 % [3].

In the largest series of MIE done by Luketich et al. using the lateral thoracoscopy with lung block, they reported a combined respiratory complication rate of 12.6 % defined as pneumonia and/or ARDS, being this complication rate in the series of Palanivelu et al., using the prone thoracoscopy of less than 7 % [4, 5]!

The only randomized study on this subject, the TIME trial, compared the thoracoscopic in prone position (and laparoscopy) versus the conventional transthoracic (and laparotomy) with intrathoracic or cervical anastomosis. Between June 2009 and March 2011, a total of 115 patients underwent randomization in five centers. Fifty-six patients were analyzed in the open esophagectomy group (OO) and 59 in the MIO group [6].

The pulmonary infection rate holding for the first 2 weeks was 29 % (16 patients) in the OO group and 9 % (5 patients) in the MIO group ($p=0.005$). The overall in-hospital incidence of pulmonary infections was 34 % (19 patients) in the OO group and 12 % (7 patients) in the MIO group ($p=0.005$). An explanation for the lower incidence of pulmonary infections may be first of all, the prone position used in which—contrasted with the lateral position—the mediastinum hangs in its usual mid-position. A second advantage may be the absence of a total collapse of the lung during the MIO in prone position in contrast with one-lung ventilation; thereby permitting optimal visualization of mediastinum with preserved ventilation and oxygenation. A third factor may be the thoracotomy wound itself. All three factors together could explain these advantages.

In addition, it was found that the MIO procedure preserved the quality of life better than the OO procedure. After 6 weeks, all the questionnaires, the SF 36, the EORTC C30, and the specific OES 18 questionnaire, showed better scores in the MIO group than in the OO group.

Hospital stay was significantly shorter in the MIO group (14 versus 11 days, ($p=0.044$)). At 6 weeks, the postoperative quality of life was significantly better in the MIO group. The shorter hospital stay in the MIO group reflects a faster postoperative recovery. Other postoperative data including pathology parameters, major postoperative complications (anastomotic leakage, 7 % in the OO and 12 % in the MIO, ($p=0.390$)), and mortality (1.8 % versus 3.4 %) were not significantly different. Interesting is the different rate for vocal cord paralysis, being 14 % in the OO group and only 2 % in the MIO ($p=0.012$).Pneumatic dissection by CO_2 from thoracic cavity into the neck can simplify the dissection in the neck and reduce the recurrent nerve lesions.

In conclusion, this randomized trial comparing open esophagectomy for cancer with minimally invasive esophagectomy shows that MIO results in a lower incidence of pulmonary infections, a shorter hospital stay, and a better short-term quality of life without compromise of the quality of the resected specimen.

Regarding esophageal benign pathology, it is interesting to take notice of the recent meta-analysis by Broeders et al. They compared with a systematic review and meta-analysis, the laparoscopic Nissen—considered the standard approach for reflux disease (GERD)—versus Toupet partial fundoplication, which has been said to reduce troublesome dysphagia and gas-related symptoms [7].

Four electronic databases (MEDLINE, Embase, Cochrane Library, and ISI Web of Knowledge CPCI-S) were searched by them, and the methodological quality of the included trials was evaluated. Outcomes included recurrent pathological acid exposure, esophagitis, dysphagia, dilatation for dysphagia, and reoperation rate.

The findings were that seven eligible randomized controlled trials (RCT) comparing LNF ($n=404$) with LTF ($n=388$) could be identified. LNF was associated with a significantly higher prevalence of postoperative dysphagia (RR 1.61 (95 % confidence interval [CI] 1.06–2.44; $p=0.02$)) and dilatation for dysphagia (RR 2.45 (CI 1.06–5.68); $p=0.04$). There were more surgical reinterventions after LNF (RR 2.19 (CI 1.09–4.40); $p=0.03$), but no differences regarding recurrent pathological acid exposure (RR 1.26 (CI 0.82–1.95); p=0.29), esophagitis (RR 1.20 (CI 0.78–1.85); $p=0.40$), subjective reflux recurrence, patient satisfaction, operating time, or in-hospital complications. Inability to belch (RR 2.04 (CI 1.19–3.49); $p=0.009$) and gas bloating (RR 1.58 (CI 1.21–2.05); $p<0.001$) were more prevalent after LNF.

Broeders et al. concluded that LTF reduces postoperative dysphagia and dilatation for dysphagia compared with LNF. Reoperation rate and prevalence of gas-related symptoms were lower after LTF, with similar reflux control. These results provide level 1a support for the use of LTF as the posterior fundoplication of choice for GERD.

Moreover, the treatment of achalasia has been analyzed extensively in a recently published randomized study comparing the pneumatic dilatation with the laparoscopic Heller myotomy [8].

Many experts consider laparoscopic Heller myotomy (LHM) to be superior to pneumatic dilation for the treatment of achalasia, and LHM is increasingly considered to be the treatment of choice for this disorder.

Patients with newly diagnosed achalasia were randomly assigned to pneumatic dilation or LHM with Dor's fundoplication. Symptoms, including weight loss, dysphagia, retrosternal pain, and regurgitation, were assessed with the use of the Eckardt score (which ranges from 0 to 12, with higher scores indicating more pronounced symptoms). The primary outcome was that of therapeutic success (a drop in the Eckardt score to ≤ 3) established at the yearly follow-up assessment. The secondary outcomes included the need for retreatment, pressure at the lower esophageal sphincter, esophageal emptying on a timed barium esophagogram, quality of life, and the rate of complications.

A total of 201 patients were randomly assigned to a pneumatic dilation (95 patients) group or to a LHM (106) group. The mean follow-up time was 43 months (95 % CI, 40–47). Abiding by an intention-to-treat analysis, the primary outcome revealed no significant difference between the two groups; the rate of therapeutic success with pneumatic dilation was 90 % after 1 year of follow-up and 86 % after 2 years, as compared with a rate with LHM of 93 % after 1 year and 90 % after 2 years ($p=0.46$). After 2 years of follow-up, there was no significant between-group difference in the pressure at the lower esophageal sphincter (LHM, 10 mmHg [95 % CI, 8.7–12]; pneumatic dilation, 12 mmHg [95 % CI, 9.7–14]; $p=0.27$); esophageal emptying, as assessed by the height of barium-contrast column (LHM, 1.9 cm [95 % CI, 0–6.8]; pneumatic dilation, 3.7 cm [95 % CI, 0–8.8]; $p=0.21$); or quality of life. Similar results were obtained in the per-protocol analysis. Perforation of the esophagus occurred in 4 % of the patients during pneumatic dilation, whereas mucosal tears occurred in 12 % during LHM. Abnormal exposure to esophageal acid was observed in 15 % and 23 % of the patients in the pneumatic dilation and LHM groups, respectively ($p=0.28$).

After 2 years of follow-up, LHM, as compared with pneumatic dilation, was not associated with superior rates of therapeutic success.

Gastric Surgery

In 2005, Hulscher et al. published the randomized study titled: "Laparoscopic versus open subtotal gastrectomy for distal gastric cancer: five-year results of a randomized prospective trial" [9].

The aim of this study was to compare technical feasibility and both early and 5-year clinical outcomes of laparoscopic-assisted and open radical subtotal gastrectomy for distal gastric cancer.

The role of laparoscopic surgery in the treatment of gastric cancer has not yet been defined, and much doubt remains about the ability to satisfy all the oncological criteria that are to be met during conventional open surgery.

This study was designed as a prospective, randomized clinical trial with a total of 59 patients. Twenty-nine (49.1 %) patients were randomized to undergo open subtotal gastrectomy (OG), while 30 (50.9 %) patients were randomized to the laparoscopic group (LG). To assess outcome differences between the groups, their demographics, ASA status, pTNM stage, histological type of the tumor, number of resected lymph nodes, postoperative complications, and 5-year overall and disease-free survival rates were studied.

The findings by Hulscher et al. were that the demographics, preoperative data, and characteristics of the tumor were similar. The mean number of resected lymph nodes was 33.4 ± 17.4 in the OG group and 30.0 ± 14.9 in the LG ($p=$not significant). Operative mortality rates were 6.7 % (2 patients) in the OG and 3.3 % (1 patient) in the LG ($p=$not significant); morbidity rates were 27.6 % and 26.7 %, respectively ($p=$not significant). Five-year overall and disease-free survival rates were 55.7 % and 54.8 % and 58.9 % and 57.3 % in the OG and the LG, respectively ($p=$not significant).

Hulscher et al. concluded that laparoscopic radical subtotal gastrectomy for distal gastric cancer is a feasible and safe oncological procedure and that its short- and long-term results are similar to those obtained with an open approach. Additional benefits for the LG were reduced blood loss, shorter time to resumption of oral intake, and earlier discharge from hospital.

Kim et al. compared laparoscopy assisted and conventional open distal gastrectomy and extraperigastric lymph node dissection in early gastric cancer [10].

Laparoscopy-assisted gastrectomy with lymph node dissection for gastric cancer is considered technically more complicated than the open method. Moreover, the safety and efficacy of laparoscopy-assisted distal gastrectomy (LADG) with lymph node dissection in patients with gastric cancer have not been established yet. To evaluate short-term surgical validity, surgical outcome of the laparoscopy-assisted distal gastrectomy (LADG) with lymph node dissection was compared with that of the conventional open distal gastrectomy (CODG) in patients with early gastric cancer.

One hundred and forty-seven patients with early gastric cancer received conventional radical distal gastrectomy during 2002 and 2003, whereby 71 patients underwent LADG. The groups were compared for aspects of clinicopathological characteristics, the postoperative outcomes and courses, and the postoperative morbidities. Similar for both groups were the baseline characteristics, including gender, age, body mass index (BMI), American Society of Anesthesiology (ASA) class, tumor size, T-stage, and lymph node metastasis. No significant differences were found between the groups in terms of the number of retrieved lymph nodes with respect to D1 + alpha (D1 + no. 7) and D1 + beta (D1 + no. 7, 8a, and 9) lymphadenectomy. In the LADG group, wound size was smaller ($P < 0.0001$), but operation time was longer ($p = 0.0001$) than in the CODG group. Perioperative recovery was faster in the LADG group than in the CODG group, as reflected by a shorter hospital stay ($p = 0.0176$) and lesser time of additional analgesics ($p = 0.0370$). Serum albumin level in LADG was higher ($p = 0.0002$) on day 7 than that in CODG, and the leukocyte count in LADG lowers ($p = 0.0445$) on day 1 than that in CODG. Postoperative morbidities and mortalities were not significantly different between the two groups.

This data confirmed that LADG with no. 7, 8, and 9 lymph node dissections proved to be a feasible and acceptable surgical technique for early gastric cancer. From a surgical point of view, LADG with lymph node dissection at least suggests being preferred surgical option for patients with early gastric cancer. Its oncological validity awaits larger and prospective multicenter trials.

Colon Cancer Surgery

The first published randomized study comparing laparoscopic versus open approach for segmental colon cancer was the “Barcelona trial” by Lacy et al., published in the Lancet in 2002 [11].

The astonishing result was that a stage III colon cancer showed a better survival rate in the laparoscopic group than in the open group. This finding positively triggered an increasing use of laparoscopic colon approach to colon cancer in daily surgery all over the world. Moreover, in this trial also important short-term advantages were observed in favor of the laparoscopically operated patients.

Since then, additional multicentric trials have been published, such as the CLASSIC study, the COST study, the COLOR I study, and the Transatlantic study.

A review of the outcome of these trials, starting with the initial study, can be given:

1. In the Barcelona trial, 111 laparoscopic patients versus 108 open patients were compared. Findings were that patients recovered quickly in the laparoscopic group for their hospital stay was shorter. Also the morbidity was significantly lower (12 pts versus 31 pts) in the laparoscopic group; although laparoscopy did not influence the perioperative mortality. Other findings were that morbidity included 8 pts with wound infection versus 18; persistent ileus, 3 versus 9 patients; 2 eviscerations in the open group; 1 postoperative bleeding in open group; 2 anastomotic leaks in the open group; and the perioperative mortality of 1 patient versus 3 patients, all respectively [11].
2. The short-term end points of the MRC CLASICC study were published in 2005. They included colon and rectum cancers. This multicenter, randomized trial involved 794 patients of 27 British centers. Allocation of patients was laparoscopic-assisted 526 and open surgery 268 patients. Hundred forty-three patients (29 %) were converted to open surgery. Patients with complications were for colon and rectum not different in laparoscopic (35 % and 59 %) and open surgery (35 % and 50 %), respectively. Specific complications such as wound infection, chest infection, anastomotic dehiscence, and deep vein thrombosis were also not different between the two groups. Moreover mortality, 5 % versus 4 %, was not different as well. They concluded that laparoscopic-assisted surgery for cancer of the colon is as effective as open in the short term and is likely to produce similar long-term outcomes [12].
3. The COST study included 435 laparoscopic patients versus 428 patients assigned to open surgery. The conversion rate was 21 %. Concerning complications, the conclusions for the two groups showed that the rates of intraoperative complications (4 % and 2 %), the 30-day postoperative mortality rate, the complications at discharge and at 60 days (19 % and 19 %), the hospital readmission rate, and reoperation rates were very similar for both groups. Mortality for the groups was less than 1 % and 1 %, respectively [13].
4. The COLOR I study included 536 laparoscopic patients versus 546 open patients. Findings were that in the short term, even if the blood loss was less and the operating time longer, and the hospital stay significantly shorter, yet the morbidity and mortality of the segmental colonic resection did not differ between the two groups. Other findings were the overall complication rate was 21 % (laparoscopic) and 20 % (open), wound infection 4 % and 3 %, wound dehiscence less than 1 %, bleeding 2 % and 2 %, anastomotic failure 3 % and 2 %, intestinal obstruction 2 % and 3 %, and reinterventions 7 % and 5 %, all respectively [14].
5. The Transatlantic study entailed the cooperative study of the Barcelona group, CLASSIC study, COST study, and COLOR I study regarding their long-term results for the laparoscopic and open groups of patients. No differences were found in being disease-free, their overall survival rate, and the local recurrences for patients between both groups of patients [15].

6. The study of Leung et al. on rectosigmoid cancers included 203 laparoscopic patients versus 200 open operated patients, respectively. They concluded that for the laparoscopic group, the operative time was longer, the recovery of patients was significantly better, but that the morbidity did not differ between the two groups: being 40 versus 45 pts, respectively. Other findings regarding aspects of the laparoscopic group and open groups were the differences in intra-abdominal bleeding 0 and 1 pt; anastomotic bleeding 2 and 3 patients; rectovaginal and rectovesical fistula 2 versus 0 patients; anastomotic leakage, 1 versus 4 patients; wound infection, 9 versus 15 patients; and presence of the incisional hernia as delayed complication in 8 versus 4 patients, all respectively. Finally, the operative mortality was found to be 0.6 % versus 2.4 %, respectively [16].

Interesting are the outcomes of randomized trials on benign colonic diseases, such as IBD and diverticulitis.

In 2009, Klarenbeek et al. published the results of the SIGMA trial that compared the laparoscopic and open approach for elective sigmoid resection after complicated diverticulitis [17].

Previously, no randomized controlled trial had compared laparoscopic sigmoid resection (LSR) to open sigmoid resection (OSR) for symptomatic diverticulitis of the sigmoid colon. Hence, this study tested the hypothesis that LSR is associated with decreased postoperative complication rates as compared with OSR.

This was a prospective, multicenter, double-blind, parallel-arm, randomized controlled trial. Eligible patients were randomized to either LSR or OSR. End points included postoperative mortality, and complications were classified as major and minor. The generator of the allocation sequence was separated from the executor. Blinding was ensured by using an opaque wound dressing to cover the abdomen. Symptomatic diverticulitis of the sigmoid colon was defined as recurrent disease Hinchey I, IIa, IIb, symptomatic stricture, or severe rectal bleeding. The decision to discharge patients was made by independent physicians held blind to the allocation sequence. Data were analyzed according to the "intention to treat" principle.

From 2002 to 2006, 104 patients were randomized in five centers. All patients underwent the allocated intervention. Fifty-two LSR patients were held comparable to 52 OSR patients for gender, age, BMI, ASA grade, comorbid conditions, previous abdominal surgery, and indication for surgery. Findings showed that LSR took longer ($p=0.0001$) but caused less blood loss ($p=0.033$). Conversion rate was 19.2 %. Mortality rate was 1 %. There were significantly more major complications in OSR patients (LSR 9.6 % versus OSR 25.0 %; $p=0.038$). Minor complication rates were similar (LSR 36.5 % versus OSR 38.5 %; $p=0.839$). LSR patients had less pain (Visual Analog Scale 1.6; $p=0.0003$), systemic analgesia requirement ($p=0.029$), and returned home earlier ($p=0.046$) than OSR patients did. The Short Form-36 health questionnaire (SF-36) showed a significantly better quality of life for the group undergoing LSR. The overall conclusion was that LSR was associated with a 15.4 % reduction in major complication rates, less pain, an improved quality of life, and a shorter hospitalization at the cost of a longer operating time.

Maartense et al. published in 2004 and 2006 two randomized studies on IBD, ulcerative colitis (UC) and Crohn's disease, thereby comparing the outcome of an open approach and laparoscopic approach in each [18, 19].

The aim of the first study was to evaluate postoperative recovery after hand-assisted laparoscopic or open-restorative proctocolectomy with ileal pouch anal anastomosis (IAPA) for ulcerative colitis and familial adenomatous polyposis (FAP), and that was done in a randomized controlled trial.

Sixty patients were randomized for hand-assisted laparoscopic ($n=30$) or open surgery ($n=30$). Primary outcome parameter was postoperative recovery in the 3 months after surgery, measured by quality of life questionnaires (SF-36 and GIQLI). Secondary parameters were postoperative morphine requirements and surgical parameters, viz., operating time, morbidity, hospital stay, and costs.

They found no difference between the two procedures in terms of quality of life assessment in the 3 months after surgery. In the first two postoperative weeks, there had been a significant decline in quality of life on all scales of the SF-36 ($P<0.001$) and total GIQLI score ($P<0.001$) in both groups (no significant difference between the groups). Quality of life returned to baseline levels after 4 weeks in the two groups. Operating times were longer in the laparoscopic group as compared with the open group (210 and 133 min, respectively; $p<0.001$). No significant differences were found in morphine requirement. Neither morbidity nor postoperative hospital stay differed between the laparoscopic and open groups (20 % versus 17 %, in 10 versus 11 days, respectively). Median overall costs were 16.728 euros for the hand-assisted laparoscopic procedure and 13.406 for the open procedure ($p=0.095$).

Patient recovery rates, as measured by quality of life questionnaires, were found comparable for hand-assisted laparoscopic as well as for open-restorative proctocolectomy with ileal pouch anal anastomosis. The laparoscopic approach can be held to be as safe, but more costly than the open procedure.

The question arose about what would happen if the operation should be completely performed laparoscopically and not done so hand assisted. Case–control study compared the group hand-assisted operated on and the group having a total laparoscopic proctocolectomy and IAPA. The only differences were regarding disadvantages holding for the last group, because the operative time was longer, and this group also experienced more reoperations during the early postoperative period [20].

In a follow-up study, Maartense et al. focused on the cosmetic long-term effect of this trial [21]. Comparing the cosmetic scores and the body imaging scores between the laparoscopic and open groups, they concluded that scores for male patients were not different after a 2-year follow-up, whereas the scores for female patients demonstrated significant differences.

In their second study Maartense et al., using a randomized trial, compared the postoperative outcome of laparoscopic-assisted approach with an open ileocolic resection for Crohn's disease [19].

Sixty patients were randomized for laparoscopic-assisted or open surgery. Primary outcome parameter was the postoperative quality of life (QoL) during 3 months of follow-up, measured by SF-36 and GIQLI questionnaires. Secondary parameters were the operating time, morbidity, hospital stay, postoperative morphine requirement, pain level, and costs.

Patient characteristics were found not to be different. Conversion rate was 10 % ($n = 3$). Median operating time was longer in the laparoscopic approach as compared with open surgery (115 versus 90 min; $p < 0.003$). Hospital stay was shorter in the laparoscopic group (5 versus 7 days; $p = 0.008$). The number of patients with postoperative morbidity within the first 30 days differed between the laparoscopic and open group (10 % versus 33 %; $p = 0.028$). There was no statistically significant difference in quality of life between the groups during follow-up. Significant time effects were found on all scales of the SF-36 ($P < 0.001$) and the GIQLI score ($P < 0.001$). Quality of life declined in the first week, returned to baseline levels after 2 weeks, and saw improvement at 4 weeks and 3 months after surgery. Median overall costs during the 3 months follow-up were significantly different: Euro 6,412 for laparoscopic and Euro 8,196 for open surgery ($p = 0.042$).

Although quality of life measured by SF-36 and GIQLI questionnaires was not different for the laparoscopic-assisted group as compared with the open group, yet, the ileocolic resection, morbidity, hospital stay, and costs were significantly lower.

Rectal Cancer Surgery

Concerning the surgical treatment of rectal cancer, there is only one randomized protocol, namely, the CLASSIC trial [12], in which a part of the group of included patients underwent an operation because of rectal cancer. In the CLASSIC trial, 381 patients with rectal cancer were randomized for either open approach or laparoscopic total mesorectal excision (TME). One-third of the laparoscopic procedures had to be converted to open surgery. Findings were that patients who had laparoscopic anterior resections for cancers located in the upper rectum were found to have positive circumferential margins in 11 % of the cases, although disease-free survival was no worse than in those who had undergone open surgery. These findings led to questions concerning the safety of laparoscopic surgery in those patients having rectal cancer.

Therefore the COLOR II trial, with more than 1,000 patients included, has been carried out. It was designed for determining the safety of minimally invasive surgery for patients with rectal cancer. Primary goal of the study was to observe if there were differences in local recurrence between the laparoscopic and open group at 3 years postoperatively. Moreover, all the data of the departments of Pathology, including the resection and circumferential margins, as well as the operative data and short-term data were studied [22]. Currently, short-term results have been calculated, and a pertaining paper has been sent to a renowned medical journal for publication.

References

1. Smithers BM, Gotley DC, Martin I, Thomas JM. Comparison of the outcomes between open and minimally invasive esophagectomy. Ann Surg. 2007;245:232–40.
2. Butler N, Collins S, Memon B, Memon MA. Minimally invasive oesophagectomy: current status and future direction. Surg Endosc. 2011;25:2072–83.
3. Hulscher JB, van Sandick JW, de Boer AG, et al. Extended transthoracic resection compared with limited transhiatal resection for adenocarcinoma of the esophagus. N Engl J Med. 2002;347:1662–9.
4. Luketich JD, Alvelo-Rivera M, Buenaventura PO, et al. Minimally invasive esophagectomy: outcomes in 222 patients. Ann Surg. 2003;238:486–94.
5. Palanivelu C, Prakash A, Senthilkumar R, et al. Minimally invasive esophagectomy: Thoracoscopic mobilization of the esophagus and mediastinal lymphadenectomy in prone position-experience of 130 patients. J Am Coll Surg. 2006;203:7–16.
6. Biere SS, van Berge Henegouwen MI, Maas KW, et al. Minimally invasive versus open oesophagectomy for patients with oesophageal cancer: a multicentre, open-label, randomised controlled trial. Lancet. 2012;379:1887–92.
7. Broeders JA, Bredenoord AJ, Hazebroek EJ, et al. Reflux and belching after 270 degree versus 360 degree laparoscopic posterior fundoplication. Ann Surg. 2012;255:59–65.
8. Boeckxstaens GE, Annese V, des Varannes SB, et al. Pneumatic dilatation versus laparoscopic Heller's myotomy for idiopathic achalasia. N Engl J Med. 2011;364:1807–16.
9. Huscher CG, Mingoli A, Sgarzini G, et al. Laparoscopic versus open subtotal gastrectomy for distal gastric cancer: five year results of a randomized prospective trial. Ann Surg. 2005;241:232–7.
10. Kim HH, Hyung WJ, Cho GS, et al. Morbidity and mortality of laparoscopic gastrectomy versus open gastrectomy for gastric cancer: an interim report-a phase III multicenter, prospective, randomized Trial (KLASS Trial). Ann Surg. 2010;251:417–20.
11. Lacy AM, Garcia-Valdecasas JC, Delgado S, et al. Laparoscopy-assisted colectomy versus open colectomy for treatment of non-metastatic colon cancer: a randomised trial. Lancet. 2002;359:2224–9.
12. Guillou PS, Quirke P, Thorpe H, et al. Short term endpoints of conventional versus laparoscopic assisted surgery in patients with colorectal cancer (MRC CLASICC trial), randomised controlled trial. Lancet. 2005;365:1718–26.
13. The Clinical Outcomes of Surgical Therapy Study Group. A comparison of laparoscopically assisted and open colectomy for colon cancer. N Engl J Med. 2004;350:2050–9.
14. Veldkamp R, Kuhry E, Hop WC, et al. Laparoscopic surgery versus open surgery for colon cancer: short term outcomes of a randomised trial. Lancet Oncol. 2005;6:477–84.
15. Bonjer HJ, Hop WC, Nelson H, et al. Transatlantic laparoscopically assisted vs Open Colectomy Trials Study Group. Arch Surg. 2007;142:298–303.
16. Leung KL, Kwok SPY, Lam SCW, et al. Laparoscopic resection of recto-sigmoid carcinoma: prospective randomized trial. Lancet. 2004;363:1187–92.
17. Klarenbeek BR, Veenhof AA, Bergamaschi R, et al. Laparoscopic sigmoid resection for diverticulitis decreases major morbidity rates: a randomised control trial: short term results of the Sigma trial. Ann Surg. 2009;249:39–44.
18. Maartense S, Dunker MS, Slors JF, et al. Laparoscopic assisted versus open ileocolic resection for Crohn's disease: a randomized trial. Ann Surg. 2006;243:143–9.
19. Maartense S, Dunker MS, Slors JF, et al. Hand-assisted laparoscopic versus open restorative proctocolectomy with ileal pouch anal anastomosis: a randomized trial. Ann Surg. 2004;240:984–91.
20. Polle SW, Dunker MS, Slors JF, et al. Body image, cosmesis, quality of life, and functional outcome of hand assisted laparoscopic versus open restorative proctocolectomy: long term results of a randomized trial. Surg Endosc. 2007;21:1301–7.

21. Polle SW, van Berge Henegouwen MI, Slors JF, et al. Total laparoscopic restorative proctocolectomy: are there advantages compared with the open and hand assisted approaches ? Dis Colon Rectum. 2008;51:541–8.
22. Color II Study Group, Buunen M, Bonjer HJ, Hop WC, et al. COLOR II. A randomised clinical trial comparing laparoscopic and open surgery for rectal cancer. Dan Med Bull 2009; 56:89–91.

Chapter 7
Is There Less Morbidity After Fast-Track Surgery?

Christine Vermeulen, Willem A. Bemelman, and Miguel A. Cuesta

Keywords Morbidity • Fast track surgery • Laparoscopic surgery • Open surgery • Recovery • Postoperative care • ERAS • Colonic surgery

Introduction

In the past decades, there have been important developments in surgical care programs. Hospital stay after conventional major abdominal (colorectal) surgery used to be long for all patients, and this was accompanied by a high morbidity rate of 20 %. Most patients are elderly and have a substantial prevalence of comorbidity. The question is if an accelerated recovery program including good information to the patient, rapid oral intake, and fast mobilization would result in shorter hospital stay and concomitantly in decreased morbidity. Such fast-track surgical programs were implemented with positive results regarding length of hospital stay. Large series and randomized studies comparing conventional with fast-track perioperative care had demonstrated superior outcome concerning hospital stay with no differences in morbidity. Different factors for the perioperative care are implemented to achieve an optimal enhanced recovery after surgery (ERAS) outcome. Additionally, the introduction of laparoscopic surgery has accelerated postoperative recovery and reduced hospital stay. An important question is if the introduction of fast-track programs can decrease complications. Moreover, the role of laparoscopic surgery in a fast-track program is important to investigate.

C. Vermeulen • M.A. Cuesta, MD (✉)
Department of Surgery, VU University Medical Center, Amsterdam,
The Netherlands
e-mail: ma.cuesta@vumc.nl

W.A. Bemelman, MD
Department of Surgery, Academic Medical Center, Amsterdam, The Netherlands

M.A. Cuesta, H.J. Bonjer (eds.), *Treatment of Postoperative Complications after Digestive Surgery*, DOI 10.1007/978-1-4471-4354-3_7,

In this chapter, we will discuss several leading studies involving the impact of fast-track surgical programs in open and laparoscopic surgery, offering the most recent evidence-based knowledge.

Fast Track in Complex Elective Open Surgery

Nowadays, many straightforward surgical procedures are routinely performed in day care. In addition, more complex procedures are more often performed in an accelerated perioperative multimodality care program, stimulating enhanced postoperative recovery and a shorter hospital stay. The pioneer in fast-track surgery programs was Kehlet, who investigated the implementation in several studies [1–4]. Fast-track programs aim at a faster recovery after surgery by reducing surgical stress.

Length of hospital stay can be reduced from 6 to 10 days in conventional surgical care programs to 5 days after implementation of such a program [5–7]. It was even observed that the length of hospital stay, in the vast majority of open colonic resection patients (excluding low anterior resection patients), could be reduced to 2–3 days after implementation of a fast-track program [8]. This consists of providing detailed and repeated information to patient and family concerning the fast-track program to follow preoperatively and postoperatively including sufficient pain management, prompt normal enteral feeding, laxation, and enforced mobilization. Although it is hypothesized and expected that the morbidity concurrently decreases, there is no real evidence in those earlier studies due to small study populations and lack of randomization.

Laparoscopic Versus Open Surgery with a Fast-Track Program

In addition to the introduction of fast-track surgery, the introduction of laparoscopic surgery has reduced the length of hospital stay in gastrointestinal surgery [9–12]. Recently, several study groups investigated whether a difference could be established between patients undergoing laparoscopic and patients undergoing open surgery, both implemented with the fast-track surgical care program. In a double-blind randomized controlled trial, 60 patients underwent either laparoscopic or open elective colon surgery with accelerated rehabilitation. A rapid recovery was observed with a median hospital stay of 2 days [13]. No difference in length of stay or recovery to normal activities was detected in either of the two groups. Moreover, there were no significant differences in postoperative morbidity, mortality, or readmissions, although three patients died in the open versus nil in the laparoscopic group.

Their conclusion was that recovery was rapid and without differences between open and laparoscopic operation.

King et al. performed a randomized trial in similar groups (2/1 randomization laparoscopic versus open colectomy) and found a 32 % shorter hospital stay in the laparoscopic group compared to the open surgery group, with no difference in morbidity [14]. Convalescence was also significantly shorter, and readmission less, in the laparoscopic group. Moreover morbidity, costs, and quality of life were not different between groups [14]. It seems likely that the detected difference in outcome between both studies is based on the different inclusion criteria. Basse et al. excluded patients undergoing low anterior resections and patients not living independently, whereas King et al. included those patients and observed the largest difference in those groups. Both studies are comprised of relatively small study populations though, which could have been an influence on the results. They did not report on the number of actual, implemented elements of the fast-track program, which could be an influence on the outcome as well.

Key Features of the Enhanced Recovery Program

(From PM King, *Br J Surg* 2006, 93:300–8)

Before admission

Conditioning and expectations
Counseling with patient and carer
Provision of written information
Meeting with stoma nurse if anticipated
Comorbid risk assessment
Optimized premorbid health status

Day before

Nutrition: three high-protein/high-calorie drinks
Bowel preparation: two enemas, evening before and morning of surgery for left colon, sigmoid, and rectum

Day of surgery

Thoracic epidural with Bupivacaine® T8–T9 level
Intraoperative fluid standardized and limited
Local anesthesia infiltration to the largest wound in minimally invasive surgery (MIS)

Surgery

MIS or transverse curved incisions
No nasogastric tubes or surgical drains

Postoperative care

Pain relief: continuous epidural anesthesia 48 h, regular paracetamol and nonsteroidal anti-inflammatory drug or equivalent
Fluids: high-protein/high-calorie drinks on day of surgery (+ diet if tolerated)
Stop IV fluids on morning after surgery

Mobilization, from arrival on ward

Laxative from day 1

Discharge

Aim for discharge on fixed day

Follow-up

Provision of telephone numbers to allow discussion of problems
Expected review if problems occur within 2 weeks
Review on patient clinic on day 12 after surgery

The LAFA Trial

The hypothesis of combining the two important developments, focusing on accelerated recovery as best perioperative strategy, needed more evidence [15]. A randomized multicenter clinical study, the LAFA trial, was initiated. Patients undergoing segmental colonic surgery were randomized into four arms: open with conventional care, open with a fast-track program, laparoscopic with conventional care, and laparoscopic with a fast-track program [16]. Thus, four study groups were created, with each comprised of approximately a hundred patients. Protocol compliance was measured and reported on in all groups. In addition to the length of hospital stay, multiple secondary outcomes were investigated: morbidity rate among others. Length of hospital stay was significantly shorter in patients that underwent laparoscopic surgery with a fast-track perioperative care program compared to all of the other combinations. The combination of open surgery with a conventional care program resulted in the longest hospital stay. In a postoperative hospital stay, both laparoscopy and a fast-track program are significant factors of influence in reducing the length of the stay. If readmissions are taken into account, laparoscopy is the only hospital-stay-reducing factor. Regression analysis showed that laparoscopy was the only independent predictive factor to reduce hospital stay. With all of the results taken into account, it seems that an optimal fast-track surgery program is comprised of the abovementioned factors (pain relief, good information, immediate oral intake, and rapid mobilization) in combination with laparoscopic surgery [16]. Obviously, this is not always possible due to pathological features of the disease or physical condition of the patient. In these cases, the open procedure should preferentially be accompanied by an enhanced recovery program.

There was no significant difference in morbidity between the four study groups, but a trend towards less overall morbidity and major complications in the laparoscopic surgery groups was observed. Indeed, logistic regression analysis showed a significantly lower overall and major morbidity rate for laparoscopy.

The fast-track surgery program, including laparoscopy, significantly reduces length of hospital stay. Discharge should be based on multiple, objectified, and predefined criteria to minimize the readmission rate [16].

Hormonal and stress response studied as substudy of the LAFA trial has confirmed the advantages of the laparoscopic fast-track surgery [17].

Conclusions

The best perioperative strategy in colonic surgery patients seems to be laparoscopy embedded in a fast-track surgical care program. When open surgery is the favorable option, accelerated recovery is best achieved in a fast-track program. Overall morbidity rate does not differ significantly between any of the perioperative strategy combinations, but seems to be decreased in laparoscopic surgery.

References

1. Wilmore DW, Kehlet H. Management of patients in fast track surgery. BMJ. 2001;322:473–6.
2. Fearon KC, Ljungqvist O, Von MM, et al. Enhanced recovery after surgery: a consensus review of clinical care for patients undergoing colonic resection. Clin Nutr. 2005;24:466–77.
3. Kehlet H. Fast track colorectal surgery. Lancet. 2008;371:791–3.
4. Kehlet H, Wilmore DW. Evidence-based surgical care and the evolution of fast track surgery. Ann Surg. 2008;248(2):189–98.
5. Möiniche S, Bülow S, Hesselfeldt P, et al. Convalescence and hospital stay with balanced analgesia, early oral feeding and enforced mobilisation. Eur J Surg. 1995;161:283–8.
6. Liu SS, Carpenter RL, Mackey DC, et al. Effects of perioperative analgesic technique on rate of recovery after colon surgery. Anesthesiology. 1995;83:757–65.
7. Bradshaw BGG, Liu SS, Thirlby RC. Standard perioperative care protocols and reduced length of stay after colon surgery. J Am Coll Surg. 1998;186:501–6.
8. Basse L, Jakobsen DH, Billesbølle P, et al. A clinical pathway to accelerate recovery after colonic resection. Ann Surg. 2000;232(1):51–7.
9. Jacobs M, Verdeja JC, Goldstein HS. Minimally invasive colon resection (laparoscopic colectomy). Surg Laparosc Endosc. 1991;1:144–50.
10. Nelson H, et al. from the Clinical Outcomes of Surgical Therapy Study Group. A comparison of laparoscopically assisted and open colectomy for colon cancer. NEJM. 2004;350(20):2050–9.
11. Bonjer HJ, et al. from Transatlantic Laparoscopically Assisted vs Open Colectomy Trials Study Group. Laparoscopically assisted vs open colectomy for colon cancer – a meta-analysis. Arch Surg. 2007;142:298–303.
12. Jayne DG, Thorpe HC, Copeland J, et al. Five-year follow-up of the Medical Research Council CLASICC Trial of laparoscopically assisted vs open surgery for colorectal cancer. Br J Surg. 2010;97:1638–45.

13. Basse L, Jakobsen DH, Bardram L, et al. Functional recovery after open vs laparoscopic colonic resection – a randomized, blinded study. Ann Surg. 2005;241(3):416–23.
14. King PM, Blazeby JM, Ewings P, et al. Randomized clinical trial comparing laparoscopic and open surgery for colorectal cancer within an enhanced recovery programme. Br J Surg. 2005;93:300–8.
15. Kehlet H. Fast track surgery – an update on physiological care principles to enhance recovery. Langenbecks Arch Surg. 2011;396:585–90.
16. Vlug MS, Wind J, Hollmann MW, et al. Laparoscopy in combination with fast track multimodal management is the best perioperative strategy in patients undergoing colonic surgery – an RCT (LAFA-study). Ann Surg. 2011;254:868–75.
17. Veenhof AA, Vlug MS, vd Pas MH, et al. Surgical stress response and postoperative immune function after laparoscopy or open surgery with fast track or standard perioperative care; a randomized trial. Ann Surg. 2012;255:216–21.

Chapter 8
Prevention and Treatment of Major Complications After Esophageal Surgery

Rachel L.G.M. Blom, Donald L. van der Peet, and Mark I. van Berge Henegouwen

Keywords Esophageal carcinoma • Esophagectomy • Complications • Treatment • Anastomotic leakage

Esophageal Surgery for Cancer

Introduction

Esophageal carcinoma is an aggressive disease with early lymphatic and hematogenous dissemination [1]. The incidence of esophageal carcinoma has been rising steadily over the past decades, which seems mainly to be a result of the sixfold increase in the number of patients with esophageal adenocarcinoma [2]. Surgical resection remains the most important part of a potentially curative treatment; however, even after esophagectomy, a substantial proportion of patients will develop local or distant recurrent disease, [3, 4] and 5-year survival rates rarely exceed 40 % [5, 6]. Esophagectomy can be performed by means of a transthoracic or transhiatal resection. Over the past few years, minimally invasive techniques for esophagectomy have been developed in an attempt to decrease invasiveness without compromising the extent of dissection and consequent survival.

R.L.G.M. Blom
Department of Surgery, Atrium Medical Center, Heerlen, The Netherlands

D.L. van der Peet, MD
Department of Surgery, VU University Medical Center, Amsterdam, The Netherlands

M.I. van Berge Henegouwen, MD, PhD (✉)
Department of Surgery, Academic Medical Center, Amsterdam, The Netherlands
e-mail: m.i.vanbergehenegouwen@amc.uva.nl

M.A. Cuesta, H.J. Bonjer (eds.), *Treatment of Postoperative Complications after Digestive Surgery*, DOI 10.1007/978-1-4471-4354-3_8,

Table 8.1 Complication rate in 940 patients who underwent esophagectomy at the Academic Medical Center

	All patients N (%)
No. of patients	940 (100)
Overall complications	636 (68)
Non-surgical complications	
Pulmonary total[b]	285 (30)
Pneumonia	262 (28)
Cardiac	97 (10)
Surgical complications	
Anastomotic leakage	
Clinical	103 (11)
Subclinical[a]	80 (9)
Chylous leakage	51 (5)
Recurrent laryngeal nerve paralysis	98 (10)
In-hospital mortality	31 (3)

Adapted from van Heijl et al. [10]
[a]Only on radiological examination
[b]Pulmonary: pneumonia, atelectasis, pleura-empyema

Centralization of surgical resections, advances in surgical techniques, and improvements in perioperative care have reduced the risk of esophagectomy to an acceptable level [7]. Esophageal surgery is however still associated with substantial morbidity. Early postoperative complication rates vary between 40 and 80 %, depending on the applied criteria and the type of resection [5, 8]. Centralization of esophageal surgery in high-volume centers has reduced in-hospital mortality to approximately 1–4 % [9].

This chapter will discuss the incidence, diagnosis, and treatment of the most important complications that are associated with surgical resection of the esophagus.

Complications: Classification and Prognostication

The overall incidence of complications after esophagectomy as reported in the literature varies between 40 and 80 %. In one of the largest series regarding esophagectomy for esophageal carcinoma, the incidence of individual complications that are associated with surgical resection of the esophagus was described. This series included almost 1,000 patients over a period of 16 years (Table 8.1) [10].

Classification of complications facilitates the evaluation and comparison of surgical outcomes among different surgeons, centers, and therapies. The severity of postoperative complications can be graded according to the morbidity scale proposed by Dindo et al. [11]. This classification system is based on the therapy used to treat the complication, and it consists of five grades (Table 8.2).

Predicting the severity of complications can reveal important information for both patient and surgeon, and individualized risk assessment may help deciding the optimal extent of surgery. Recently, a nomogram was developed based on preoperative risk factors to predict the severity of complications in esophageal cancer patients who undergo surgical resection (Fig. 8.1) [12].

Table 8.2 Dindo classification

Grade	Definition
Grade I	Any deviation from the normal postoperative course without the need for treatment
Grade II	Requiring pharmacological treatment
Grade III	Requiring surgical, endoscopic or radiological intervention
IIIa	Intervention not under general anesthesia
IIIb	Intervention under general anesthesia
Grade IV	Life-threatening complication requiring ICU management
IVa	Single organ dysfunction
IVb	Multiorgan dysfunction
Grade V	Death of a patient

Adapted from Dindo et al. [11]
ICU intensive care unit

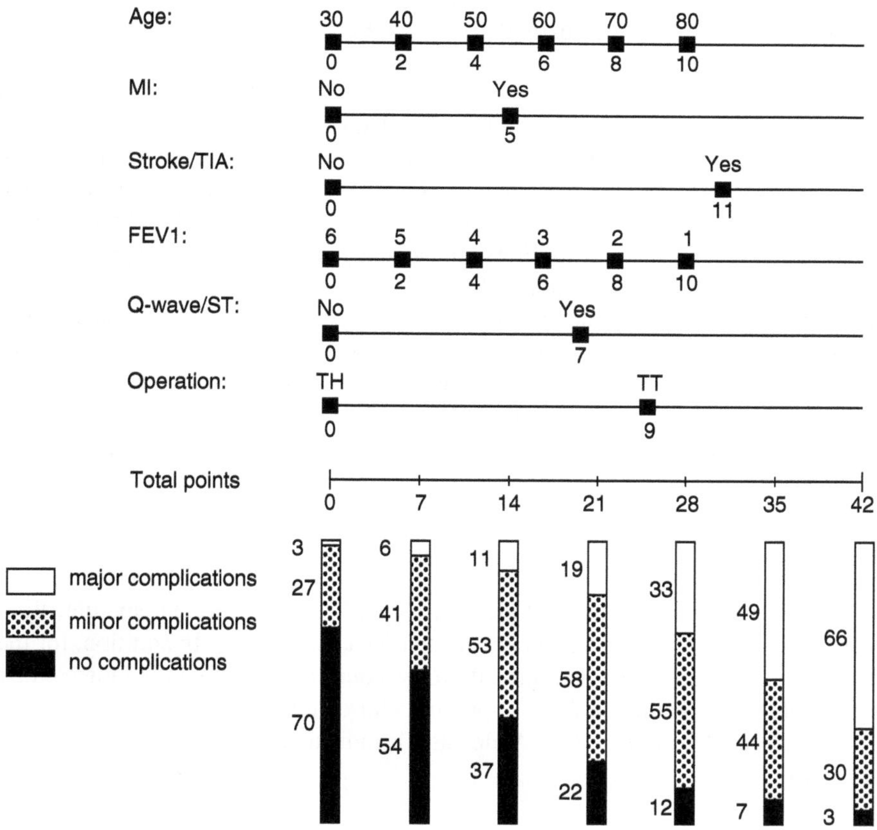

Fig. 8.1 Nomogram for the prediction of severity of complications with use of preoperative risk factors. *Instruction*: Locate the age on the axis. Determine how many point the patient receives. Repeat this for each axis. Sum the points for all predictors and locate the sum on the total points axis. Draw a line straight down to the bar graphs. Bar graphs represent the chance for an individual patient after esophagectomy for cancer to develop major, minor-to-moderate, or no complications. *FEV1* forced expiratory volume in the first second, *MI* myocardial infarction, *TIA* transient ischemic attack (Adapted from Lagarde et al. [12])

Treatment and Incidence of Specific Complications

Nonsurgical Complications

Pulmonary Complications

Incidence and Definition

Surgical resection of the esophagus is considered to be one of the most extensive and traumatic gastrointestinal surgical procedures. Transthoracic resections are associated with higher postoperative complication rates compared to transhiatal esophagectomies [5]. Transthoracic esophagectomy includes a two-field lymphadenectomy that leads to pulmonary complications in a relatively large number of patients. Furthermore, one-lung ventilation can cause alveolar damage, and breathing may be impaired due to pain after thoracotomy. Risk factors for the development of pulmonary complications are advanced age, a history of smoking, and chronic obstructive pulmonary disease (COPD). Preoperative lung function test is performed to exclude patients with an inadequate lung function from surgical resection. Pulmonary complications are defined as pneumonia, acute respiratory distress syndrome (ARDS), and atelectasis [5]. ARDS is defined according to the American-European consensus conference on ARDS criteria [13]. The incidence of pulmonary complications after esophagectomy depends on the type of procedure; generally it varies between 30 % and 57 % [5, 10]. Epidural analgesia leads to less postoperative pain and is therefore associated with a lower pulmonary complication rate [14]. With the introduction of minimally invasive esophageal surgery (MIE), pulmonary complication rates have further decreased. Several large series that have compared minimally invasive to conventional open esophagectomies have shown a lower pulmonary complication rate after MIE, ranging from 10 to 30 % [15, 16].

Diagnosis

Clinical signs of pneumonia include fever (<38.5 °C) and purulent sputum. Both pneumonia and atelectasis can be diagnosed on a chest X-ray. In addition, for the diagnosis of pneumonia a sputum culture is required. Pneumonia is indicated by the isolation of a pathogen from a sputum culture and a new or progressive infiltrate on a chest X-ray (Fig. 8.2). Atelectasis is indicated by lobar collapse on chest X-ray [5].

Treatment

Treatment of pneumonia consists of antibiotics and supportive care if needed. Supportive care includes oxygen and readmission to the intensive care unit with reintubation.

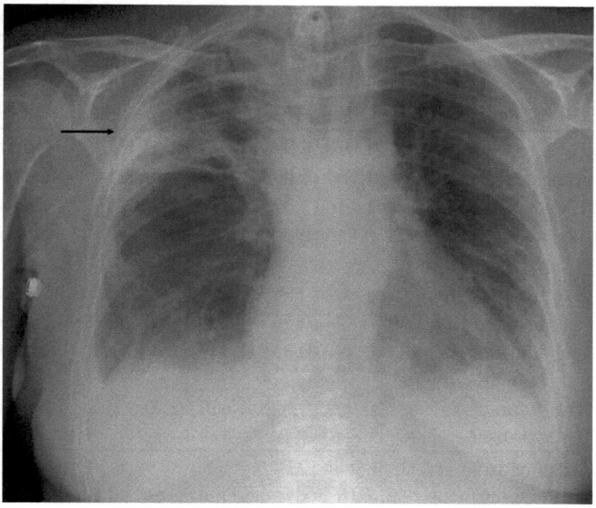

Fig. 8.2 X-ray of pulmonary infiltrate in the right upper lobe (*arrow*) in a patient 8 days after thoracolaparoscopic esophagectomy

Cardiac Complications

Incidence and Definition

Cardiac complications after esophagectomy include myocardial infarction and congestive heart failure but consist mainly of atrial fibrillation (AF). AF occurs most frequently after transthoracic esophagectomy with an incidence ranging from 13 to 46 % [5, 17]. It can also occur after transhiatal resections due to manipulation and blunt dissection, which inevitably compresses the atria [18]. AF is a complicated arrhythmia of incompletely understood pathogenesis. Ectopic foci, single-circuit reentry, and multiple-circuit reentry have been implicated in initiating and maintaining the condition [19]. Risk factors for the development of AF after esophagectomy include age older than 65 years, male sex, history of heart disease, and chronic obstructive pulmonary disease [17].

Diagnosis

Patients with AF suffer from shortness of breath and fatigue and can be hemodynamically compromised. Diagnosis is confirmed by means of electrocardiography [20].

Treatment

AF can be treated with medication that either reduces the heart rate or reverts the rhythm back to normal. Pharmacological therapy includes digoxin and calcium channel or β-blockers. Synchronized electrical cardioversion can also be used to convert AF to a normal rhythm [20].

Table 8.3 Univariate and multivariate analysis of potential predictors of anastomotic leakage

	Univariate logistic regression analysis		Multivariate logistic regression analysis	
All patients ($n=828$)	OR (95 % CI)	p-value	OR (95 % CI)	p-value
Age	1.010 (0.990–1.029)	0.332	Not in model	–
Male sex	**1.797 (1.093–2.954)**	**0.021**	**1.675 (1.002–2.801)**	**0.049**
BMI > 27 kg/m^3	**1.616 (1.074–2.430)**	**0.021**	**1.548 (1.027–2.335)**	**0.037**
Squamous cell carcinoma	0.886 (0.600–1.307)	0.540	Not in model	–
Stapled anastomosis	1.002 (0.999–1.004)	0.235	Not in model	–
Tumor stage III or IV	0.824 (0.565–1.200)	0.312	Not in model	–
Neoadjuvant chemo (radiotherapy)	0.897 (0.555–1.449)	0.656	Not in model	–
Transthoracic approach	0.964 (0.656–1.417)	0.853	Not in model	–

Adapted from van Heijl et al. [23]
CI confidence interval, *BMI* body mass index, *OR* odds ratio

Surgical Complications

Anastomotic Leakage

Incidence and Definition

Anastomotic leakage is a serious complication resulting in significant morbidity and mortality. After transhiatal esophagectomy, an anastomosis at the cervical level between the replacement conduit and the proximal esophagus is required. In case of a transthoracic procedure, cervical and intrathoracic anastomoses are possible. In general, surgeons tend to favor a cervical anastomosis, considering the hypothesis that anastomotic leakage will be confined to the neck area instead of leaking directly into the mediastinum [21, 22]. However, the performed technique seems not to be of influence on the incidence of anastomotic leakage; hand-sewn and stapled techniques show comparable leakage rates [23]. Potential predictors of anastomotic leakage were evaluated among over 800 patients who underwent esophagectomy and include male sex and a body mass index > 27 kg/m^2 (Table 8.3).

The incidence of anastomotic leakage after esophagectomy ranges from 1.6 to 20 %, depending on and the applied criteria [24]. In general, anastomotic leakage is defined as clinical evidence of salivary fistula or infection of the cervical wound which requires opening of the wound to objectify the leakage. Radiological anastomotic leakage is defined as extravasation of water-soluble contrast medium [21].

Diagnosis

Traditionally, anastomotic leakage can be diagnosed through X-ray with water-soluble contrast, generally 6–10 days after surgery [21, 23]. Although contrast

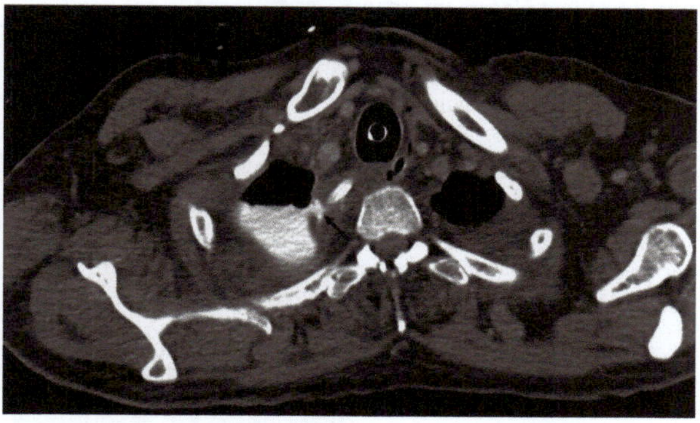

Fig. 8.3 CT of contrast leakage from the conduit into the right pleural cavity (*arrow*) in a patient 7 days after thoracolaparoscopic esophagectomy

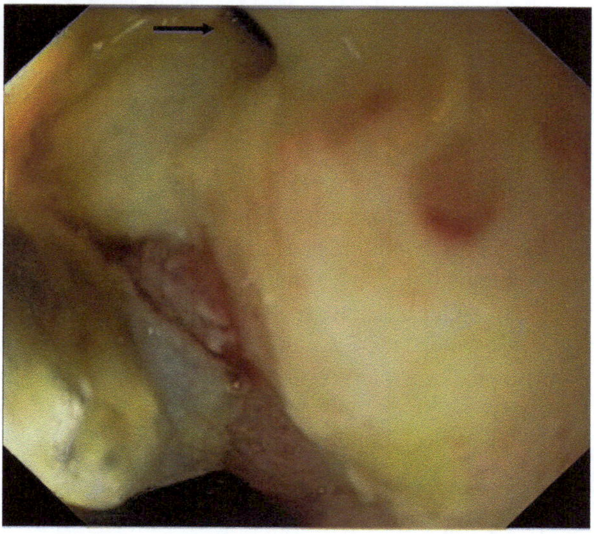

Fig. 8.4 Endoscopic view of ischemic mucosa of gastric tube with leakage site (*arrow*) in a patient 9 days after transthoracic esophagectomy

swallow examination is performed routinely in many centers throughout the world, routine examination has a low sensitivity and a low positive predictive value and therefore may not be justified in all patients after esophagectomy [25]. However, in case of clinical signs of anastomotic leakage, a swallow examination should be performed.

In patients in whom a swallow examination is not feasible, a contrast enhanced computed tomography (CT) can be performed (Figs. 8.3 and 8.4). Furthermore, upper endoscopy can be performed to rule out conduit necrosis, and moreover, during endoscopy immediate treatment is possible with stent placement [26].

Treatment

Treatment options for anastomotic leakage range from conservative treatment in case of a nonsignificant radiological leak to conduit takedown in case of severe

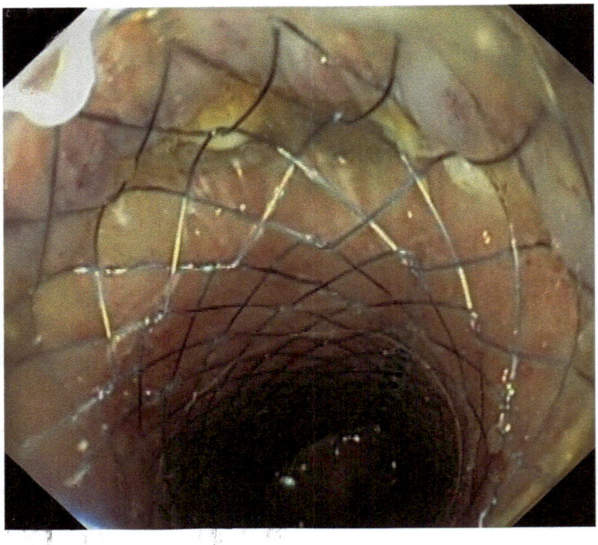

Fig. 8.5 Stent placement during esophagogastroduodenoscopy in a patient 9 days after transthoracic esophagectomy

conduit necrosis. Nonsurgical therapy for anastomotic leakage includes maintaining the patient nil by mouth, broad-spectrum antibiotics, stent placement (Fig. 8.5a and b), radiological drainage, and reinstituting transnasal drainage of the conduit [26]. In case of larger leaks, reexploration of the cervical incision or thoracoscopic drainage can be performed. Conduit necrosis requires immediate surgical therapy and breakdown of the interponate with cervical esophagostomy. Segmental necrosis can be managed with drainage and followed up with endoscopy, but in case of extensive conduit necrosis, conduit takedown is required [26].

Chylous Leakage

Incidence and Definition

Postoperative chylous leakage results from injury to the main thoracic duct or its branches, which have a close relationship with the esophagus [27]. Chylous leakage after esophagectomy is most commonly due to perioperative injury of the thoracic duct during extensive lymph node dissection and is less frequently caused by injury to the cisterna chyli in the upper abdomen. Chyle is defined as intestinal lymphatic fluid that is enriched with fat absorbed from the intestinal lumen, which is responsible for the milky appearance of chyle after enteral feeding. Lymphatic fluid consists of lymphocytes, immunoglobulins, and enzymes [27]. The incidence of chylous leakage after extended esophagectomy ranges from 1 to 4 % and occurs more frequently after transthoracic esophagectomy [28]. Extensive loss or a long duration of chylous leakage can cause loss of calories, fluids, lymphocytes, and albumin, which may lead to immunosuppression. This can result in infection-related complications [27].

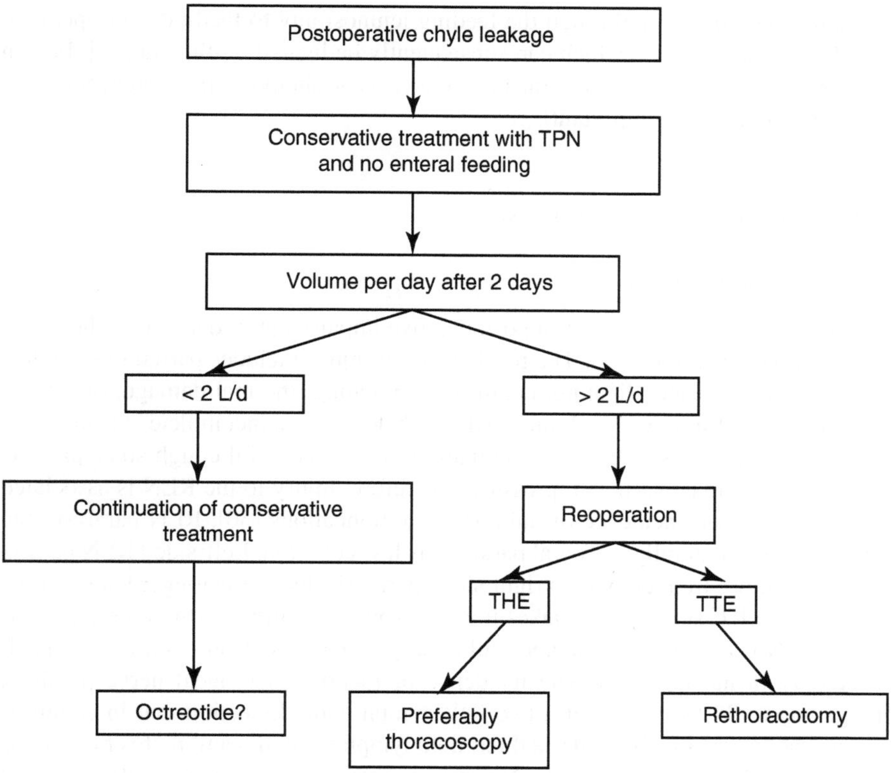

Fig. 8.6 Treatment strategy for chylous leakage after esophagectomy. This study was performed before the introduction of thoracolaparoscopic esophagectomy at the Academic Medical Center. Currently, in most cases thoracoscopic reintervention would be performed. *THE* transhiatal esophagectomy, *TPN* total parenteral nutrition, *TTE* transthoracic esophagectomy (Adapted from Lagarde et al. [27])

Diagnosis

The diagnosis of chylous leakage is based on the appearance of the drain output, which changes from clear to milky upon enteral feeding in case of chylous leakage. After discontinuation of enteral feeding, the drain output changes back to clear. The diagnosis is confirmed if the triglyceride concentration in the drain output is greater than 1.2 mmol/L [27].

Treatment

Adequate conservative management including total parenteral nutrition instead of enteral feeding is the first step in treatment of chylous leakage. In 80 % of patients, chylous leakage can be managed solely with conservative treatment [27]. A medium-chain triglyceride diet has only a limited role in case of massive chylous leakage. Therefore, if the leakage persists for more than 2 days with a drain output of more than 2 L per day, a reoperation is indicated, preferably minimally invasive (Fig. 8.6).

Cream should be given through the feeding jejunostomy to facilitate perioperative localization of the leak, which can subsequently be ligated or clipped [27]. Fusion of intrathoracic and intra-abdominal chylous leakage should be prevented; compartmentalization is very important.

Recurrent Laryngeal Nerve Paralysis

Incidence and Definition

Esophageal surgery can result in postoperative impairment or damage of the recurrent laryngeal nerve (RLN). The mechanism of injury includes partial or complete transaction, misplaced ligature, contusion, stretching, thermal damage, or a compromised blood supply [29]. Injury to the RLN leads to an incomplete closure of the vocal folds and consecutively to the inability of a successful cough since patients are unable to create sufficient pressure. Therefore, injury to the RLN is associated with an increased incidence of pulmonary complications [30]. RLN paralysis can occur uni- or bilaterally; bilateral paralysis is less common. Left-sided RLN paralysis occurs more frequently than right-sided paralysis due to the longer length of the RLN on the left side, which makes it more prone for injury. Furthermore, the left-sided RLN is at risk since the aortopulmonary window is cleared during lymphadenectomy in most centers. The incidence of recurrent laryngeal nerve paralysis ranges up to 34 % in case of a two-field lymph node dissection, but in countries where esophagectomy includes a three-field lymph node dissection, this rate can be as high as 80 %. Furthermore, RLN paralysis occurs more frequently after cervical anastomosis than intrathoracic anastomosis since the RLN is exposed during cervical dissection of the esophagus [30].

Diagnosis

The majority of RLN lesions are transient. Diagnosis of postoperative uni- or bilateral RLN paralysis is initially based on clinical symptoms such as hoarseness and a breathy voice and is proven by laryngoscopy. The patients' cough is weak, and pulmonary complications including aspiration can occur more frequently. Bilateral RLN paralysis can be a severe and life-threatening complication that manifests immediately after extubation with signs of airway obstruction such as dyspnea, tachypnea, and inspiratory stridor [29].

Treatment

Transient RLN lesions generally recover within 6–12 months after surgery [29]. Conservative therapy consists of logopedic voice and swallowing training, and in case of persistent RLN paralysis, several operative procedures can be performed depending on the position of the paralyzed vocal fold. In case of unilateral vocal fold paralysis in a lateral position with aphonia, medialization of the vocal cord allows glottal closure, which leads to an improved voice and a better swallowing function. Medialization of the vocal cord can be achieved by a titanium implant, autologous cartilage chips, and collagen or fat implantation.

Bilateral vocal cord paralysis causes a medial position of the vocal cords with a narrow glottal opening that generally requires an emergency tracheotomy. In a later stage, lateralization of one vocal fold or a cordectomy can be performed after which the tracheotomy can be closed. Since RLN paralysis often ameliorates during the first year postoperatively, surgical interventions should be withheld during this period with the exception of cases with a poor prognosis for recovery, e.g., if the nerve was resected for oncological reasons [30].

Late Complications

Fistula from Gastric Conduit to Trachea or Bronchial Tree

Incidence and Definition

A benign fistula between the gastric conduit and trachea or bronchial tree is a rare but potentially fatal complication of esophageal surgery. Risk factors include perioperative chemoradiotherapy and extensive upper mediastinal lymph node dissection, which can cause local devascularization of the membranous trachea or mainstem bronchi [31]. Tracheo-neo-esophageal fistulas are related to tracheal trauma such as direct laceration during esophagectomy, endotracheal tube-induced trauma, or anastomotic leakage. It can also be a complication caused by dilation of an anastomotic stenosis. The incidence of fistulas between the trachea and the gastric conduit varies between 0.2 and 0.3 % after both transthoracic and transhiatal approaches [31].

Diagnosis

The clinical presentation of fistulas varies; symptoms can be relatively mild consisting of a cough associated with oral intake or more severe symptoms including recurrent bronchopneumonia, respiratory failure, and mediastinitis, which can be life threatening [32].

When a fistula is suspected based on clinical symptoms, radiologic contrast studies in upright and supine positions can be used to confirm diagnosis. Fistulas can be localized during endoscopy (Fig. 8.7), but because identifying a small defect in the folded neo-esophageal mucosa can be difficult, bronchoscopy can be more informative [32].

Treatment

The severity of symptoms in combination with the site and size of the fistula is most important in determining the optimal treatment strategy. The principles of management should emphasize control of sepsis and limiting ongoing soilage of the bronchial tree [31].

In the absence of severe mediastinal or pulmonary infections, a conservative treatment (nil by mouth, enteral feeding, antibiotics) can be considered.

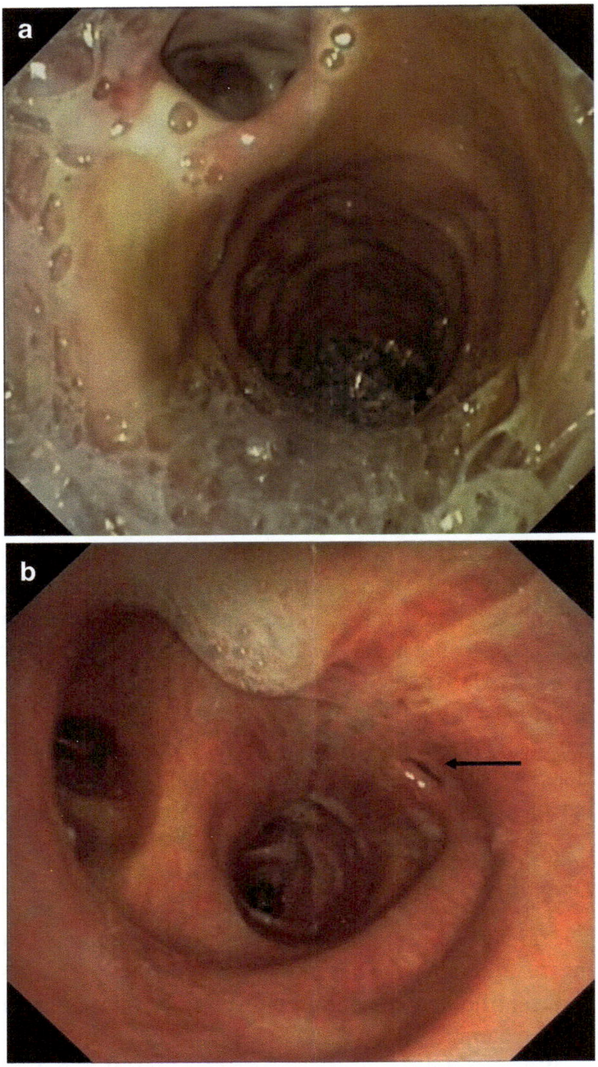

Fig. 8.7 Mediastinal leakage in a patient 24 days after a thoracolaparoscopic esophagectomy with a fistula to the right intermediate bronchus. (**a**) Endoscopy showing the leakage site. (**b**) Bronchoscopy showing the fistula at the right intermediate bronchus (*arrow*)

If the fistula persists for more than 4–6 weeks, endoscopic treatment with stent placement can be performed.

Surgical repair remains the mainstay of fistula treatment. Closure of the fistula can be achieved by using omentum, pleura, a pericardial graft or pericardial fat pad, or a muscle flap (sternohyoid, intercostal, latissimus dorsi, and pectoralis major, dependant on the position of the fistula and availability of vital tissue) [31]. If the gastric conduit cannot be preserved, continuity of the gastrointestinal tract can be reconstructed with a colonic interposition either in the same or in a later session if

Table 8.4 Risk factors for development of benign cervical stricture after esophagectomy

	Multivariate analysis	
All patients ($n=607$)	OR (95 % CI)	p-value
Transthoracic vs transhiatal	0.93 (0.58–1.49)	0.76
Colonic interposition vs gastric tube	**0.11 (0.01–0.83)**	**0.03**
Stapled vs hand sewn anastomosis	Not in model	–
Age <70 years	Not in model	–
Male vs female	Not in model	–
BMI > 25 kg/m^2	1.10 (0.77–1.57)	0.607
Smoking	Not in model	–
History of cardiovascular disease	**1.78 (1.23–2.58)**	**0.002**
Diabetes	1.82 (0.87–3.78)	0.11
% of predicted FEV1 (l/s) < 80 %	Not in model	–
Neoadjuvant chemotherapy	0.65 (0.35–1.21)	0.65
Neoadjuvant chemoradiotherapy	Not in model	–
Anastomotic leakage	**2.07 (1.30–3.29)**	**0.002**

Adapted from van Heijl et al. [33]
BMI body mass index, *FEV1* forced expiratory volume in one second

patients' condition precludes a reconstruction in the same session. The colon segment is preferably placed in the prevertebral position to reinforce the posterior wall of the trachea [32].

Strictures

Incidence and Definition

An important cause of long-term morbidity after esophagectomy is the development of benign cervical anastomotic strictures. Potential risk factors for this complication are diverse and include postoperative anastomotic leakage, neoadjuvant therapy, and a history of cardiac disease (Table 8.4). Risk factors for refractory anastomotic strictures are chemoradiotherapy, early stricture development, and anastomotic leakage [33]. End-to-side (ETS) anastomoses are associated with a lower stricture rate compared to end-to-end (ETE) anastomoses; however, anastomotic leakage occurs more frequently after ETS anastomoses [34].

Approximately 26–42 % of patients will develop strictures, which are known to be burdensome, often need frequent therapy, and lower the quality of life [35].

Diagnosis

In general, the diagnosis of benign esophageal stricture is based on clinical symptoms. Patients suffer from dysphagia and weight loss which can lead to a decreased quality of life [36].

Treatment

Several treatment modalities for benign esophageal strictures have been described including dilation with bougies or Savary dilation [36]. Endoscopic mechanical dilation is the preferred treatment of benign strictures; it is known to be a successful treatment of dysphagia [35, 37]. The majority of strictures respond well on dilation, and successful treatment in these patients is achieved in three to eight sessions. In case of refractory strictures, up to 30 dilations can be required [35, 37].

Other techniques include electrocautery incision of the stricture, intralesional steroid injections, and self-expandable metal stents (SEMS) or self-expandable plastic stents (SEPS).

Can Minimally Invasive Esophageal Surgery Decrease Short-Term Complications? Looking for Evidence-Based Surgery

Three meta-analyses comparing MIO and OO served as starting points in the quest for evidence-based surgery.

Biere et al. identified 10 studies after a comprehensive search [38]. Three comparative groups were created for analysis: (1) total MIO versus open transthoracic esophagectomy (TTE), (2) thoracoscopy and laparotomy versus open transthoracic, and (3) laparoscopy versus open transhiatal esophagectomy (THE). Our conclusion was that with MIO a faster postoperative recovery and therefore a reduction in morbidity could be achieved. Furthermore, we expect a lower mortality rate following the implementation of MIO. It was accentuated that MIO had been only investigated in case–control studies, and hence, bias may have been introduced simply by the pertaining study design.

The study of Nagpal et al. collected 12 selected studies for analysis [39]. There was no randomized study performed. They included 672 patients for MIO and hybrid MIO and 612 patients for OO. They found that MIO to be a safe alternative for use of the OO. Patients undergoing MIO may benefit from shorter hospital stay and lower respiratory complications and total morbidity as compared to OO.

In the meta-analysis of Sgourakis et al, also published in 2010, they pooled the effects of the outcomes of 1,008 patients enrolled into eight comparative studies [40]. They performed two comparisons: (1) open thoracotomy versus all MIO procedure and (2) open thoracotomy versus only MIO thoracoscopic phase. In comparison 1, both procedures report equally comparable outcomes (removed lymph nodes, 30-day mortality, 3-year survival) with the exception of overall mortality and anastomotic stricture in favor of the open thoracotomy arm. In comparison 2, no differences were noted between treatment arms concerning postoperative outcomes and survival.

These three meta-analyses generated the initiative for further prospective comparative or randomized controlled trials focusing on the short-term and oncological impact of MIO. Following this quest, we went on to assess the reduction of pulmonary infections and improved quality of life associated with MIE. We conducted a multicenter, randomized trial comparing open with minimally invasive esophagectomy in patients with esophageal cancer.

After a long period of practicing both the transhiatal and the thoracoscopic esophagectomy for cancer, we designed a prospective randomized study for comparison of MIO and OO in 2008. The study was in the end called the TIME trial (Traditional Invasive versus Minimally invasive Esophagectomy). The TIME trial is a prospective, multicenter, randomized study comparing traditional transthoracic esophageal resection with minimally invasive resection for esophageal cancer [41]. The primary endpoint of the study concerned the respiratory complications, especially the postoperative bronchopneumonia confirmed by thorax X-ray or CT scan, and positive sputum culture.

Secondary endpoints were operation-related events, complications, ICU and hospital stay, quality of life as determined by questionnaires (SF-36 and EORTC C30-OES18), and the quality of specimen resected (length of specimen, number and location of lymph nodes resected, and circumferential resection margins). Also, hospital mortality and readmissions were recorded.

The pulmonary infection rate within the first two weeks was 29 % (16 patients) in the OO group and 9 % (5 patients) in the MIO group, $p=0.005$. The overall in-hospital incidence of pulmonary infections was 34 % (19 patients) in the OO group and 12 % (7 patients) in the MIO group, $p=0.005$. Explanation for the lower incidence of pulmonary infections may be, first of all, the used prone position in which in contrast with the lateral position the mediastinum hangs in its usual midposition; a second advantage may be the absence of total collapse of the lung during the MIO in prone position in contrast with one-lung ventilation and this permits optimal visualization of mediastinum with preserved ventilation and oxygenation; and a third factor may be the thoracotomy wound itself. All factors together could explain these advantages.

Other postoperative data included major postoperative complications (anastomotic leakage, 7 % in the OO and 12 % in the MIO, $p=0.390$) and mortality (1.8 % versus 3.4 %) that were not significantly different. Interesting is the different rate for vocal cord paralysis, 14 % in the OO group and only 2 % in the MIO, $p=0.012$. Pneumatic dissection by CO_2 from thoracic cavity into the neck can simplify the dissection in the neck and reduce the recurrent nerve lesions.

In conclusion, this randomized trial comparing open esophagectomy for cancer with minimally invasive esophagectomy shows that MIO results in a lower incidence of pulmonary infections, less rate of recurrence nerve lesions, and a better short-term quality of life without compromise of the quality of the resected specimen.

Esophageal Surgery for Benign Disease

Introduction

Benign esophageal disorders that can be treated surgically include gastroesophageal reflux disease (GERD), achalasia, and paraesophageal herniation.

GERD is a common disorder that affects 20–40 % of the Western population [42]. Frequent or long-lasting reflux of acidic gastric contents can lead to the development of GERD. The main symptoms include heartburn, retrosternal pain, regurgitation, and chronic cough. The most widely performed surgical technique for treatment of GERD is the Nissen or Toupet fundoplication during which the distal esophagus is brought into the abdominal cavity. Subsequently, the hiatus is approximated posteriorly and either a 360° (Nissen) or a 270° (Toupet) fundoplication is created [43].

Achalasia is an esophageal motor disorder that is characterized by the absence of esophageal peristalsis combined with a defective relaxation of the lower esophageal sphincter. Clinical symptoms include dysphagia, chest pain, and regurgitation of undigested food. Surgical treatment of achalasia consists of a Heller's myotomy, mainly performed laparoscopically (laparoscopic Heller's myotomy; LHM). A myotomy is performed extending from above the level of the gastroesophageal junction down to the proximal 1–1.5 cm of the stomach. To prevent reflux, an anterior fundoplication (Dor) can be performed subsequently [44].

Paraesophageal or hiatal hernias are a common disorder of the digestive tract that are characterized by a protrusion of the stomach into the thoracic cavity through a widening of the right crus of the diaphragm [45]. Hiatal hernias are classified into four subtypes: type I, sliding hernias, in which the gastroesophageal junction is herniated into the thorax; type II, true paraesophageal hernias where the gastroesophageal junction maintains its position posteriorly with anterior herniation of the gastric fundus; type III, a combination of types I and II; and type IV, in which the stomach migrates completely into the thoracic cavity (upside-down stomach), sometimes accompanied by other visceral organs [45]. Type I hernias are the most common type of hiatal hernias and occur in 95 % of patients with diaphragmatic herniation. This type may predispose to gastroesophageal reflux. Only 5 % of hiatal hernias are true paraesophageal hernias (type II), but these hernias are important due to the potentially life-threatening complications such as obstruction, acute dilation, or perforation [45]. In general, no conservative treatment options are available for the treatment of type II hernias. Surgical treatment consists of complete excision of the peritoneal sac from the mediastinum and reduction of the herniated stomach and distal esophagus into the abdominal cavity and subsequent repair of the hiatus; there is still debate about the need for a fundoplication [45]. Surgery can be performed by either a conventional open procedure or a laparoscopic procedure.

Fundoplication and Its Complications

Most frequent complications after Nissen or Toupet fundoplication are depicted in Fig. 8.8. In general 90 % of fundoplications are successful. Most frequent complications are dysphagia and recurrence of reflux symptoms.

Dysphagia is a common problem early after either Nissen or Toupet fundoplication but will disappear in the majority of patients. It is persistent, however, in

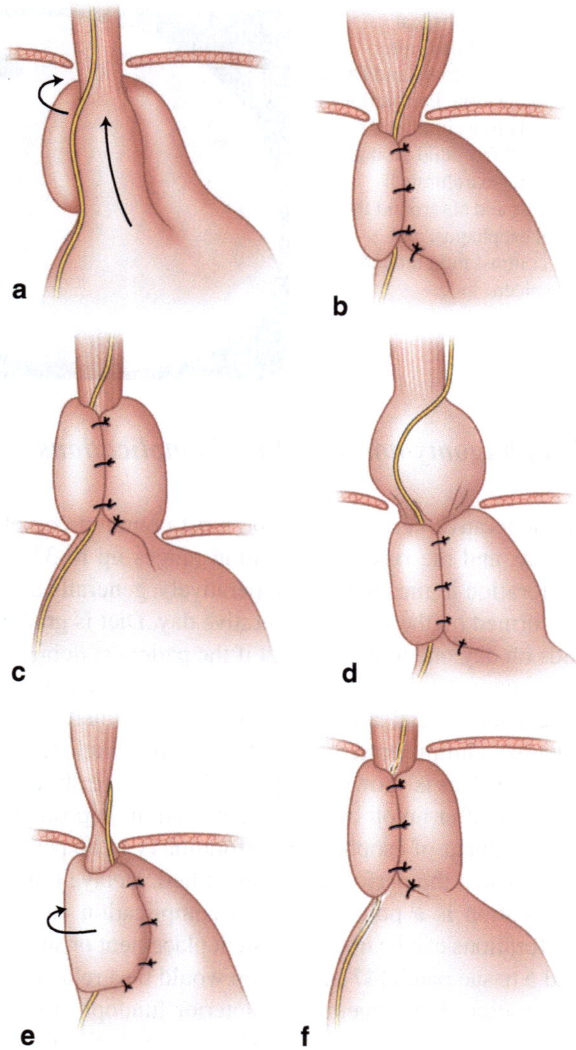

Fig. 8.8 Failures after Nissen fundoplication. (**a**) The fundoplication has given way, leading to recurrent GERD. (**b**) Fundoplication is too tight (and/or too long) leading to dysphagia. (**c**) Intrathoracic herniation of the complete wrap. (**d**) Telescoping of the esophagogastric junction through the wrap. (**e**) Torsion due to tension of the wrap. (**f**) Vagus nerve lesion in combination with an otherwise intact fundoplication (Adapted from van Lanschot et al. [43])

5–10 % of patients. Recurrent reflux may occur in up to 5 % of patients. Disruption or migration, either into the chest or down the stomach, occurs in up to 7 % of patients (Fig. 8.8). Wrap disruption or migration, a too tight fundoplication, telescoping of the esophagogastric junction through the wrap, and torsion (complications A, B, D, and E in Fig. 8.8) are best treated by relaparoscopy or relaparotomy. Intrathoracic herniation is best treated by thoracotomy, but there is no surgical solution for delayed gastric emptying due to damage of the vagus nerve (Fig. 8.8f), which is probably the most severe complication after Nissen fundoplication [43].

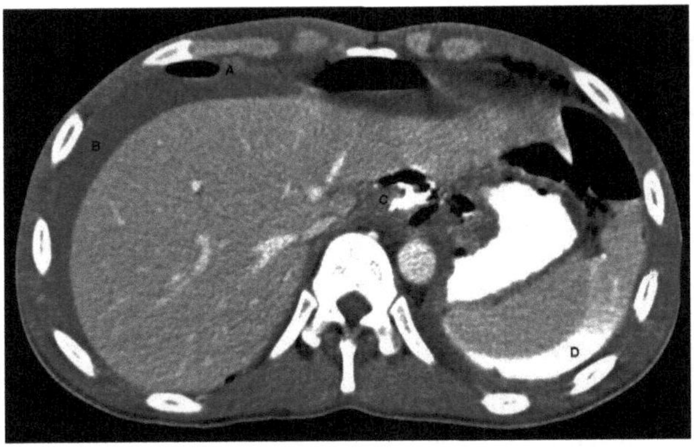

Fig. 8.9 Esophageal perforation 5 days after esophagomyotomy and DOR fundoplication. Perforation with (*A*) free air around the liver, (*B*) free fluid around the liver, (*C*) extraluminal contrast and air around the distal esophagus, and (*D*) contrast fluid around the spleen

Esophagomyotomy and Its Complications

Intraoperative perforation is the most common complication during esophagomyotomy, and the risk of perforation ranges up to 33 % [46]. To visualize mucosal perforation immediately postoperatively, generally an X-ray with soluble contrast is performed on the first postoperative day. Diet is gradually advanced from clear liquids on day one to normal diet if the patient is doing clinically well.

In case of clinical deterioration (abdominal pain, signs of sepsis), additional diagnostic investigations have to be performed including CT with water-soluble contrast administered orally. In case of perforation, free fluid/contrast and air is visible on CT as is shown in Fig. 8.9. This image shows free contrast, fluid, and air in a patient after myotomy with a perforation on postoperative day 4.

Treatment of esophageal perforations can be performed immediately perioperatively when the perforation is identified. Delayed diagnosis of a clinically relevant perforation is a potentially fatal complication and can lead to fistula formation. Perforations can be treated by stent placement or surgically through primary closure and a tissue patch [47]. First step would be a relaparoscopy and suture repair of the perforation. Subsequently, an anterior fundoplication should be performed to seal off the repaired mucosal site which has a high risk of repeated leakage. Adequate drainage is also advised.

Paraesophageal Hernia Repair and Its Complications

Complications of paraesophageal hernia repair include visceral injury, vagal nerve injury, pneumothorax, hemorrhage, and pulmonary complications. The most important complication after hernia repair, however, is recurrent herniation [48]. Postoperative recurrence occurs in up to 44 % of patients, depending on the applied criteria (radiological versus clinical). Risk factors for the development of hiatal hernia recurrence include postoperative vomiting, obesity, coughing, and heavy lifting.

Dilation can be performed in patients with dysphagia as sole symptom of recurrent hiatal hernia. Indications for reoperation are regurgitation, dysphagia without response to dilation, and persistent chest pain [49].

References

1. Pohl H, Welch HG. The role of overdiagnosis and reclassification in the marked increase of esophageal adenocarcinoma incidence. J Natl Cancer Inst. 2005;97(2):142–6.
2. Kamangar F, Dores GM, Anderson WF. Patterns of cancer incidence, mortality, and prevalence across five continents: defining priorities to reduce cancer disparities in different geographic regions of the world. J Clin Oncol. 2006;24(14):2137–50.
3. Hulscher JB, van Sandick JW, Tijssen JG, Obertop H, van Lanschot JJ. The recurrence pattern of esophageal carcinoma after transhiatal resection. J Am Coll Surg. 2000;191(2):143–8.
4. Mariette C, Balon JM, Piessen G, Fabre S, Van Seuningen I, Triboulet JP. Pattern of recurrence following complete resection of esophageal carcinoma and factors predictive of recurrent disease. Cancer. 2003;97(7):1616–23.
5. Hulscher JB, van Sandick JW, de Boer AG, Wijnhoven BP, Tijssen JG, Fockens P, et al. Extended transthoracic resection compared with limited transhiatal resection for adenocarcinoma of the esophagus. N Engl J Med. 2002;347(21):1662–9.
6. Omloo JM, Lagarde SM, Hulscher JB, Reitsma JB, Fockens P, van Dekken DH, et al. Extended transthoracic resection compared with limited transhiatal resection for adenocarcinoma of the mid/distal esophagus: five-year survival of a randomized clinical trial. Ann Surg. 2007;246(6):992–1000.
7. Wu PC, Posner MC. The role of surgery in the management of oesophageal cancer. Lancet Oncol. 2003;4(8):481–8.
8. Swisher SG, Deford L, Merriman KW, Walsh GL, Smythe R, Vaporicyan A, et al. Effect of operative volume on morbidity, mortality, and hospital use after esophagectomy for cancer. J Thorac Cardiovasc Surg. 2000;119(6):1126–32.
9. Wouters MW, Wijnhoven BP, Karim-Kos HE, Blaauwgeers HG, Stassen LP, Steup WH, et al. High-volume versus low-volume for esophageal resections for cancer: the essential role of case-mix adjustments based on clinical data. Ann Surg Oncol. 2008;15(1):80–7.
10. van Heijl M, van Lanschot JJ, Blom RL, Bergman JJ, Ten Kate FJ, Busch OR, et al. Outcomes of 16 years of oesophageal surgery: low postoperative mortality and improved long-term survival. Ned Tijdschr Geneeskd. 2010;154:A1156.
11. Dindo D, Demartines N, Clavien PA. Classification of surgical complications: a new proposal with evaluation in a cohort of 6336 patients and results of a survey. Ann Surg. 2004; 240(2):205–13.
12. Lagarde SM, Reitsma JB, Maris AK, van Berge Henegouwen MI, Busch OR, Obertop H, et al. Preoperative prediction of the occurrence and severity of complications after esophagectomy for cancer with use of a nomogram. Ann Thorac Surg. 2008;85(6):1938–45.
13. Bernard GR, Artigas A, Brigham KL, Carlet J, Falke K, Hudson L, et al. The American-European Consensus Conference on ARDS. Definitions, mechanisms, relevant outcomes, and clinical trial coordination. Am J Respir Crit Care Med. 1994;149(3 Pt 1):818–24.
14. Zingg U, Smithers BM, Gotley DC, Smith G, Aly A, Clough A, et al. Factors associated with postoperative pulmonary morbidity after esophagectomy for cancer. Ann Surg Oncol. 2011;18(5):1460–8.
15. Schoppmann SF, Prager G, Langer FB, Riegler FM, Kabon B, Fleischmann E, et al. Open versus minimally invasive esophagectomy: a single-center case controlled study. Surg Endosc. 2010;24(12):3044–53.

16. Zingg U, McQuinn A, DiValentino D, Esterman AJ, Bessell JR, Thompson SK, et al. Minimally invasive versus open esophagectomy for patients with esophageal cancer. Ann Thorac Surg. 2009;87(3):911–9.
17. Tisdale JE, Wroblewski HA, Wall DS, Rieger KM, Hammoud ZT, Young JV, et al. A randomized, controlled study of amiodarone for prevention of atrial fibrillation after transthoracic esophagectomy. J Thorac Cardiovasc Surg. 2010;140(1):45–51.
18. Malhotra SK, Kaur RP, Gupta NM, Grover A, Ramprabu K, Nakra D. Incidence and types of arrhythmias after mediastinal manipulation during transhiatal esophagectomy. Ann Thorac Surg. 2006;82(1):298–302.
19. Nattel S. New ideas about atrial fibrillation 50 years on. Nature. 2002;415(6868):219–26.
20. Murthy SC, Law S, Whooley BP, Alexandrou A, Chu KM, Wong J. Atrial fibrillation after esophagectomy is a marker for postoperative morbidity and mortality. J Thorac Cardiovasc Surg. 2003;126(4):1162–7.
21. Walther B, Johansson J, Johnsson F, Von Holstein CS, Zilling T. Cervical or thoracic anastomosis after esophageal resection and gastric tube reconstruction: a prospective randomized trial comparing sutured neck anastomosis with stapled intrathoracic anastomosis. Ann Surg. 2003;238(6):803–12.
22. Boone J, Livestro DP, Elias SG, Borel Rinkes IH, Van HR. International survey on esophageal cancer: part I surgical techniques. Dis Esophagus. 2009;22(3):195–202.
23. van Heijl M, van Wijngaarden AK, Lagarde SM, Busch OR, van Lanschot JJ, van Berge Henegouwen MI. Intrathoracic manifestations of cervical anastomotic leaks after transhiatal and transthoracic oesophagectomy. Br J Surg. 2010;97(5):726–31.
24. Urschel JD, Blewett CJ, Bennett WF, Miller JD, Young JE. Handsewn or stapled esophagogastric anastomoses after esophagectomy for cancer: meta-analysis of randomized controlled trials. Dis Esophagus. 2001;14(3–4):212–7.
25. Boone J, Rinkes IB, van Leeuwen M, van Hillegersberg R. Diagnostic value of routine aqueous contrast swallow examination after oesophagectomy for detecting leakage of the cervical oesophagogastric anastomosis. ANZ J Surg. 2008;78(9):784–90.
26. Low DE. Diagnosis and management of anastomotic leaks after esophagectomy. J Gastrointest Surg. 2011;15:1319–22.
27. Lagarde SM, Omloo JM, de Jong K, Busch OR, Obertop H, van Lanschot JJ. Incidence and management of chyle leakage after esophagectomy. Ann Thorac Surg. 2005;80(2):449–54.
28. Omloo JM, Lagarde SM, Vrouenraets BC, Busch OR, van Lanschot JJ. Compartimentalization for chylothorax originating from the abdomen after extended esophagectomy. Report of two cases and review of the literature. Dig Surg. 2006;23(1–2):86–92.
29. Gelpke H, Grieder F, Decurtins M, Cadosch D. Recurrent laryngeal nerve monitoring during esophagectomy and mediastinal lymph node dissection. World J Surg. 2010;34(10):2379–82.
30. Gockel I, Kneist W, Keilmann A, Junginger T. Recurrent laryngeal nerve paralysis (RLNP) following esophagectomy for carcinoma. Eur J Surg Oncol. 2005;31(3):277–81.
31. Bakhos C, Alazemi S, Michaud G, DeCamp MM. Staged repair of benign tracheo-neo-esophageal fistula 12 years after esophagectomy for esophageal cancer. Ann Thorac Surg. 2010;90(6):e83–5.
32. Buskens CJ, Hulscher JB, Fockens P, Obertop H, van Lanschot JJ. Benign tracheo-neo-esophageal fistulas after subtotal esophagectomy. Ann Thorac Surg. 2001;72(1):221–4.
33. van Heijl M, Gooszen JA, Fockens P, Busch OR, van Lanschot JJ, van Berge Henegouwen MI. Risk factors for development of benign cervical strictures after esophagectomy. Ann Surg. 2010;251(6):1064–9.
34. Nederlof N, Tilanus HW, Tran TC, Hop WC, Wijnhoven BP, de Jonge J. End-to-end versus end-to-side esophagogastrostomy after esophageal cancer resection: a prospective randomized study. Ann Surg. 2011.
35. Honkoop P, Siersema PD, Tilanus HW, Stassen LP, Hop WC, van Blankenstein M. Benign anastomotic strictures after transhiatal esophagectomy and cervical esophagogastrostomy: risk factors and management. J Thorac Cardiovasc Surg. 1996;111(6):1141–6.

36. van Hooft JE, van Berge Henegouwen MI, Rauws EA, Bergman JJ, Busch OR, Fockens P. Endoscopic treatment of benign anastomotic esophagogastric strictures with a biodegradable stent. Gastrointest Endosc. 2011;73(5):1043–7.
37. Pierie JP, de Graaf PW, Poen H, van der Tweel I, Obertop H. Incidence and management of benign anastomotic stricture after cervical oesophagogastrostomy. Br J Surg. 1993;80(4):471–4.
38. Biere SS, Cuesta MA, van der Peet DL. Minimally invasive versus open esophagectomy for cancer: a systematic review and meta-analysis. Minerva Chir. 2009;64:121–33.
39. Nagpal K, Ahmed K, Vats A, et al. Is minimally invasive surgery beneficial in the management of esophageal cancer ? A meta-analysis. Surg Endosc. 2010;24:1621–9.
40. Sgourakis G, Gockel I, Radtke A, et al. Minimally invasive versus open esophagectomy: meta-analysis of outcomes. Dig Dis Sci. 2010;55:3031–40.
41. Biere SS, van Berge Henegouwen MI, Maas KW, et al. Minimally invasive versus open oesophagectomy for patients with oesophageal cancer: a multicentre, open-label, randomised controlled trial. Lancet. 2012;379:1887–92.
42. Locke III GR, Talley NJ, Fett SL, Zinsmeister AR, Melton III LJ. Prevalence and clinical spectrum of gastroesophageal reflux: a population-based study in Olmsted County, Minnesota. Gastroenterology. 1997 May;112(5):1448–56.
43. van Lanschot JJ, Gouma DJ, Jansen PLM, Jones EA, Pinedo HM, Schouten WR, et al. Integrated medical and surgical gastroenterology. Houten: Bohn Stafleu Van Loghum; 2004.
44. Boeckxstaens GE, Annese V, des Varannes SB, Chaussade S, Costantini M, Cuttitta A, et al. Pneumatic dilation versus laparoscopic Heller's myotomy for idiopathic achalasia. N Engl J Med. 2011;364(19):1807–16.
45. Draaisma WA, Gooszen HG, Tournoij E, Broeders IA. Controversies in paraesophageal hernia repair: a review of literature. Surg Endosc. 2005;19(10):1300–8.
46. Iqbal A, Haider M, Desai K, Garg N, Kavan J, Mittal S, et al. Technique and follow-up of minimally invasive Heller myotomy for achalasia. Surg Endosc. 2006;20(3):394–401.
47. Erdogan A, Gurses G, Keskin H, Demircan A. The sealing effect of a fibrin tissue patch on the esophageal perforation area in primary repair. World J Surg. 2007;31(11):2199–203.
48. Trus TL, Bax T, Richardson WS, Branum GD, Mauren SJ, Swanstrom LL, et al. Complications of laparoscopic paraesophageal hernia repair. J Gastrointest Surg. 1997;1(3):221–7.
49. Haider M, Iqbal A, Salinas V, Karu A, Mittal SK, Filipi CJ. Surgical repair of recurrent hiatal hernia. Hernia. 2006;10(1):13–9.

Chapter 9
Prevention and Treatment of Major Complications After Gastroduodenal Surgery

Jose Luis Garcia Sabrido and Wenceslao Vasquez Jimenez

Keywords Gastric surgery • Leakage • Duodenal stump • Peptic ulcer • Rebleeding • Benign stricture

Gastric surgery involves different types of interventions, such as gastric resection for cancer and gastrojejunostomy for gastric cancer palliation. Also we know of surgically treated complications of peptic ulcer, such as the closure of a perforation or the suturing of a bleeding ulcer, and it is increasingly used in bariatric surgery. Complications after bariatric surgery will be treated extensively in Chap. 10; our focus in this chapter is on postoperative complications after gastric and benign duodenal surgery.

Concerning gastric cancer, two new therapeutic methods have recently been implemented: the use of neoadjuvant therapy for locally invasive cancer and the use of the laparoscopic approach. Moreover, use of the surgical approach for complicated peptic ulcers has declined dramatically since the discovery of Helicobacter pylori and the proton pump inhibitors. If an intervention has to be performed, the perforated ulcer is closed laparoscopically, and the primary treatment for abating the bleeding is the endoscopic/angiographic approach. All of these therapeutic procedures can lead to complications—each difficult to approach by surgery.

The rule remains to prevent, as much as possible, postoperative complications by establishing a correct surgical indication and by using an appropriate operative technique. Furthermore, in the case of postoperative complications, it is important to recognize these as early as possible and to treat each adequately. Diagnosis and

J.L.G. Sabrido
Department of General Surgery III and Liver Transplant Unit,
Hospital General Universitario Gregorio Marañón, Madrid, Spain

W.V. Jimenez, MD, PhD (✉)
Department of Surgery III, Gregorio Marañon Hospital, Madrid, Spain
e-mail: tumi100@yahoo.com

M.A. Cuesta, H.J. Bonjer (eds.), *Treatment of Postoperative Complications after Digestive Surgery*, DOI 10.1007/978-1-4471-4354-3_9,

treatment of complications are a multidisciplinary effort, involving the coordinated work of the gastroenterologist, the intervention radiologist, and the surgeon.

Most postoperative complications are simply due to errors of indication or in using surgical technique, such as when the wrong procedure is used for the situation at hand. Others can be due to the consequences of underlying disease or by the presence of a patient's associate diseases or because of medication.

The most frequent as well as major postoperative complications are the following: (1) postoperative bleeding, either intraluminal or intra-abdominal; (2) leakage of the duodenal stump; (3) leakage of the esophagojejunostomy; (4) stenosis and obstruction of any anastomosis; (5) leakage after closure of a perforated ulcer; and (6) rebleeding after suturing a bleeding peptic ulcer.

General Complications

Yasuda et al. analyzed the risk factors for complications following the resection of a large gastric (>10 cm) cancer. Overall morbidity and mortality rates were 39 and 7 %, respectively. The most frequent complication was pleural effusion (17 %), followed by anastomotic leakage (14 %), abdominal abscess (12 %), wound infection (12 %), pancreatic leakage (8 %), and general peritonitis (6 %). Risks factors associated with postoperative complications were found to be operating time, blood loss, and the pancreatic invasion by tumor. Complications were independent of patient age, nutritional status, type of gastrectomy, splenectomy or pancreatectomy, extent of lymph node dissection, tumor location, tumor size, and stage of disease [1].

Cuschieri et al. published the short-term results of the Medical Research Council (MRC) gastric cancer trial. In a prospective randomized controlled trial, D1 resection (level 1 lymphadenectomy) was compared with D2 resection (levels 1 and 2 lymphadenectomy). Central randomization (200 patients in each arm) followed a staging laparotomy.

The D2 group was found to have a greater postoperative hospital mortality (13 % vs 6.5 %; $p=0.04$), a higher overall postoperative morbidity (46 % vs 28 %; $p<0.001$), and their hospital stay was longer. The excess postoperative morbidity and mortality in the D2 group as established for this study were accounted for by distal pancreaticosplenectomy and splenectomy [2].

In 1995, Bonenkamp et al. published the short-term outcome of the randomized Dutch D1 versus D2 study. Among the 711 patients (380 in D1, 331 in D2) judged to have curable lesions, the D2 patients had a higher operative mortality rate than did the D1 patients (10 % vs 4 %; $p=0.004$) and had incurred more complications (43 % vs 25 %; $p<0.001$). They also needed longer postoperative hospital stays (median 25 [range 7–277] vs 18 [7–143] days; $p<0.001$). The morbidity and mortality differences persisted in almost all subgroup analyses. They concluded that "While we await survival results, D2 dissection should not be used as standard treatment for Western patients" [3, 4].

Sasako et al. analyzed the risk factors holding for surgical treatment in the Dutch gastric cancer trial. Using the database of the abovementioned randomized trial, they evaluated the risk factors for hospital death and complications in the 711 patients treated with curative intent, by engaging in multivariate analysis and using stepwise regression analysis. Sasako et al. came to the following findings regarding risk factors. Having an age higher than 65 years, male gender, and the particular extent of nodal dissection involved were considered the most important risk factors for mortality. For overall complications, splenectomy was the most important risk factor, while pancreatectomy and the type of gastrectomy were the only factors significantly found influencing the occurrence of major surgical complications. The cumulative mortality risk of these factors should be carefully considered when planning surgery for individual patients [5].

Brady et al. studied the effect of the splenectomy during gastrectomy on the morbidity rate by a retrospective analysis of 392 patients who underwent curative resection of gastric adenocarcinoma. Their aim was to evaluate the impact of splenectomy on postoperative morbidity and survival from gastric cancer. Using univariate analysis, 12 factors, including that of splenectomy, were associated with a poor prognosis. Remarkably, their multivariate analysis identified six of these factors, but not splenectomy being independently predictive of death due to gastric cancer. The apparent adverse effect of splenectomy was because of its association with other significant risk factors. Postoperative complications occurred more commonly in patients who underwent splenectomy than in those who did not (45 % vs 21 %), and patients in the splenectomy group also had a higher percentage of infectious complications than those in the non-splenectomy group (75 % vs 47 %). Their conclusion was that splenectomy has no direct influence on survival but that it increases the morbidity of curative gastrectomy and should be avoided unless the spleen is close to or invaded by the tumor [6].

Wu et al. analyzed the morbidity and mortality after gastrectomy for cancer in a prospective study of 474 patients who underwent radical gastrectomy [7]. Their findings were that the overall morbidity and mortality rates were 20.1 and 3.0 %, respectively. After the first 200 cases, the morbidity and mortality rates fell significantly from 27.0 to 15.7 % ($p=0.003$) and 5.5 to 1.1 % ($p<0.001$), respectively. By logistic regression analysis, it was found that male gender, combined organ(s) resection, extended lymphadenectomy, respiratory tract disease, and tumor location were significantly related to postoperative morbidity. Having an age older than 65 years, total gastrectomy, combined organ(s) resection, and respiratory tract disease were considered factors that negatively affected operative mortality and increased postoperative morbidity.

Bozzetti et al. analyzed the role of the amount of gastrectomy for treating cancer on the occurrence of postoperative morbidity and mortality by a multicenter randomized trial held in Italy [8]. This study treats the controversy whether the optimal surgery holding for gastric cancer in the distal half of the stomach is to be subtotal or total gastrectomy. A cluster of 624 patients with cancer in the distal half of the stomach were randomized into a group of 320 subtotal gastrectomy D2 lymphadenectomy cases and a group of 304 total gastrectomy D2 lymphadenectomy cases.

The end points applied were the occurrence of a postoperative event, the complication rate, the mortality rate, and the length of postoperative stay.

Bozzetti et al.'s findings were that nonfatal complications and death occurred in 9 and 1 % of subtotal gastrectomy patients and in 13 and 2 % of total gastrectomy patients, respectively. Multivariate analysis of postoperative events showed that splenectomy or resection of adjacent organs was associated with a twofold risk of postoperative complications. The mean length of stay—adjusted for extension of surgery—was 13.8 days for subtotal gastrectomy and 15.4 days for total gastrectomy.

These data show that D2 subtotal and total gastrectomies, performed as an elective procedure, have similar postoperative complication rates and surgical outcomes. Consequently, a conclusive long-term evaluation of the two sorts of operations and an accurate estimate of the oncologic impact of surgery on long-term survival, which is not penalized by excess surgical risk of one of the two operations, can be considered feasible.

The consequences of the anastomotic complications for long-term survival were analyzed by Sierzega et al on behaf of the Polish gastric cancer study group. Anastomotic leakage was diagnosed in 41 (5.9 %) of 690 patients who underwent total gastrectomy. Two Cox proportional hazard models, which included all the patients were used to identify anastomotic leakage as an independent predictor of survival with hazards ratios of 3.47 and 3.14 respectively. An important finding was the occurrence of anastomotic leakage as major independent prognostic factor for long-term survival [9].

Complications After Laparoscopic Gastrectomy

Hu compared and described the development of surgery-related complications after laparoscopic gastrectomy. This approach has developed rapidly for both early and advancer gastric cancer. Most studies showed that the operation-related complication rate is comparable between laparoscopic and open surgery. The common complications related to laparoscopic gastrectomy were found to be anastomotic leakage, stenosis, intra-abdominal bleeding, pancreatic leakage, and bowel obstruction [10].

Kim et al. described 753 patients who underwent a laparoscopic gastrectomy for gastric cancer. There were 69 cases of total gastrectomy, 682 subtotal gastrectomies, and two cases were proximal gastrectomies. According to the TNM stage, 8 patients were in stage 0, 619 in stage I, 88 in stage II, and 38 in stage III. The operation-related complications occurred in 77 cases (10.2 %). The number of postoperative complications and survival rates provided in Kim et al.'s series are comparable to the results found in other reports, as treated above [11].

Nagasako et al. described 400 patients who were operated on laparoscopic because of a T1 adenocarcinoma. All patients underwent a gastrectomy with regional lymphadenectomy. Anastomotic complications included anastomotic leakage, stricture, and remnant gastric stasis. Anastomotic complications occurred in 37 (9.3 %) of 400 patients. Multivariable analysis indicated surgeon experience to be the only independent predictor of anastomotic complications. Patients with anastomotic complications had a significantly worse overall 5-year survival rate than those without (81 % vs 94.2 %) [12].

Specific Complications

Intraluminal and Intra-abdominal Postoperative Bleeding

Intraluminal bleeding following elective gastric surgery occurs usually at the anastomoses—whereas intra-abdominal bleeding is caused by a splenic tear or by an unsecured vessel. Both complications happen during the first 24 h after operation.

Many anastomoses are being performed by staplers, and although it is not always possible to control the anastomosis for bleeding, if possible, it should be done (Fig. 9.1).

Bleeding of the staple line is associated with the administration of high doses of low molecular weight heparin (LMWH) for thromboprophylaxis. Therefore, high doses of LMWH should be avoided within 12 h prior to the procedure.

If anastomosis is performed manually, a continuous suture will penetrate all layers of the stomach, and the assistant should adequately maintain the tension. Any visible bleeding should be fixed separately during an operation. Furthermore, the anesthesiologist should discern whether the patient is unstable at the end of the

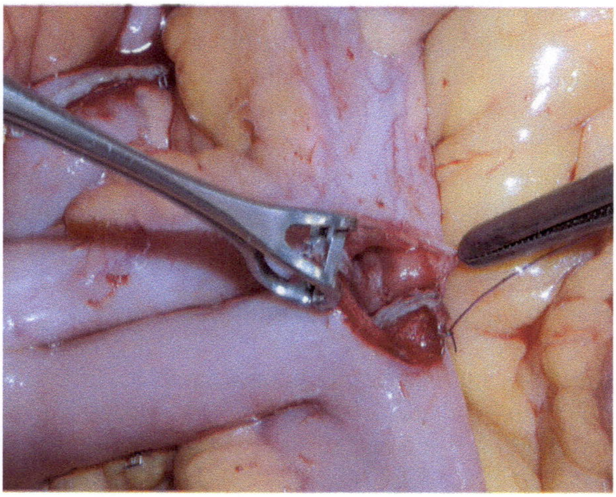

Fig. 9.1 Review of the suture line with stapler after jejunojejunostomy

operation, if hemoglobin has been decreased or if fresh blood is present in the nasogastric tube. These observations can be important for avoiding a reoperation.

During the laparoscopic approach, either using mechanical or manual anastomosis, it is necessary to control the intraluminal suture line in order to assure hemostasis. To control the bleeding, bipolar electrocoagulation, hemostatic stitches, or clips can be used.

Clinical Manifestations

Hematemesis, hematochezia, and melena are the most important signs along with decrease of hemoglobin. Absence of blood in the drains never excludes an intra-abdominal bleeding, and it does not assure the end of bleeding, as clots may obstruct the drain.

Placement or replacement of the nasogastric tube to diagnose the bleeding can help the surgeon to treat the patient. However, risk for perforation is always present at the level of the anastomosis and also the nasogastric tube can be obstructed by clots.

Laboratory

Low hemoglobin and high levels of urea due to the metabolism of blood without increase of the levels of creatinine.

Imaging

Abdominal Angiography CT Scan

Positive findings are in relation to the mL/min of bleeding. During arterial or late venous phase, active bleeding can be seen as a blush at the level of the anastomosis.

CT angiography may confirm bleeding inside the lumen and also intra-abdominal bleeding. Other causes of bleeding can also be ruled out—including bleeding at the level of the spleen, trocar ports, and at the level of the mesentery and omentum (Figs. 9.2 and 9.3).

The presence of intraperitoneal fluid with blood density (>25 U Hounsfield) will confirm the possibility of hemoperitoneum.

How to Approach This Complication

Bleeding can be caused by an unsecured bleeding point at the anastomosis, technical failure of applied stapler, or a coagulation disorder. Incidence is less than 4 %, and more than the half of the patients can be treated conservatively [13]. If the

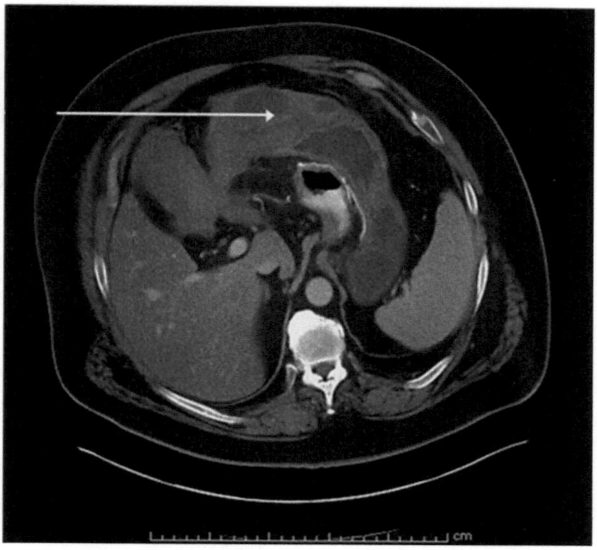

Fig. 9.2 *Arrow* showing intra-abdominal hematoma at the level of the suture line of the gastric wall

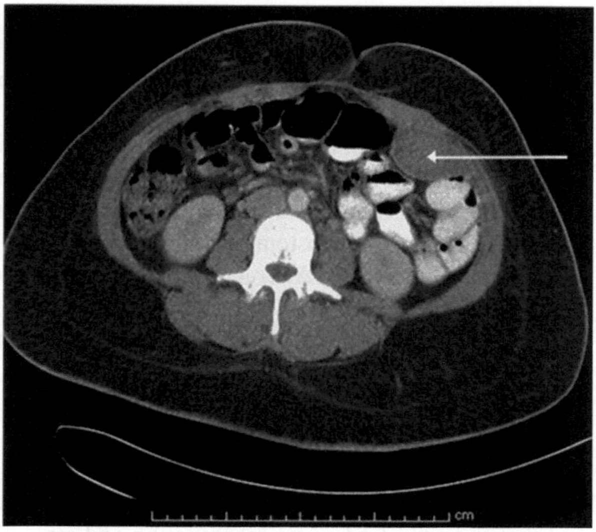

Fig. 9.3 *Arrow* showing hematoma of the abdominal wall associated with the trocar entrance

patient is hemodynamically stable, coagulation should be corrected, prophylactic coagulation should be stopped, the rest of the stomach should be kept empty by a good patent nasogastric tube, and blood transfusions will be given when necessary. If a slow decrease of hemoglobin is found, a careful gastroscopy can help to establish a diagnosis and fix the problem.

Initial Resuscitation

Initial management includes ensuring peripheral IV lines of good caliber (14F) to administer saline/colloids and to replace blood loss. If coagulation disorders are present, these should be corrected.

Patients with early postoperative bleeding—being hemodynamically unstable in spite of adequate resuscitation—should be reoperated.

Endoscopic Treatment

Endoscopic treatment is the first choice if the patient is hemodynamically stable, because it allows for identifying and controlling of the bleeding at the level of the anastomosis, either by means of electrocoagulation or by clips. The combined use of epinephrine, electrocoagulation, and/or clips is recommended. These procedures are not associated with a higher risk of dehiscence due to ischemia of the anastomosis line [14, 15].

The problem is how to approach the unstable patient. Endoscopic examination by gastroscopy is not without risks, whereas a CT angiography scan may, in the case of a clear blush, help to establish the diagnosis and to treat it by means of coiling [13–15].

However, if the patient remains unstable in spite of initial resuscitation and use of other therapeutic options or failure of coiling, the patient should be reoperated without delay.

During reoperation, the stomach should be opened in the longitudinal direction above anastomosis rather than through it. The stomach should be emptied of clots and blood, and anastomosis inspected from within. If cause of bleeding is not in the stomach, the jejunojejunostomy should be inspected, and if bleeding is found, it must be fixed by stitches. After a total gastrectomy under anesthesia, the esophagojejunostomy should be first inspected by gastroscopy before laparotomy takes place. In this case, a stent may be a good alternative for solving the problem.

Intra-abdominal Bleeding

A patient who in the early period after the operation is hemodynamically unstable and that in spite of adequate resuscitation and reposition of blood loss should be directly operated on. Splenic bleeding should be treated by conservative measures if possible (e.g., hemostasis devices, splenic mesh), but if not resolved, then splenectomy should be done. Hemostasis will be optimal. Other found causes of bleeding (such as mesenteric and omental bleeding or trocar port bleeding) should be fixed by stitches. Failure to observe bleeding of epigastric vessels during laparoscopic surgery is an important cause of postoperative shock, and the patient should be operated on without delay. Ligature of epigastric vessels on both sides should then be done.

Peritonitis After Gastrectomy

Peritonitis is the most common complication following gastroduodenal surgery. Also, fluid collections and abscesses are common, mostly due to contamination at the time of surgery. Leakage may occur early because of a failure to obtain a watertight anastomosis or occur late because of ischemia/necrosis of the suture line. If leakage is limited, the fluid can be walled off and controlled, as abscesses, by adjacent viscera. Such inflammatory lesions or plastron may also result in early or late anastomosis or in intestinal obstruction.

Prevention of peritonitis involves the decompression of the dilated stomach before operation, the proper use of prophylactic antibiotics to minimize any contamination during resection, and performing a watertight anastomosis in vital tissues. Moreover anastomosis will need to be patent, not twisted, and without tension. After partial gastrectomy, the gastrojejunostomy should be fixed to the mesocolon in order to avoid stenosis, or a twist of the jejunal loop, or an internal herniation.

Diagnosis of Postoperative Peritonitis

What if the patient fails to improve or is worsening? The suspicion for peritonitis can be high in the case of fever, abdominal pain, tachycardia, increased drain production, or with suspect aspect such as bile or intestinal contents, leukocytosis being present, and CRP being increased. Engaging a CT scan with double contrast (IV and oral) will diagnose the leakage and the peritonitis, followed by an explorative laparotomy. Surgeon should always think about possible leakage locations, in this succeeding order: duodenal stump, gastrojejunostomy or esophagojejunostomy anastomoses, jejunojejunal anastomosis, and inadvertent lesion of a hollow organ and/or biliary tract.

In the case of presence of fluid collections without leakage of anastomosis, a CT scan-guided percutaneous drainage and culture of the fluid will entail the initial treatment. Amylase should be determined if leakage of pancreas or duodenum is suspected. In the case of leakage, the only option for conservative treatment is if, on the CT scan, no intra-abdominal collections are visible and the leakage comes out completely as a canalized fistula through the drains.

Management of General Peritonitis Following Partial Gastrectomy

After diagnosis and initial resuscitation, relaparotomy should be performed. The cause of peritonitis, such as leakage of the duodenal stump of other anastomosis (such as gastrojejunostomy or jejunojejunostomy), accidental lesion of small bowel, or ischemia of transverse colon, should be detected and treated. Treatment consists of reinforcement stitches with omentoplasty, rinsing of the abdomen and leaving of drains, or, in the case of colonic ischemia, doing a transverse colectomy and colostomy. The detection and treatment of leakage of duodenal stump will be treated separately, below.

Management of General Peritonitis Following Total Gastrectomy

The policy discussed above should be applied for treating peritonitis after total gastrectomy. The leakage problems at esophagojejunostomy will be treated more specifically below.

Leakage of Duodenal Stump

The main cause of peritonitis following gastrectomy is the leakage of duodenal stump. In the past, surgeons learned how to deal with a difficult duodenum during the surgery of complicated peptic ulcers. Many ingenious ways have been described to deal with this problem, but none will completely prevent a significant incidence of stump leakage. Nowadays, this kind of surgery is incidental. While treating gastric cancer, the only indication to divide the duodenum is when there is no inflammation or fibrosis of the duodenum. Moreover, invasive gastric cancer is generally treated by neoadjuvant chemotherapy, and immunosuppression may increase the rate of duodenal stump leakage after gastrectomy.

Approach to This Complication

Local Duodenal Conditions

The closure of the duodenal stump has to be safe; it is usually performed with linear stapler with triple staple lines. Reinforcement of the stump by sutures is not recommended, because the duodenal wall is thick but weak.

Closure Techniques

In those cases where the stump closure is considered unsafe, a lateral duodenotomy is recommended; this creates duodenal decompression, which can also be achieved with the placement of a nasogastric/transjejunal tube up to the end of the duodenal stump. Lateral duodenotomy implies the introduction of a Foley-like tube through a purse string suture, being exteriorized and sealed by wrapping omentum around it. The lateral duodenotomy will emerge through the upper-right abdominal wall, above the level of the duodenum, to assure adequate drainage. The tube should remain for 3 or 4 weeks before removal, in order to assure a good canalized fistula and thereby reducing the possibility of a peritoneal leakage. Adequate use of the external drains left in subhepatic area is also important [16, 17].

In the infrequent case of gastrectomy used because of a complicated peptic ulcer, we specify two maneuvers that are useful for the closure of a difficult stump:

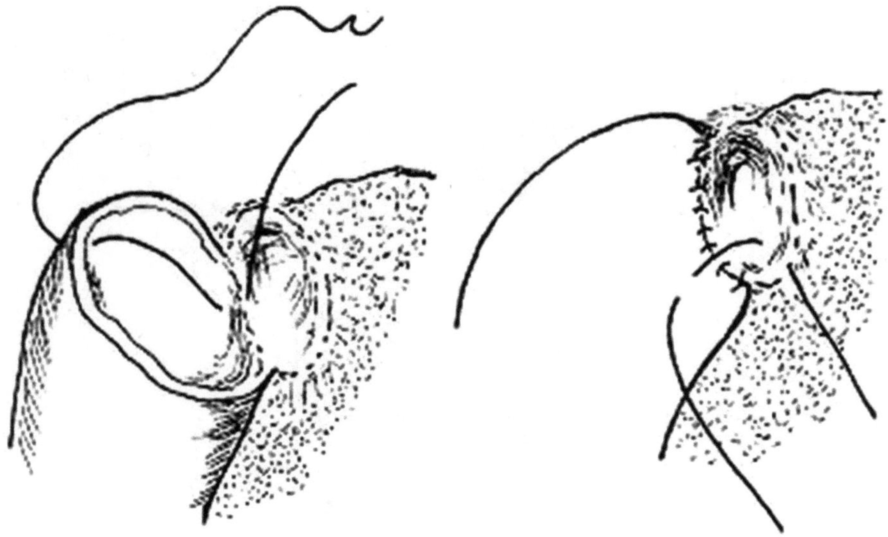

Fig. 9.4 Nissen procedure. A first layer has been completed and a second layer is being done where the callous edge of the ulcer is taken, with the anterior side at some distance, as shown in the *second figure* to the *right*

1. The Nissen closure is performed in those cases with a difficult-to-manage duodenum in which the duodenal stump is closed by means of separated stitches of the anterior wall of the duodenum with the fibrotic posterior wall plus omentoplasty (Fig. 9.4).
2. The Finsterer-Bancroft-Plenk closure is a good alternative to the Nissen closure (see Fig. 9.5). It consists of three procedures: (a) the division of the antrum 6 cm from the pylorus, keeping its irrigation from the pyloric and gastroepiploic arteries; (b) the mucosa cuff being resected following the submucous layer up to the pylorus, which is closed with stitches that take the pyloric muscular layer; and (c) the completed procedure. The anterior and posterior antrum walls have been attached with internal stitches and a second continuous suture layer (Fig. 9.5).

Diagnosis of This Complication

Clinical Manifestations

This complication occurs postoperatively rather early, usually between the fourth and seventh postoperative days. The most important signs and symptoms are fever, abdominal pain, tachycardia, and (if a drain is still in situ) the presence of biliary and duodenal leakage through it.

Moreover, the presence of duodenal leakage in the abdominal cavity is associated with symptoms and signs of systemic inflammatory response syndrome (SIRS)

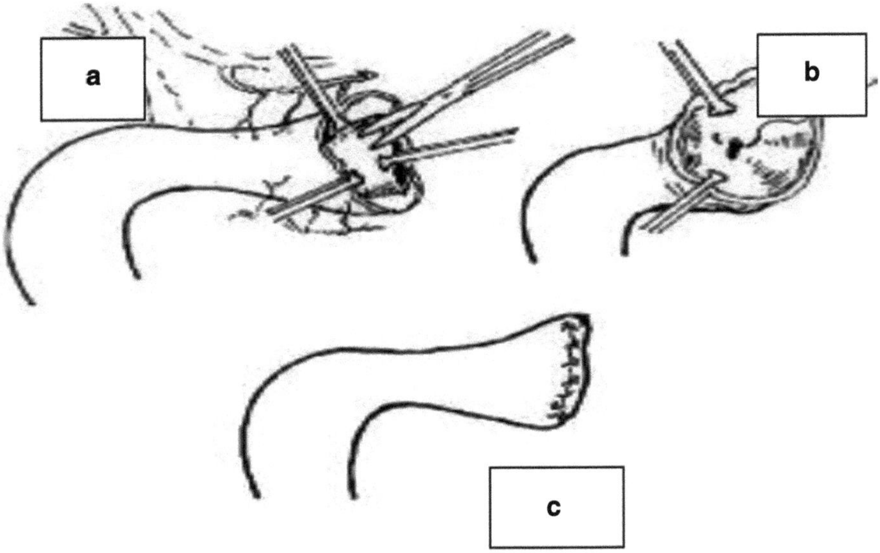

Fig. 9.5 Finsterer-Bancroft-Plenk procedure. (**a**) The antrum has been sectioned at 8 cm of the pylorus keeping its irrigation from the pyloric and gastroepiploic arteries. The mucosa is being resected following the submucous layer. (**b**) The mucous cuff has been completely resected until the pyloric hole, which is closed with points that take the pyloric sphincter. (**c**) Completed procedure. The anterior and posterior antral sides have been attached with internal points and the section borders sutured

or sepsis. At physical exploration, the patient may appear as septic, hemodynamically unstable, and dyspneic, and the abdomen may show signs of distension and peritonitis. The patient should then be admitted to the medium care or intensive care department for initial resuscitation.

Such clinical symptoms and signs, together with the findings of the CT scan, will form the indications for emergency surgical exploration.

Imaging

The CT scan of the abdomen with IV and oral preparation will show the duodenal leakage but also signs of local or general peritonitis, such as free air and fluid collections.

Treatment of This Complication

The leakage of the duodenal stump appears in 1–3 % of gastric resections. Nowadays, the mortality associated with this complication is, due to improvements in postoperative critical care, between 0 and 12 % [12].

Initial Resuscitation

- Fluid reposition of losses associated to SIRS syndrome and the losses of the biliopancreatic leakage.
- Antibiotic treatment applies in cases of abdominal sepsis and is always associated with adequate drainage of the duodenal leakage. Broad-spectrum antibiotics IV are to be administered. Blood cultures are also important for identifying the cause of sepsis and modifying the treatment accordingly. Empirical treatment with antifungals is recommended in patients with prolonged hospitalization and in case of following broad-spectrum antibiotic treatment for less than 15 days.

Surgical Treatment

In the majority of cases, relaparotomy is indicated. The most commonly used technique is the terminal duodenotomy. A 22- or a 24-French Petzer or Foley catheter is introduced through the duodenal leakage at the stump, and a purse string is made with nonabsorbable material. This procedure can be complemented with wrapping and fixation of the major omentum around the suture (Wu technique), which contributes to closing it. A Penrose and a sump drain are left subhepatic and in the Morrison pouch. A temporary gastrostomy for suction and a jejunostomy for feeding are created. The abdomen should be rinsed and drained. Skin should be left open.

The only option for conservative approach will be the situation in which the duodenal leakage is fistulized and drained totally through a drain. Moreover, the patient should be hemodynamically stable, and no intra-abdominal collections are allowed to be present on the CT scan. But also in this situation, if the flow is persistent and higher than 500 mL/24 h (high-flow biliopancreatic fistula), then surgical exploration could be indicated. In this case, the high flow may be associated with distal obstruction (afferent loop syndrome) or the presence of local abscess.

Total parenteral nutrition (TPN) through a central venous access should be initiated early after reoperation because these patients have an increased catabolism and do not get enteral food for several days.

The use of octreotide or somatostatin analogues (e.g., Lanreotide®) has demonstrated the efficacy of decreasing the fistula production during the first week; however, its share in the closure of the fistula is still controversial [18].

Acute Pancreatitis

After extensive D2-type lymphadenectomy, lesion to the pancreas during dissection may lead to acute pancreatitis, pancreatic fluid collection, or abscess. If an abscess is suspected on the CT scan, percutaneous drainage should be done. Acute pancreatitis should be treated conservatively.

Postoperative Jaundice

In the case of postoperative jaundice, differential diagnosis should be done immediately for distinguishing between the obstructive type and the rest. An ultrasonography (or CT scan) and laboratory examination will establish the diagnosis. If obstructive jaundice with dilated intrahepatic biliary ducts occurs, an MRCP (magnetic resonance cholangiopancreatography) should be done. If the proximal biliary duct is dilated and its distal part is not visible, a PTC should be done for diagnosis and temporarily drainage of the biliary tract. Reconstruction will follow afterwards. In cases of very distal gastric cancer in which a relatively long segment of post-pyloric duodenum has to be resected, it is important during resection to identify the common bile duct (CBD) and papilla of Vater by means of a thin catheter introduced through the cystic duct into the duodenum. This is a safe method to avoid inadvertent lesion to the distal CBD or papilla during an extended gastrectomy.

Esophagojejunostomy Leakage

Esophagojejunostomy leakage is a much-feared postoperative complication, occurring in 4–27 % of cases after total gastrectomy and being associated with a mortality of 60 %. Moreover, thirty to fifty percent of patients with leakage of an esophagojejunal anastomosis will later develop a stenosis at that level [19].

Factors Involved in the Prevention

a. Optimization of the nutritional status before surgery

   Patients with an esophageal and gastric cancer usually have a poor oral intake and enteral nutrition should be given through a nasojejunal tube. If not possible because of obstruction, total parenteral nutrition (TPN) should be administered at least 2 weeks prior to surgery. This extra nutrition must be given longer if the oral intake is not adequate, and the patient should be treated by neoadjuvant chemotherapy.

   Some groups systematically create a feeding jejunostomy or leave a long nasojejunal feeding tube in order to give patients an adequate caloric and protein intake during the immediate postoperative period. This may be associated with low morbidity and mortality rates [20, 21].

b. Surgical technique

   Distal esophageal margins should be well perfused and free of cancer. In most cases, free margins will be assured by means of an intraoperative frozen-section evaluation. Many times, it is necessary to divide the hiatus anteriorly to get an optimal esophageal margin for a safe anastomosis. The jejunal loop to be anastomosed needs to have enough length and a good perfusion, being the jejunal vessels evaluated by means of palpation and transillumination. The best way to reach the esophagus, without any tension of the jejunal loop, is the transmesocolic route. The esophagojejunal Roux-en-Y anastomosis is usually performed in an

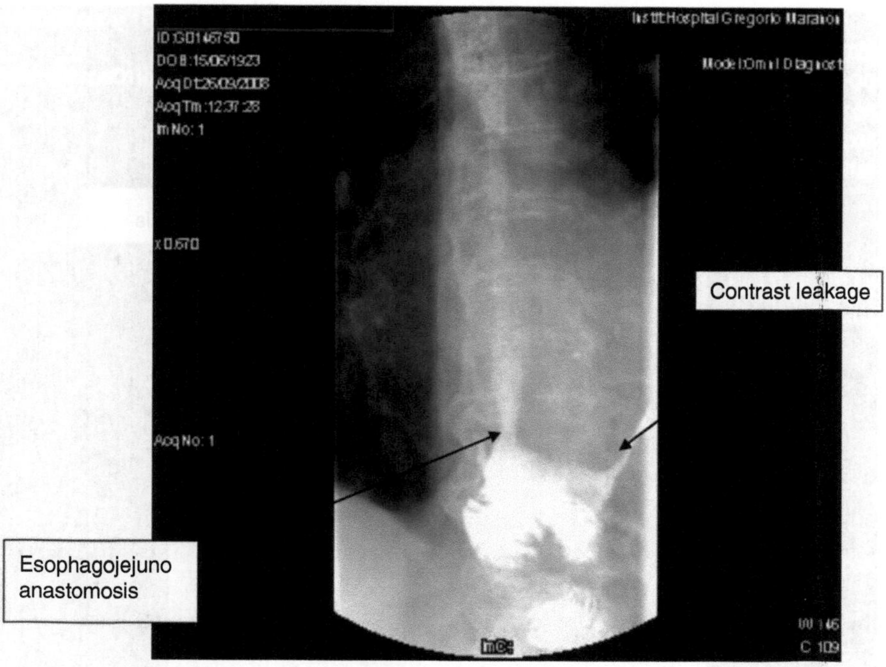

Fig. 9.6 Leakage of contrast from the esophagojejunal anastomosis

end-to-side fashion by means of a 21- to 25-mm circular stapler. Another alternative is to manually perform the anastomosis in one layer with interrupted stitches.

Intraoperative anastomosis control is recommended by inspection of the donuts and administration of methylene blue through the nasogastric tube.

Placement of a drain does not diminish the incidence of anastomotic leak but may decrease the immediate clinical impact of such a complication and may allow the possibility of a less invasive treatment such as the placement of a stent [22].

Diagnosis of This Complication

Clinical: Upper abdominal pain, fever, and presence of suspect fluids through drains usually happen between the 7th and 10th postoperative day.

a. Imaging: The oral swallowing of Gastrografin® usually shows the contrast leakage (Fig. 9.6). It is not recommended to use barium-containing contrast due to the risk of chemical peritonitis. A CT scan of thorax and abdomen, with oral and IV contrast, will provide sufficient information about the anastomotic leakage and the presence of peri-anastomotic abscesses, mediastinitis, or general peritonitis.

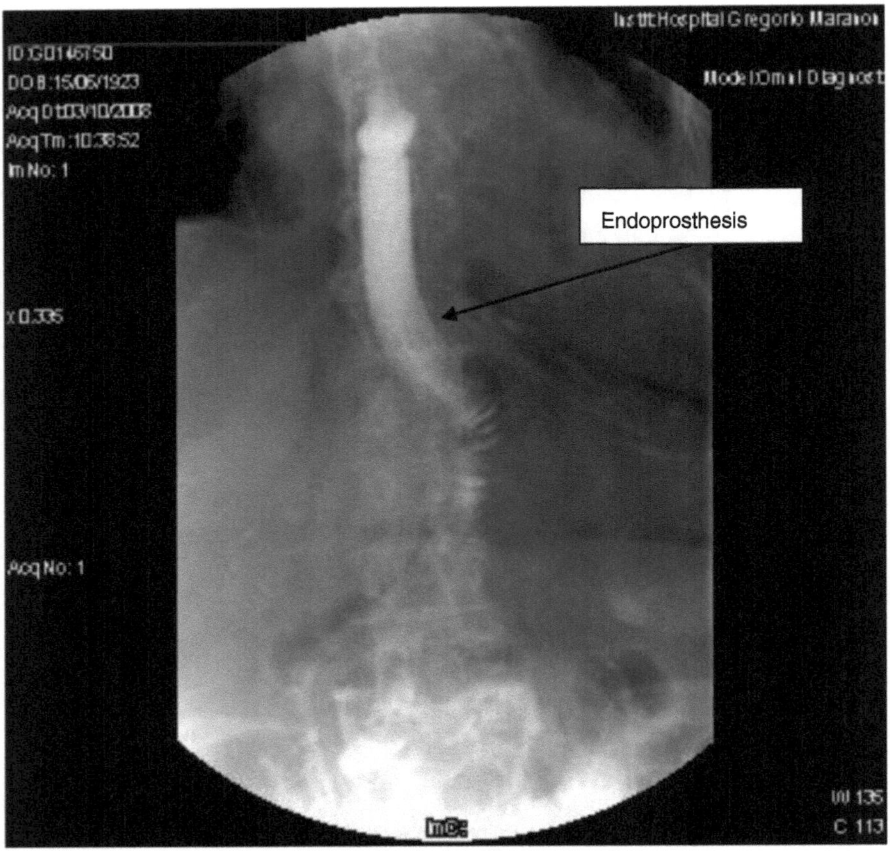

Fig. 9.7 Control of the leakage of the esophagojejunostomy by means of stent

b. Endoscopic: in those cases without a clear diagnosis after clinical and radiological evaluation or in a case whereby the possibility of treatment by means of a stent is being considered, an endoscopic study is indicated to determine the localization and extension of the anastomotic leakage. In most of the cases during endoscopic evaluation, a stent should be placed (Fig. 9.7).

Treatment

a. The patient should be admitted to intensive care or medium care. Resuscitation measures: fluids are to be repositioned to achieve an optimal mean arterial pressure ≥90 mmHg, CVP 8–12 mmHg, and urinary flow ≥0.5 mL/kg/h. Eventually, noradrenalin should be used.

b. Broad-spectrum IV antibiotics should, according to protocol, be started immediately after diagnosis.
c. Control of anastomotic leakage:

    1. In case a hemodynamically unstable patient is in critical septic condition despite resuscitation measures, the patient should be operated on urgently, including either:

        - Closure of the distal esophageal stump plus cervical esophagostomy and jejunostomy for feeding
          or
        - Esophagojejunal dismantling and placement of drains in the distal esophagus and in the jejunum

    2. In case of a hemodynamically stable patient, time is available to perform a quick study of anastomotic leakage. If the leakage is <30 % of the circumference, treatment may be conservative, including sepsis control, adequate local drainage of fluid collections, stent placement, and enteral feeding by microtube through the anastomosis or TPN [23, 24]. If the leakage is >30 %, then the esophagojejunostomy should be dismantled and adequately drained. A reconstruction may be performed 6–12 weeks later in order to redo the anastomosis.

Stenosis-Obstruction of Anastomosis

Gastric-outlet obstruction and intestinal obstruction are relatively frequently occurring complications after gastrectomy. Five percent of all gastrectomies are complicated with stenosis/obstruction of any anastomoses [25].

The main cause of the obstruction is an area of inflammatory adhesions adjacent to the anastomosis, probably as consequence of small suture-line leakages and bleeding. Clearly, these complications are preventable. Moreover, functional paralysis of the stomach, common in patients after long-standing gastric dilatation as resulting from pyloric stenosis, may mimic gastric-outlet obstruction. Gastric peristalsis may also be reduced by postoperative hypopotassemia.

Obstruction After a Partial Gastrectomy

There are many mechanical problems related to the gastrojejunostomy, whether ante- or retrocolic. Gastric outlet occurs in about 5 % of all retrocolic anastomoses. A retrocolic anastomosis can be stenosed by the transverse mesocolon. In order to prevent this, the defect in the mesocolon should be sutured to the stomach at least 2 cm above the anastomosis. If this is not performed, the mesocolon may slide down resulting in mechanical obstruction of one or both jejunal loops. In making the anastomosis, it does not matter if it is isoperistaltic or antiperistaltic, but it is important that the anastomosis is not twisted or obstructed.

Following a total gastrectomy, another cause of obstruction may become the torsion of the long loop of the jejunum used for the esophagojejunostomy. Furthermore, if antecolic anastomosis is performed, an internal hernia between the loop and colon may be the cause of obstruction.

Prevention of This Complication

Benign stenosis after esophagojejunostomy occurs in 26–42 % of patients, which is of significant influence on the nutritional status and quality of life [20, 21]. Despite the technical and postoperative improvements, the incidence of benign stenosis has not changed in the last 15 years.

Stenoses are associated with anastomotic leakages and cardiovascular disease. Stenoses after anastomotic leakage may be due to (a) initial local ischemia manifested as a leakage and/or (b) local inflammatory reaction.

Also, cardiovascular disease may have an important influence on the anastomosis healing process due to poor irrigation, as consequence of atherosclerosis or a low cardiac output.

Diagnosis of This Complication

If transit through the anastomosis is impaired for longer than 5 days, involving the necessity of emptying the gastric remnant by means of nasogastric tube, then diagnostic assessment is indicated by means of a CT scan using oral contrast. It will help diagnosing the level of the obstruction but also ruling out abscesses or leakages that should be treated first. Stenosis may be found at the level of the esophagojejunostomy, at the level of the gastrojejunostomy, or after a Billroth II anastomosis at the afferent or efferent loop. Gastroscopy is the next step in order to assess the stenosis/obstruction and to evaluate the possibility for dilatation therapy. If possible, progressive balloon dilatation done in several sessions will be the treatment of choice.

Decompression of the stomach is the initial step, along with adequate feeding by means of intestinal feeding tube introduced by the gastroscopist distal of the stenosis or by TPN.

Treatment depends on the diagnosis.

If abscesses are present, these must first be drained percutaneously before the dilatation program can be started. If there is only stenosis, a dilatation program will be scheduled. Dilatation by means of a balloon will frequently lead to optimal results [25].

If dilatation is not possible or obstruction is complete because of a technical problem, such as internal hernia or torsion, then reoperation will need to be planned.

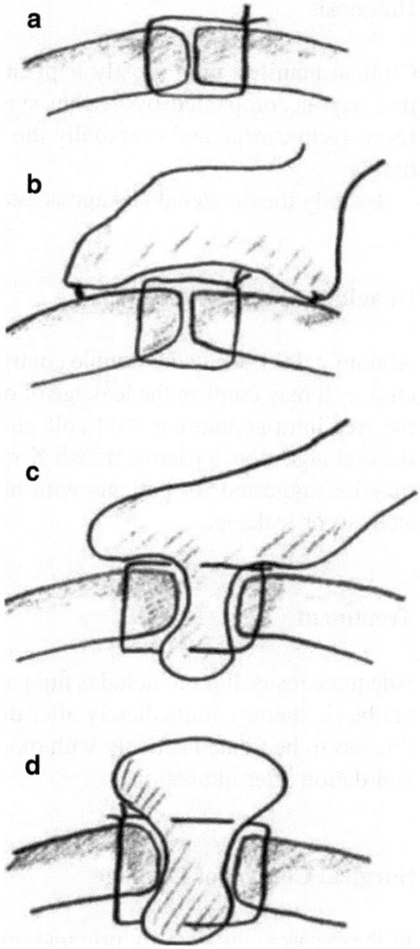

Fig. 9.8 Closure techniques of perforated duodenum. (**a**) Primary closure with interrupted sutures. (**b**) Primary closure with interrupted sutures covered with pedicled omentoplasty. (**c**) Cellan Jones repair: plugging the perforation with omentoplasty. (**d**) Graham Patch: plugging the perforation with free omental plug

Leakage After Closure of Duodenal Perforation

Prevention starts with a good operative treatment of the perforation. Perforated duodenal ulcers that cover more than one third of the pyloric circumference are not suitable for primary suture reparation, due to the high risk of leakage [26]. In this situation, perforation should be closed and a protective gastrojejunostomy must be performed. Methylene blue may be used through the nasogastric tube to ascertain the containment of the primary suture. Perforations equal to or less than one third of the circumference are suitable for primary suture and omentoplasty (Fig. 9.8) [27–29].

Diagnosis

Clinical manifestation mostly happens between the third and seventh postoperative day, accompanied by certain symptoms and signs such as abdominal pain, fever, tachycardia, and eventually the leakage of gastrointestinal contents through drains.

Usually the duodenal leakage is associated with signs of SIRS or sepsis.

Imaging

Abdominal CT scan with double contrast (oral and IV) is the complementary test of choice. It may confirm the leakage of oral contrast through duodenum and visualize the free intra-abdominal fluid collections and pneumoperitoneum. Before starting the oral ingestion, a routine transit X-ray on the second and third postoperative days may be suggested for patients with high-risk closure of duodenum for ruling out stenosis or leakage.

Treatment

Adequate resuscitation includes fluid and electrolyte reposition and broad-spectrum antibiotic therapy immediately after diagnosis. If there is respiratory insufficiency, this has to be treated actively with oxygen therapy and, if needed, with mechanical ventilation after intubation.

Surgical Control of Leakage

In these cases, the antropyloric and duodenal bulb resection and reconstruction by means of gastrojejunal Roux-en-Y anastomosis is recommended [28].

Rebleeding After Repair of a Bleeding Duodenal Ulcer

Acute bleeding is the most common complication of peptic ulcer disease, and its mortality rate lies between 5 and 10 %. Currently, endoscopic treatment is adequate in the majority of patents; however, 5–10 % of them may experience rebleeding and require embolization or surgery. After surgery, the risk of rebleeding is about 5 %.

The factors that increase the risk of rebleeding are having an ulcer larger than 2 cm localized in the lesser curvature or posterior side of the duodenal bulb and being in shock [30–31].

General Principles of Repair of Bleeding Ulcer

Primary suture of the ulcer bed consists of duodenotomy through the pylorus and visualization of the ulcer and a bleeding point, followed by suture of the four cardinal points to control bleeding from the gastroduodenal artery or any of its branches. Some authors also recommend the selective ligation of the gastroduodenal artery. However, this has been studied in series with a limited number of patients, and hence, the conclusions on lower rebleeding rates are inconclusive.

In 1952, Dorton reported that suture of the bleeding ulcer, pyloroplasty, and truncal vagotomy reduced the rebleeding to 4 % in duodenal and 7 % in gastric ulcers.

Furthermore, a comparative study was performed in the beginning of the 1990s to compare both procedures, the ulcer treatment plus truncal vagotomy and the pyloroplasty versus ulcer treatment alone. The first procedure has less risk of rebleeding than only ulcer treatment (3 % vs 17 %). However, this study was made at the beginning of the 1990s when neither PPI treatment nor Helicobacter pylori eradication therapy existed. Nowadays, the use of vagotomy in those cases is exceptional [32].

The most important cause of rebleeding is a failure to control the initial bleeding. Insufficient or failed attempts to manage the bleeding point by sutures, with or without ligation of the vessels around the duodenum (e.g., gastroduodenal artery), may lead to rebleeding.

Prevention of This Complication

Coagulation disorders should be corrected and treatment with proton pump inhibitors (PPI) at high doses should be initiated. PPIs have demonstrated the efficacy of diminishing the risk of rebleeding and mortality [33].

Diagnosis

Clinical Diagnosis

The most important signs for bleeding are hematemesis and melena or fresh blood through the nasogastric tube, along with a decrease in hemoglobin values. Hemodynamic instability and poor peripheral perfusion are frequently found.

Laboratory

The presentation of anemia can take up to 6 h after bleeding.

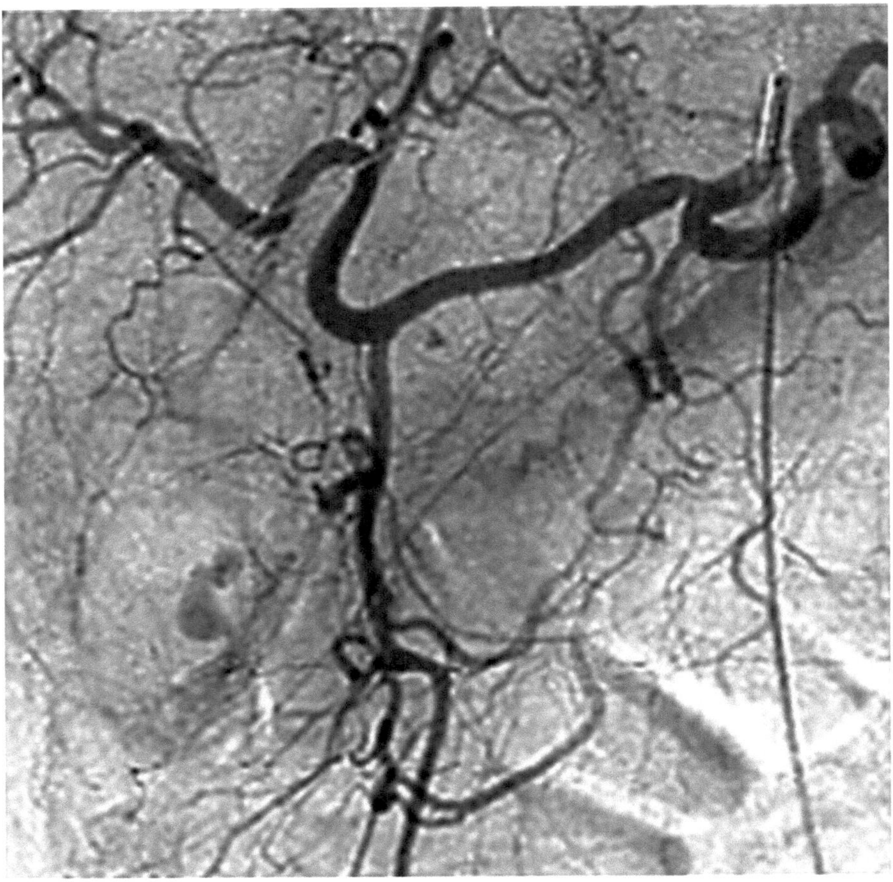

Fig. 9.9 Celiac trunk angiography shows active bleeding at gastroduodenal artery after surgery

Endoscopy

This is the most frequently used diagnostic tool; it may be hazardous because of the fragility of the suture.

Angiography

The evaluation of the celiac trunk and the superior mesenteric artery is the best strategy to diagnose the rebleeding and potentially treat it by means of embolization. It may also be performed in hemodynamically unstable patients. Evaluation of both arteries is necessary because of the risk of rebleeding from one of the collateral branches (Fig. 9.9).

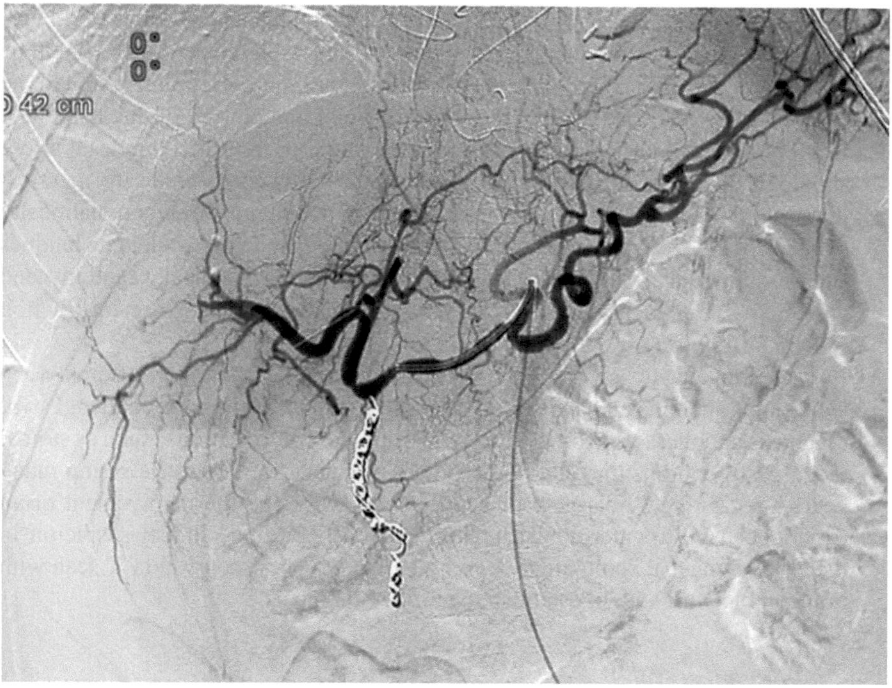

Fig. 9.10 Selective embolization by coiling of the gastroduodenal artery

How to Treat This Complication

1. New endoscopy and use of combined methods (epinephrine injection plus heat-energy application plus clips) have demonstrated certain efficacy to control bleeding. However, the rate of failure with this strategy is 10 %.
2. Angiography and embolization.

   Celiac trunk and superior mesenteric artery angiography and selective embolization (coiling) of the gastroduodenal artery are efficacious, with a 95 % technical success (absent radiologic bleeding) and a 72 % clinical efficacy. The outcomes are comparable to the ones reached with rebleeding surgery.

   Angioembolization proximal of Treitz ligament has a low risk of ischemia due to the presence of important collateral circulation. New catheters and material to embolize are available: detachable microcoils, absorbable particles, and cyanoacrylate rubber (Fig. 9.10).

   Even if morbidity seems lower after angioembolization, the risk for rebleeding and mortality is similar with an outcome after redo operations 29 % versus 23 % and 26 % versus 21 %, respectively [33–39].

3. Relaparotomy and Surgery. If a patient is hemodynamically unstable and unresponsive to resuscitation maneuvers or after coiling, then relaparotomy should be performed. During laparotomy, duodenum suture or pyloroplasty should be opened followed by suturing of the bleeding point and closure of duodenotomy. If not performed during the first operation, ligature of the gastroduodenal artery should be done. If the reclosure of the duodenum is not considered safe, a gastrojejunostomy should be added in order to bypass the duodenum. In hemodynamically stable patients, the control of bleeding may be associated with antacid techniques such as (a) truncal vagotomy and pyloroplasty and (b) truncal vagotomy and antrectomy (ulcer resection) with gastrojejunal Roux-en-Y reconstruction [30, 33, 40].

Less frequent postoperative complications such as dumping, afferent loop syndrome, anemia, and nutritional disorders remain important challenges for diagnosis and therapy. Moreover, diagnosis of late complications (such as stomal ulcer, gastrocolic fistula, and development of cancer in the gastric stump many years after surgical treatment of peptic ulcer) will need the involvement of an experienced gastroenterologist having acumen regarding clinical suspicion in the case of unusual complaints. A combination of gastroscopy and CT scan with oral contrast will help to establish the proper diagnosis.

References

1. Yasuda K, Shiraishi N, Adachi Y, et al. Risk factors for complications following resection of large gastric cancer. Br J Surg. 2001;88:873–7.
2. Cuschieri A, Fayers P, Fielding J, et al. Postoperative morbidity and mortality after D1 and D2 resections for gastric cancer: preliminary results of the MRC randomised controlled surgical trial. The Surgical Cooperative Group. Lancet. 1996;347:995–9.
3. Bonenkamp JJ, Songun I, Hermans J, et al. Randomised comparison of morbidity after D1 and D2 dissection for gastric cancer in 996 Dutch patients. Lancet. 1995;345:745–8.
4. Hartgrink HH, van de Velde CJ, Putter H, et al. Extended lymph node dissection for gastric cancer: who may benefit? Final results of the randomized Dutch gastric cancer group trial. J Clin Oncol. 2004;22:2069–77.
5. Sasako M, Saka M, Fukagawa T, et al. Surgical treatment of advanced gastric cancer: Japanese perspective. Dig Surg. 2007;24:101–7.
6. Brady MS, Rogatko A, Dent LL, Shiu MH. Effect of splenectomy on morbidity and survival following curative gastrectomy for carcinoma. Arch Surg. 1991;126:359–64.
7. Wu CW, Chang IS, Lo SS, et al. Complications following D3 gastrectomy: post hoc analysis of a randomized trial. World J Surg. 2006;30:12–6.
8. Bozzetti F, Marubini E, Bonfanti G, et al. Total versus subtotal gastrectomy: surgical morbidity and mortality rates in a multicenter Italian randomized trial. The Italian Gastrointestinal Tumor Study Group. Ann Surg. 1997;226:613–20.
9. Sierzega M, Kolodziejczk P, Kulig J, et al. Impact of anastomotic leakage on long-term survival after total gastrectomy for carcinoma of the stomach. Br J Surg. 2010;97:1035–42.
10. Hu WG. Complications of laparoscopic gastrectomy for gastric cancer and the management. Zhonghua Wei Chang Wai Ke Za Zhi. 2012;4:325–7.

11. Kim KH, Kim MC, Jung GJ, Kim HH. Long-term outcomes and feasibility with laparoscopy-assisted gastrectomy for gastric cancer. J Gastric Cancer. 2012;12:18–25.
12. Nagasako Y, Satoh S, Isogaki J, et al. Impact of anastomotic complications on outcome after laparoscopic gastrectomy for early gastric cancer. Br J Surg. 2012;99:849–54.
13. Bakhos C, Alkhoury F, Kyriakides T, et al. Early postoperative hemorrhage after open and laparoscopic Roux-en-Y gastric by-pass. Obes Surg. 2009;19:153–7.
14. Jamil LH, Krause KR, Chengelis DL, et al. Endoscopic management of early upper gastrointestinal hemorrhage following laparoscopic Roux-en-Y gastric by-pass. Am J Gastroenterlol. 2008;103:86–91.
15. Kirschniak A, Stierle D, Philipp F, et al. Current management of upper gastrointestinal bleeding. Minerva Chir. 2011;66(6):573–87.
16. Isik B, Yilmaz S, Kirimlioglu V, et al. A life-saving but inadequately discussed procedure: tube duodenostomy. Known and unknown aspects. World J Surg. 2007;31:1616–24.
17. Tsuei BJ, Schwartz RW. Management of the difficult duodenum. Curr Surg. 2004;61: 166–71.
18. Gayral F, Campion JP, Regimbeau JM, et al. Randomized, placebo-controlled, double-blind study of the efficacy of lanreotide 30 mg PR in the treatment of pancreatic and enterocutaneous fistulae. Ann Surg. 2009;250:872–7.
19. Lang H, Piso P, Stukenborg C, et al. Management and results of proximal anastomotic leaks in a series of 1114 total gastrectomies for gastric carcinoma. Eur J Surg Oncol. 2000;26:168–71.
20. Kight CE. Nutrition considerations in esophagectomy patients. Nutr Clin Pract. 2008;23:521–8.
21. Deguchi Y, Fukagawa T, Morita S. Identification of risk factors for esophagojejunal anastomotic leakage after gastric surgery. World J Surg. 2012;36:1617–1622.
22. Takeyoshi I, Ohwada S, Ogawa T, et al. Esophageal anastomosis following gastrectomy for gastric cancer: comparison of hand-sewn and stapling technique. Hepatogastroenterology. 2000;47:1026–9.
23. Blackmon SH, Santora R, Schwarz P, et al. Utility of removable esophageal covered self-expanding metal stents for leak and fistula management. Ann Thorac Surg. 2010;89: 931–6.
24. Dai YY, Gretschel S, Dudeck O, et al. Treatment of oesophageal anastomotic leaks by temporary stenting with self-expanding plastic stents. Br J Surg. 2009;96:887–91.
26. Gupta S, Kaushik R, Sharma R, Attri A. The management of large perforations of duodenal ulcers. BMC Surg. 2005 Jun 25;5:15.
25. Fukagawa T, Gotoda T, Oda I, et al. Stenosis of esophago-jejuno anastomosis after gastric surgery. World J Surg. 2010;34:1859–63.
27. Lo HC, Wu SC, Huang HC, et al. Laparoscopic simple closure alone is adequate for low risk patients with perforated peptic ulcer. World J Surg. 2011;35:1873–8.
28. Di Carlo I, Toro A, Sparatore F, et al. Emergency gastric ulcer complications in elderly. Factors affecting the morbidity and mortality in relation to therapeutic approaches. Minerva Chir. 2006;61:325–32.
29. Bertleff MJ, Lange JF. Laparoscopic correction of perforated peptic ulcer: first choice? A review of literature. Surg Endosc. 2010;24:1231–9.
30. Chiu PW. Bleeding peptic ulcers: the current management. Dig Endosc. 2010;22 Suppl 1:S19–21.
31. Kawamura T, Yasuda K, Morikawa S, et al. Dig Endosc. 2010;22 Suppl 1:S26–30.
32. Dorton HE. Vagotomy, pyloroplasty, and suture for bleeding gastric ulcer. Surg Gynecol Obstet. 1966;122:1015–20.
33. Wilkins T, Khan N, Nabh A, Schade RR. Diagnosis and management of upper gastrointestinal bleeding. Am Fam Physician. 2012;85:469–76.
34. Loffroy R, Guiu B. Role of transcatheter arterial embolization for massive bleeding from gastroduodenal ulcers. World J Gastroenterol. 2009;21(15):5889–97.

35. Loffroy R, Guiu B, Mezzetta L, et al. Short- and long-term results of transcatheter embolization for massive arterial hemorrhage from gastroduodenal ulcers not controlled by endoscopic hemostasis. D Can J Gastroenterol. 2009;23:115–20.
36. Rudler M, Cluzel P, Massard J, et al. Optimal nonsurgical management of peptic ulcer bleeding, including arterial embolization is associated with a mortality below 1%. Clin Res Hepatol Gastroenterol. 2012;37:64–71.
37. Loffroy RF, Abualsaud BA, Lin MD, Rao PP. Recent advances in endovascular techniques for management of acute nonvariceal upper gastrointestinal bleeding. World J Gastrointest Surg. 2011;3:9–100.
38. Wong TC, Wong KT, Chiu PW, et al. A comparison of angiographic embolization with surgery after failed endoscopic hemostasis to bleeding peptic ulcers. Gastrointest Endosc. 2011;73:900–8.
39. Loffroy R. Transcatheter arterial embolization should be the salvage treatment of choice in all patients with bleeding from duodenal ulcers resistant to endoscopic hemostasis. Scand J Gastroenterol. 2010;45:1003–4.
40. Songür Y, Balkarli A, Acartürk G, Senol A. Comparison of infusion or low-dose proton pump inhibitor treatments in upper gastrointestinal system bleeding. Eur J Intern Med. 2011;22: 200–4.

Chapter 10
Prevention and Treatment of Major Complications After Bariatric Surgery

Frits J. Berends and Ignace M.C. Janssen

Keywords Bariatric surgery • Obesity • Preoperative considerations • Postoperative complications • Laparoscopic adjustable band • Laparoscopic gastric bypass • Erosion band

Introduction

Obesity is a serious problem of global public health affecting developed and undeveloped countries. People with body mass index (BMI) > 30 kg/m^2 represent 7 % of the world's population. However, in some of the developed countries, the prevalence of morbid obesity (BMI > 40 kg/m^2) is as high as 5 %. Bariatric surgery is one of the fastest growing hospital procedures in the USA and in Europe. It is estimated that in the USA 220,000 weight loss surgeries were performed in 2008 [1].

The operations that surgeons use today to treat severe obesity are modifications of procedures that were designed to save lives requiring removal of the stomach or intestine. For example, one of the well-known side effects of the Billroth II operation is weight loss. The empiric use of bypass and restrictive procedures proved to be very effective in reducing excess weight but also introduced new complications in itself. Some of these were related to the procedure, others to metabolic changes induced by the new anatomic situation. During the last 50 years, the 30-day mortality risk of bariatric surgery has decreased from 4 to less than 0.5 %. Operative times have diminished from more than 4 h to 60 min, and hospital stay is reduced from a week to 1 or 2 days.

Obesity surgery began in 1954 when the first intestinal bypass was performed at the University of Minnesota in an attempt to treat a patient with morbid obesity [2].

F.J. Berends • I.M.C. Janssen (✉)
Department of Surgery, Rijnstate Hospital, Arnhem, The Netherlands
e-mail: ijanssen@alysis.nl

M.A. Cuesta, H.J. Bonjer (eds.), *Treatment of Postoperative Complications after Digestive Surgery*, DOI 10.1007/978-1-4471-4354-3_10,

This event marks a change in attitude towards obesity as it demonstrated that obesity could be considered a disease and treated successfully. Earlier, morbid obesity was looked upon as a behavioral problem that was to be managed with conservative therapies such as dietary coaching and psychotherapy.

Although the intestinal bypass led to significant weight loss, it came clear that it was associated with an unacceptable high rate of complications. Bacterial overgrowth in the excluded small intestine and migration of protein breakdown products and bacteria in the portal circulation led to liver damage and autoimmune disease in kidneys and joints. Reeking diarrhea was one of the unpleasant side effects. Precipitation of calcium oxalate in the kidney led to formation of stones, adding to kidney damage. In all about 7 % of patients died of liver failure or developed liver cirrhosis.

The disadvantages of the intestinal bypass drove surgeons to search for alternative procedures that either led to restriction of the food intake or to modify the intestinal tract through a bypass or a combination of these. In 1966 the gastric bypass was introduced as a modification of the original Billroth operation. It combined a stomach reduction with a bypass of a certain part of the proximal jejunum. Because of bile reflux and ulcer formation, a Roux-Y reconstruction was added later on. Thereafter a large number of procedures and modifications were developed and in a lot of cases abandoned again. To date only a handful of bariatric procedures represent the vast majority of weight loss surgeries among which the Roux-Y gastric bypass (RYGB) is the gold standard (Fig. 10.1). The adjustable gastric band (AGB) (Fig. 10.2) and the sleeve gastrectomy (SG) (Fig. 10.3) represent the most performed restrictive procedures now that the vertical banded gastroplasty is mostly abandoned because of complications on the long term. The sleeve gastrectomy with duodenal switch (DS) (Fig. 10.4) and the biliopancreatic diversion (BPD) (Fig. 10.5), originally designed by Scopinaro, represent the malabsorptive side of the weight loss surgery specter.

Preoperative Considerations

Many comorbid conditions like metabolic, cardiovascular, psychological, orthopedic, neurological, hepatic, pulmonary, and renal disorders are seen in association with obesity. These conditions add to the risk of surgical procedures in general and bariatric surgery in particular. Evidence has accumulated suggesting that obesity is a state of chronic, low-grade inflammation; it may represent a potential mechanism whereby obesity leads to the metabolic derangements that may hamper healing and recovery after surgery [3]. The development of insulin resistance in mouse models of obesity and type 2 diabetes mellitus (DM) is characterized by progressive accumulation of inflammatory macrophages and subpopulations of T cells in the visceral adipose. Regulatory T cells may play a critical role in modulating tissue inflammation via their interactions with both adaptive and innate immune mechanisms. Furthermore it is important to recognize nondiagnosed underlying conditions that may influence the operative and postoperative course. Undiagnosed sleep apnea may lead to postoperative hypoventilation especially when opiates are

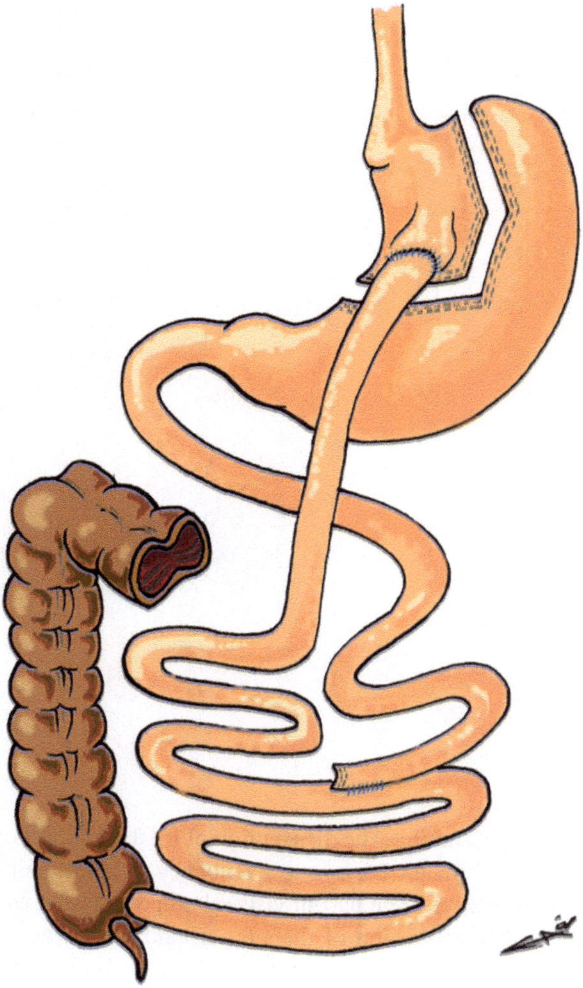

Fig. 10.1 Roux-Y gastric bypass

administered for analgesia. Before surgery in each patient, individual risk factors have to be assessed, and the potential benefits and risks of weight loss surgery have to be balanced. Several well-known risk factors have to be taken into consideration [4] (Table 10.1).

Older Age – As the incidence of comorbidities rises with age, so does the operative risk. Mortality rates are three times higher in patients over 65 years compared to younger patients. This raises the question if bariatric surgery should be performed on older patient especially since life expectancy remains unchanged in the elderly. However, the effects of weight loss and increase in quality of life scores are similar compared to younger patients which may justify bariatric surgery in selected older patients.

Fig. 10.2 Adjustable gastric band

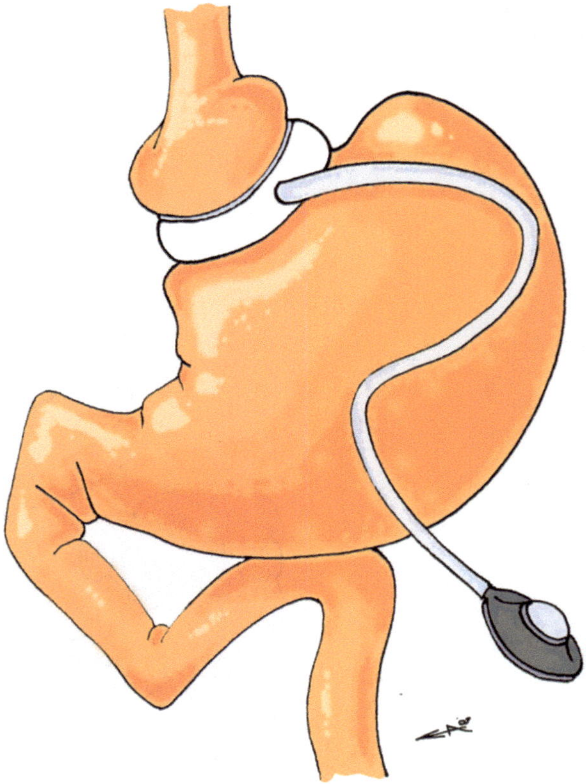

Male Gender – The distribution of total body fat is often different in males compared to females. Men have a tendency to store their excess fat around the waist, with a relative large part in visceral adipose tissue, whereas a lot of women have a relative large portion of their fat around the lower body especially the hips, buttocks, and legs. This typical fat distribution is depicted as an apple- or pear-shaped body composition and is associated with a different metabolic profile. Apple-shaped patients have a higher risk of the metabolic syndrome and consequently a higher risk of death from stroke and myocardial infarction. From a surgical point of view, a large amount of visceral fat makes the surgical exposure of the upper gastrointestinal tract more difficult and in that way adds to the operative risk. A large study among Medicare beneficiaries in 2006 demonstrated that the 1 year mortality after surgery that was two times higher in males compared to females.

Chronic Disease and Super Obesity – It is understandable that chronic disease adds to the complication risk of any surgical procedure. However, in daily practice, it is hard to estimate relative risks of chronic diseases, especially when multiple chronic conditions are involved, and relate them to surgical outcome. Superobese patients (BMI > 50 kg/m^2) are more likely to have chronic disease and are averagely more difficult to operate because of a higher change of visceral adiposity. In a

Fig. 10.3 Sleeve gastrectomy

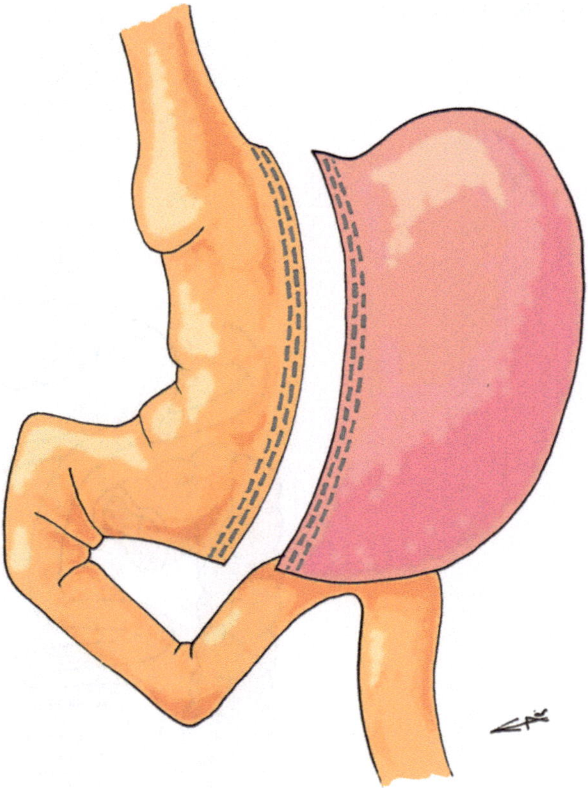

review of 856 bariatric Veteran patients in the USA, a Diagnostic Cost Group (DSG) risk adjustment measure was used to reflect the level of comorbidities. A DSG score of ≥2 was associated with a significant increase in risk of death. [5]

Low-Volume Surgeons and Hospitals – As in almost every surgical procedure, the risk of adverse events is associated with the volume of operations performed. This is especially the case for high-complex procedures such as malabsorptive laparoscopic bariatric surgeries. The Longitudinal Assessment of Bariatric Surgery (LABS) study examined the relationship between surgeons' annual RYGB volumes and 30-day patient outcomes at 10 centers within the USA. The study demonstrates that the patient's risk of an adverse outcome after RYGB decreased significantly with the increase in surgeon RYGB volume (cases performed annually >50) [6].

Type of Surgery – The introduction of the laparoscopic approach in weight loss surgery has demonstrated a benefit in perioperative mortality compared to open surgery. Also both morbidity and mortality are dependent on the type of procedure. The 30-day mortality rate is lower for laparoscopic adjustable gastric banding (LAGB) then for laparoscopic gastric bypass. In the longer term however after LAGB, more reoperations are necessary.

Fig. 10.4 Duodenal switch

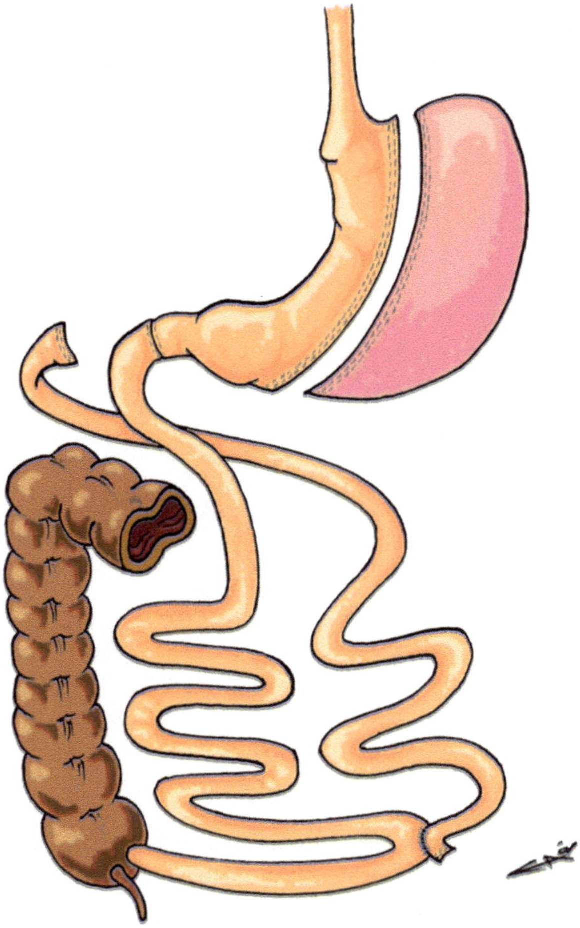

Predicting Mortality – The Obesity Surgery Mortality Risk Score (OS-MRS) is a scoring system to assess the risk of perioperative death in patients that undergo bariatric surgery. It classifies patients in three categories with increasing risk: Class A, low risk; Class B, intermediate risk; and Class C, high risk. Several studies have shown significant differences in perioperative death between the three different risk classes. [7]

Operative Complications

The physical properties of obese patients sometimes form a challenge for the bariatric surgeon. The thick abdominal wall often hampers maneuverability, thus limiting subtle handling of instruments. The often large liver and abundant visceral adipose tissue further complicate visualization and access in both open and laparoscopic

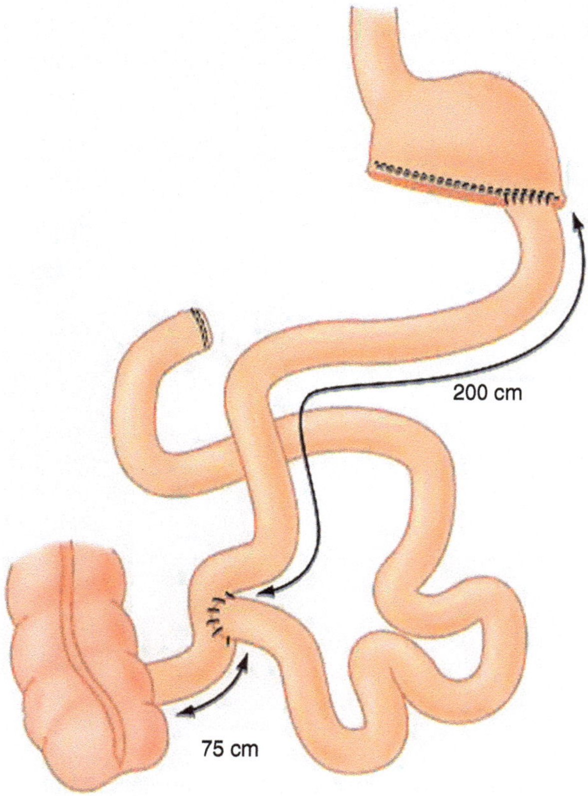

Fig. 10.5 Biliopancreatic diversion

Table 10.1 Risk factors in bariatric surgery

Age >50 years
Male gender
BMI >50 kg/m^2
Redo surgery
Comorbidities such as hypertension and diabetes

surgery. Furthermore, the excess visceral fat, the thick mesentery, and large greater omentum can be the cause of traction, for example, when the alimentary limb in gastric bypass surgery is pulled up to the gastric pouch on the ventral side of the transverse colon. As stated before, the implications of any complication are often more serious in bariatric patients. Therefore, the bariatric surgeon must in all cases stick to the basic principles of (laparoscopic) surgery, even when the conditions are often less than ideal. Optimal camera equipment, state-of-the-art instruments and stapling, gentle manipulation of tissues, and timely conversion to open surgery can prevent complications.

Trocar Injuries – Both Veress needle and Hasson trocar can be safely used in the obese patient. Probably the safest place for introducing a Veress needle is the left upper quadrant of the abdomen. The often large overlying omentum forms a relative

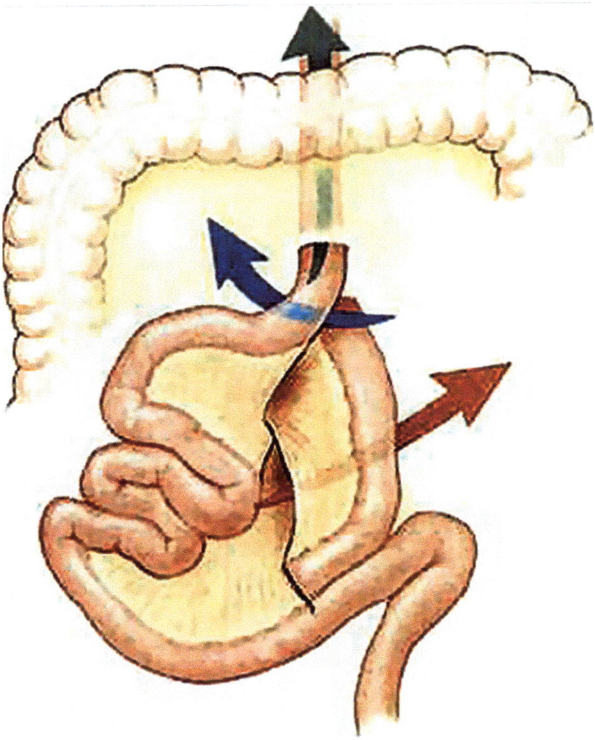

Fig. 10.6 Petersen's defect and other internal herniation sites

protective shield against serious organ injury. Although the enlarged left liver lobe is often punctured with a Veress needle, this seldom leads to serious hemorrhage. Modern optical bladeless trocars further help in safe access. In the past especially pyramid-shaped trocar blades were a cause of sharp organ trauma and bleeding from the trocar site.

Splenic Injury – Splenic injury sometimes occurs as many of the bariatric procedures aim to staple of the gastric fundus at the angle of His. Also, in placement of laparoscopic adjustable gastric band, a route is made behind the cardia of the stomach towards the angle of His. Probably the greatest risk of bleeding from the spleen is during sleeve gastrectomy when the short gastric vessels are divided sometimes causing a hemorrhage from the spleen. Although splenic bleeding can be tedious and sometimes difficult to control, splenectomy is hardly ever necessary.

Internal Hernia – Internal herniation is a relatively rare complication mostly seen after gastric bypass surgery. A potential hernia site remains when the Roux limb is pulled up to meet the gastric cardia and crosses over the transverse colon mesentery. This so-called Petersen's space (Fig. 10.6) is the location where the small intestine can herniate, giving rise to postprandial complaints of obstruction and pain. Sometimes an acute obstruction is present needing emergency surgery.

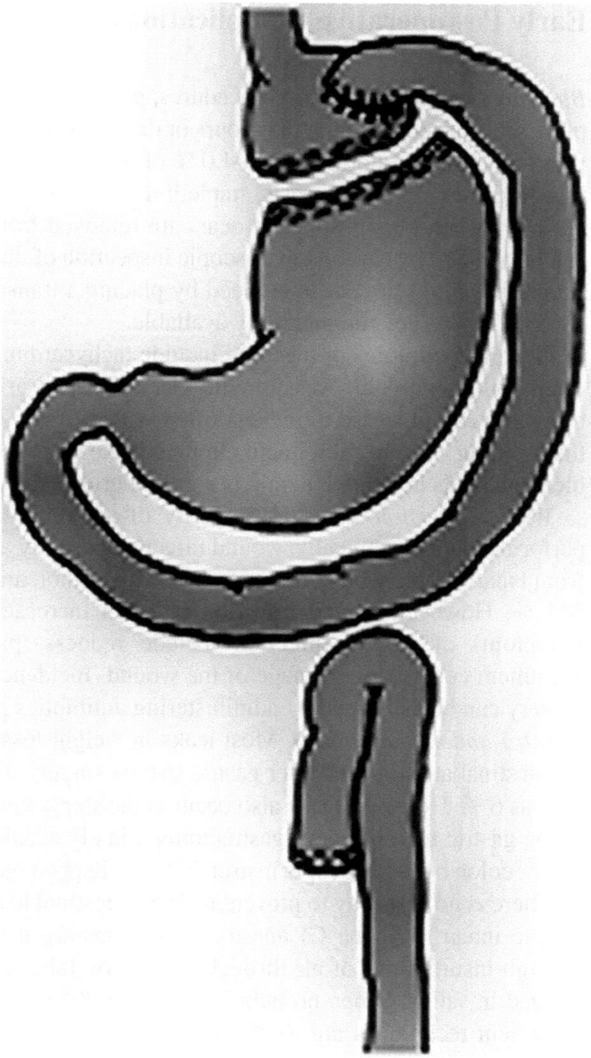

Fig. 10.7 Roux-en-"O"

The enterostomy is a second site for internal herniation after RYGB. After LAGB there are reports of small bowel obstruction caused by the tubing between the band and port that acts as an intra-abdominal adhesion.

Misconstruction – The limited space and measuring of both the biliopancreatic and alimentary limb in gastric bypass surgery can lead to wrongfully anastomosing the biliopancreatic limb to the gastric pouch, thus creating a wrongful Roux-en-"O," an absolute obstruction, leading to vomiting, gastric dilatation, and sometimes gastric blowout (Fig. 10.7). It is recommended to drain the gastric remnant during reoperation, as it takes the dilated biliopancreatic limb often a couple of days to regain function.

Early Postoperative Complications

Bleeding – As in all surgical procedures, postoperative bleeding is one of the complications that occur in the first hours or day after surgery. Significant bleeding after gastric bypass is reported in 0.6–4.0 % of patients. In weight loss surgery potential bleeding sites are anastomosis, staple lines, and trocar sites. Trocar bleeding arises typically when (sharp-tipped) trocars are removed from the abdominal wall. They can be avoided by careful laparoscopic inspection of the trocar wound on the inside. Trocar bleedings are easily stopped by placing a transabdominal suture, for which several devices are commercially available.

General symptoms of bleeding include tachycardia, decrease in hematocrit, and often abdominal pain. Anastomotic bleeding often arises from the gastrojejunostomy and can give rise to melena often without pain. Gastroscopic localization of the bleeding site and subsequent clipping is the preferred treatment. However, when bleeding leads to hemodynamic instability, urgent surgery is mandatory.

Wound Infection – As the majority of weight loss procedures nowadays are performed laparoscopically, wound infections usually are not a big issue. Morbidity from laparoscopic wound infection is usually minor, and incidence is not more than 3–4 %. However, wound infection rate can increase threefold in open surgery. Symptoms of wound infection include redness, pain, fever, and fluctuation. Treatment consists of drainage of the wound. Incidence of wound infections in GI surgery can be decreased by administering antibiotics perioperatively.

Intra-abdominal Leaks – Most leaks in weight loss surgery arise from the gastrointestinal anastomosis after gastric bypass surgery. Reported incidence can be as high as 6 %. However, leaks also occur at the staple line of the excluded stomach or of the gastric tube in sleeve gastrectomy. Finally accidental damage of small intestine or colon by laparoscopic instruments can happen outside the view of the camera.

There is no sure way to prevent a gastrointestinal leakage. Many surgeons evaluate the integrity of the GI anastomosis by testing it with methylene blue dye or through insufflations of air through the gastric tube while the anastomosis is submerged in saline. When no bubbles are seen, there is no apparent leak. Also reinforcement techniques are used for staple lines to prevent leakage, such as fibrin glue, buttressing materials, and oversewing. However, these measures add to the operative costs while there is little evidence that they can prevent leakage.

Leaving wound drains near to the gastrointestinal anastomosis obviously cannot prevent leakage but may help to detect a leak early. Furthermore having a drain in place can be very helpful in case of a leak because it is an essential part of the treatment and it may prevent needing a reoperation.

Symptoms of leak can be very discrete and sometimes merely consist of tachycardia or abdominal tenderness. Other symptoms include fever, tachypnea, and leukocytosis. Especially tachycardia > 100 bpm and respiratory distress are the most sensitive physical signs for postoperative leak. CRP is elevated after all operative procedures, and discrete elevations are therefore not very reliable. When reconvalescence after surgery is out of the ordinary, a leak must be suspected. As physical examination in the obese patient is mostly of limited value, further diagnostics can be considered [8]. Barium swallow or computed tomography can radiographically demonstrate a leak; however, a (false) negative result does not rule out the possibility of leak. Reported sensitivity and specificity of CT scan for GI leakage can be very high, even up to 100 % in some reports.

As the mortality rate after GI leakage can be as high as 15 %, it is mandatory to treat the leak as soon as possible. Therefore, it is questionable if the effort of additional diagnostic procedures should be undertaken at all. Urgent surgical intervention is probably the best response when a leak is suspected. Most often a laparoscopic approach at reoperation after initial laparoscopic weight loss surgery is feasible.

Cardiovascular Complications – Cardiac complications can occur during surgery but also happen postoperatively. Although improving morbidity is one of the goals of weight loss surgery, the weight loss in itself increases cardiac risk. In some reports cardiovascular mortality in the first year after bariatric surgery is as high as 5 %.

Pulmonary Complications – Pulmonary embolism (PE) is one of the major causes of perioperative death in bariatric surgery. The combination of high BMI, venous stasis during surgery, and hypoventilation can easily lead to deep venous thrombosis (DVT) and pulmonary emboli even weeks after surgery. Prevention of PE includes perioperative administering low-molecular heparin, compression stockings during surgery, and early mobilization.

Pulmonary infection and hypoventilation are frequently observed after weight loss surgery. Atelectasis occurs often in morbidly obese patients in the perioperative period. The obesity hypoventilation syndrome and obstructive sleep apnea syndrome (OSAS) in combination with perioperative opiates lead to desaturation and respiratory insufficiency. Positive end-expiratory pressure ventilation during anesthesia, perioperative physiotherapy support, early ambulation, and continuous positive airway pressure treatment in patients with OSAS can prevent a number of pulmonary complications.

Late Complications

After RYGB

Pouch-Related Complications – A Roux-Y gastric bypass (RYGB) consists of a small gastric pouch and a Roux-en-Y reconstruction of the jejunum, creating an alimentary limb of 75–200 cm that is attached to the pouch and a biliopancreatic limb of about 50 cm.

Stenosis of the stoma between pouch and Roux limb is especially observed when the anastomosis is created with a circular stapler, in particular when a small-sized anvil (21 mm or less) is used. Symptoms consist of dysphagia, vomiting, reflux, and excessive weight loss. Treatment consists of (repeated) gastroscopic balloon dilatation of the stoma.

Dilatation of the pouch can arise over time leading to complaints of reflux, increased intake, and weight regain. Debate remains if prophylactic placement of a Silastic ring can prevent dilatation. In extreme cases operative reduction of pouch size can help.

Marginal ulcers are observed regularly at the distal margin of the gastric pouch. Symptoms are dysphasia, food intolerance, heartburn, and in severe cases perforation or hemorrhage. Relative ischemia especially after redo surgery, presence of Helicobacter pylori, and nonsteroidal anti-inflammatory drug use can contribute to ulcer formation. Treatment consists of proton pump inhibiting (PPI) drugs.

Dumping Syndrome – Dumping syndrome is the collection of symptoms that occur after eating food that is rich in carbohydrates. The rapid passage to the jejunum leads to an increase in serum insulin and subsequently a decrease in blood glucose. Symptoms are similar with hypoglycemia: nausea, tachycardia, weakness, and dizziness. Treatment for patients with severe dumping problems entails dietary advice, avoiding large amounts of carbohydrates, and spreading meals throughout the day.

Internal Hernia – Internal hernia after gastric bypass surgery can arise at three locations: the space between the Roux limb and the transverse colon (Petersen's space), the mesenteric defect at the enterostomy, and the defect in the mesocolon when a retrocolic approach is chosen for the Roux limb. Incidence can be as high as 5 %. Complaints are typically after meals and consist of abdominal pain, colics, and obstructive symptoms. Sometimes acute obstruction is the reason for emergency surgery to prevent small bowel ischemia. The incidence of internal herniation can be decreased by closing all defects during bypass surgery (Fig. 10.6).

Diagnosing an internal hernia can be challenging. Simple contrast studies seldom reveal an internal hernia. CT scan with a typical "swirl sign" of the mesenteric vasculature is a strong sign of internal hernia. However, when everything else fails, diagnostic laparoscopy can provide the ultimate answer.

Nutritional Deficiencies – As reduced food intake is one of the aims of gastric bypass surgery, it is not surprising that deficiencies can easily occur, especially because absorption of vitamins and minerals are drastically altered after GB. Practically all patients develop in time some shortage, may that be vitamin B12, iron or calcium. In this respect it is questionable if deficiencies can be considered "complications" or rather must be considered expected side effects. Nevertheless it illustrates the necessity for all patients that underwent gastric bypass surgery to commit to lifelong vitamin supplementation and at least yearly blood testing.

Weight Loss Failure – The mean excess weight loss percentage after GB surgery ranges from 50 to 70 %. However, some patients lose only a limited amount of weight or regain weight after initial successful weight loss. Although often the surgery is blamed and for disappointing results, in reality noncompliant eating behavior and behavioral habits are responsible. Revisional surgery with conversion to more extreme bypass constructions or addition of restrictive measures (Silastic band or banded bypass) is technically feasible but should be offered with restraint.

Gallstones – A large number of patients develop gallstones during weight loss in the first year. About 40 % of these become symptomatic. However, no studies have demonstrated a benefit of prophylactic cholecystectomy. Incidence of cholecystolithiasis can be drastically reduced with prophylactic use of ursodeoxycholic acid.

After LAGB

Adjustable gastric banding is one of the most frequently performed bariatric operations in morbidly obese patients. Laparoscopic adjustable gastric banding (LAGB) is a safe and effective method of weight loss and reduction of comorbidities associated with obesity. Despite its good safety profile compared with Roux-en-Y gastric bypass, patients with LAGB can manifest unique complications that are distinctive to the LAGB and need a special assessment and treatment. The most common complications are pouch enlargement, band slip, band erosion, esophageal dilatation, reflux, port rotation, port-site infection, and breakage of the tubing [9].

Normal Situation – In the assessment of a patient with a LAGB, one should make an upper gastrointestinal radiograph series. A normal image of the upper abdomen after LAGB placement is demonstrated in Fig. 10.8. The band is placed just below the gastroesophageal junction. The pouch is hardly visible for the first year but will extend to a size of appropriately 50–80 mL. The right position of the band is seen on the radiography if it has an angle of approximately 45° towards the left shoulder.

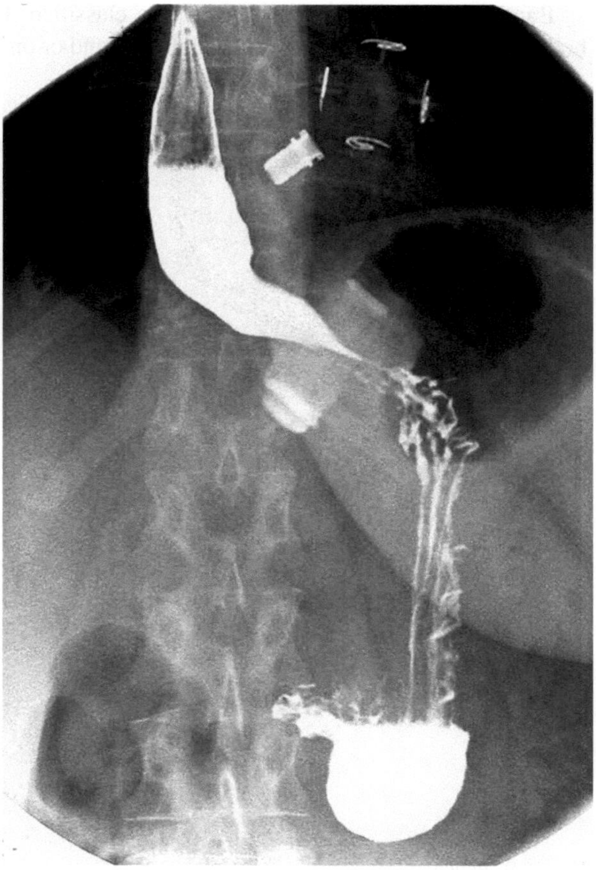

Fig. 10.8 Normal AGB

Band Slip and Pouch Dilatation – The most important cause of slippage is an increased pressure in the pouch due to vomiting. In a lot of cases, overfilling is the real cause. Most patients feel that they have the best support of the band if they can hardly eat. They will ask for filling of the band if they do not lose weight. Prevention of overfilling is prevention of pouch dilatation and helps to get a good long-term result. The patient with a band slippage and obstruction usually presents with dysphagia, vomiting, regurgitation, and food intolerance. The diagnosis is easily made by an upper gastrointestinal series. Complications related to band slip include gastric perforation, necrosis of the slipped stomach (type V prolapse), upper gastrointestinal bleeding, and aspiration pneumonia.

Pouch enlargement or prolapse is diagnosed when dilation of the proximal gastric pouch is present with or without change in the angle of the band on an upper abdominal radiograph and in the absence of signs of obstruction. The lower esophagus may or may not be dilated. Pouch enlargement is also a pressure-related phenomenon that may be surgically induced by band overinflation or overeating with vomiting, resulting high pressure in the pouch. Primary placement of the band with too much fundus above the band gives a high risk of pouch dilatation. Symptoms of pouch enlargement can be lack of satiety, heartburn, regurgitation, and occasional chest pain. The diagnosis is made with an upper gastrointestinal series (Fig. 10.9).

Band slip and pouch dilatation can be classified depending on the part of the body of the stomach that moves through the band or on the dilatation of the stomach or placement of the band (Tables 10.1 and 10.2).

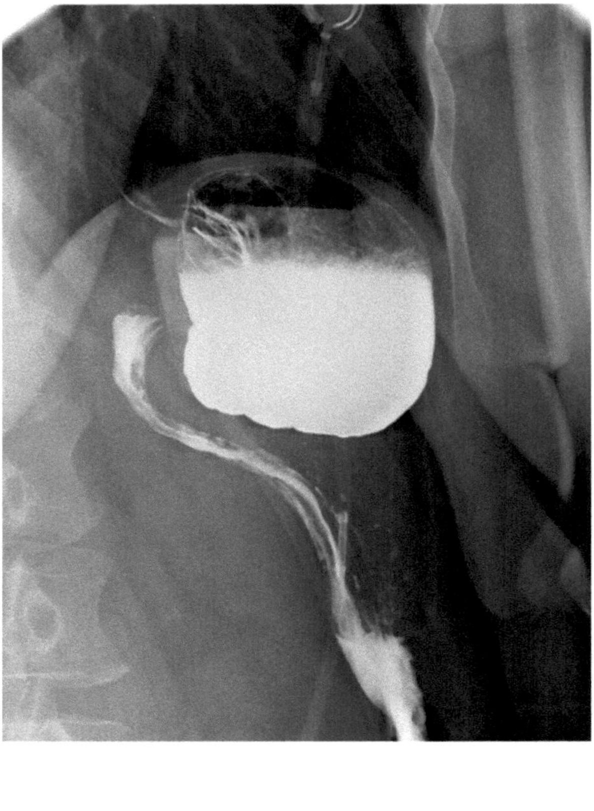

Fig. 10.9 Pouch dilatation

Table 10.2 Band slip and pouch dilatation

Type	Definition	Mechanism	Etiology	Management
I	Anterior slip	Downward migration of band	Insufficient anterior fixation	Surgical
II	Posterior slip	Posterior stomach wall herniates through band	Perigastric approach	Surgical
III	Pouch enlargement	Pouch dilatation	Tight band or overeating	Band deflation, re-education
IV	Immediate postoperative slip	Band placed too low on stomach	Inappropriate band placement	Surgical
V	Type I or II with gastric necrosis	Band slip with pouch ischemia	Acute pouch dilatation	Surgical

Incidence of slippage varies in literature. O'Brien and Dixon reported 25 % of band slip in their first 500 patients using the perigastric approach (accessing the right crus perigastrically) and only 4.8 % of slippage in the last 600 patients with the pars flaccida technique (accessing the right crus through the pars flaccida) [10]. Other published literature reports an incidence of slip of 1–22 %.

Since the amount of tissue of the stomach in the band is bigger at the body of the stomach than at the angle of His (normal band position), obstruction of the gastrointestinal tract can occur when the band slips. Band slip can be posterior or anterior, depending on whether the anterior or posterior region of the stomach herniates through the band. In all patients with obstructive complaints and pain not responding to emptying of the band, a gastroscopy is mandatory to rule out gastric ischemia or necrosis. These conditions require an immediate surgical intervention.

Laparoscopic removal or repositioning of the band is the preferred method of treatment for both slippage and pouch dilatation. In patients who were successful in losing weight with the gastric band, repositioning can be considered. If the patient did not experience significant weight loss, removing the band and creating a gastric bypass in one or two tempi is the preferred option. In situations of substantial prolapse where reduction is not possible or when evidence of intra-abdominal infection is present, the most prudent management is removal of the gastric band.

Band Erosion – Band erosion is an uncommon complication of LAGB. The band gradually erodes through the stomach wall into the gastric lumen. The reported incidence is around 1 %, with an estimated prevalence varying from 0 to 11 % [11]. Band erosion may be the result of gastric-wall injury during band placement or tight anterior fixation.

A high index of suspicion is required for diagnosis of band erosion as most patients are asymptomatic. When symptomatic, complaints related to erosion include loss of restriction, nonspecific epigastric pain, gastrointestinal bleeding, intra-abdominal abscesses, or port-site infection. The diagnosis is often made at the time of gastroscopy (Fig. 10.10).

The recommended treatment is complete removal of the eroded gastric band, gastroscopically, laparoscopically, or via laparotomy. Removing a band that has eroded into the stomach can be difficult owing to the extensive inflammatory response around the proximal stomach and left lobe of the liver. This is the rationale

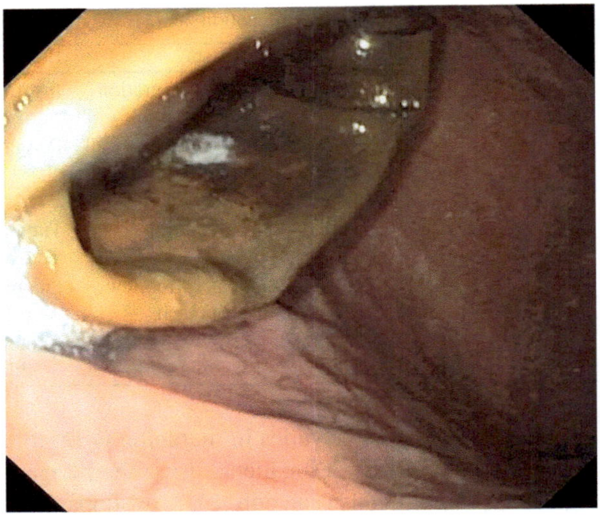

Fig. 10.10 Band erosion

for a gastroscopic approach: With the scope a thin metal wire is positioned around the band. The two ends of the wire are brought trough a thin flexible shaft which is gently brought down through the esophagus to the band. The wires are pulled with force against the flexible shaft thus cutting through the silicone band. From the outside, the port must be surgically removed and the tubing cut. After this, the band can be removed orally, most of the times. This procedure can only be performed when the band is well visible within the stomach.

Because of the difficult direct laparoscopic approach, transgastric techniques have been proposed to facilitate band removal. Using distal transgastric ports, the band can be removed with a combined laparoscopic/endoscopic approach. It is surgically easier to operate and close a gastrotomy in normal gastric tissue than near an eroded band. In the case of acute gastric perforation, laparotomy with wide drainage is necessary.

Port-Site Infection – Port-site infections can be classified as early and late. Early infections will manifest with the cardinal signs of erythema, swelling, and pain. These infections typically occur in the immediate postoperative period. These infections with cellulitis alone may be treated with oral antibiotics. If the response is inadequate, then intravenous antibiotic use is warranted. When the infection does not respond to intravenous antibiotics and is limited to the port, the port can be removed and the tubing knotted and left inside the abdomen. A new port may be placed when all signs of infection are gone. The tubing can be connected with laparoscopic guidance.

Late port-site infections are often caused by band erosion with ascending infection. This usually manifests several months after surgery and can be associated with loss of restriction. Gastroscopy must be done to confirm the diagnosis of band erosion. In each case of erosion, removal of the band is necessary.

Tube Breakage – Breakage or damage of the tube typically refers to leakage of the tubing leading into the port or a place where there is a metal connector. To prevent leakage from the port, the use of a standard coring needle is strongly discouraged, and only Huber (noncoring) needles should be used to access the port. If port access is difficult or if the tubing connected to the port is at risk of perforation, then band adjustment under fluoroscopy is advised. Tube breakage usually manifests as a slow leak with the loss of the injected fluid volume on aspiration and the absence of restriction. It can be difficult to identify the leak site but local exploration of the port site can confirm the diagnosis.

Leakage from the intra-abdominal tubing is more difficult to diagnose. Injection of dilute nonionic iodinated contrast into the port under fluoroscopy can help to identify the site of the leak. Another approach is to inject diluted methylene blue into the port under direct laparoscopic visualization of the tubing and the band. Port, tubing, or band replacement is usually necessary depending on the site of the leakage and type of band used.

Laparoscopic Sleeve Gastrectomy (LSG)

Sleeve gastrectomy is a surgical weight loss procedure in which the stomach is reduced to about 25 % of its original size, by surgical removal of a large portion of the stomach, following the major curve. The open edges are then attached together (often with surgical staples) to form a sleeve or tube with a banana shape. The procedure permanently reduces the size of the stomach. The procedure is performed laparoscopically and is not reversible.

Sleeve gastrectomy (also called gastric sleeve) is usually performed on extremely obese patients, with a body mass index of 40 or more, where the risk of performing a gastric bypass or duodenal switch procedure may be too large. A two-stage procedure is performed: the first is a sleeve gastrectomy, and the second is a conversion into a gastric bypass or duodenal switch. Patients usually lose a large quantity of their excess weight after the sleeve gastrectomy procedure alone. If weight loss ceases the second step is performed. For patients that are obese but not extremely obese, sleeve gastrectomy alone is a suitable operation with low risks. The sleeve gastrectomy currently is an acceptable weight loss surgery option for obese patients as a single procedure.

Compared to other bariatric procedures, perioperative risk of LSG appears to be relatively low even in patients considered "high risk." The overall reported mortality rate for LSG is 0.3 %. Complication rates range from 0 to 29 % (average 11.2 %) in literature. Major complications after LSG are staple line leakage 0–5.5 % and internal bleeding 0–14.5 % [12].

Staple Line Leakage – Staple line leakage after LSG typically arises in the first days after surgery. Symptoms are similar as in leakage after RYGB with tachycardia, abdominal pain, leukocytosis, and fever. Diagnosis of a leak is made via contrast (Gastrografin) swallow or abdominal computed tomography (CT) scan (Fig. 10.11). When a drain is present, ingestion of methylene blue (5 mL in 250 mL of water) can provide clear evidence of a leak. Patients can be treated depending on the onset or detection of the leak. This divides the management of leaks as to whether they were early (1–3 days) or late and whether or not sepsis is present.

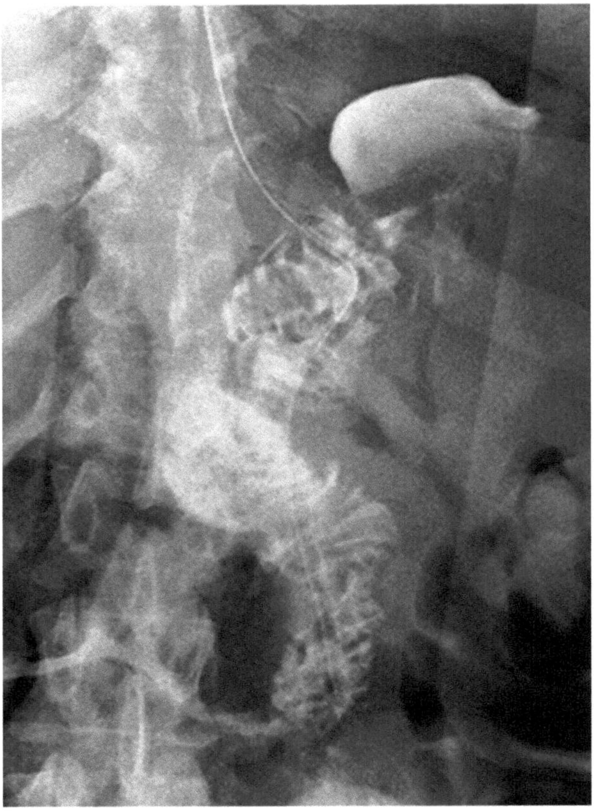

Fig. 10.11 Leakage of gastric sleeve

Early Leak – In a patient with an early leak, the patient should be taken back to the operating room for a laparoscopic or open washout and placement of drains. An attempt can be made to repair the hole in the sleeve through suturing the hole, closure with an omental patch, or insertion of a T tube through the defect [13, 14]. Intravenous antibiotics are administered. Endoscopic insertion of a nasogastric or nasojejunal tube can be considered especially when closing the leak has failed. A feeding jejunostomy is a more patient friendly alternative.

Late Leak – In case of a late leak, an attempt to repair the hole in the sleeve is usually unsuccessful; however, surgical washout of the abdomen and placement of drains are mandatory. The defect in the sleeve can be closed by gastroscopic placement of a covered stent. Care must be taken to use the right stents as they tend to get incorporated in the gastric mucosa. For that reason, stents must be exchanged or removed after 4 weeks. Intravenous antibiotics, nasogastric tube placement, and drainage of abscesses are all essential components of successful treatment.

If a leak is well controlled (drain production < 500 mL/day), conservative treatment can be continued and the drain output monitored over time. Once drain output is less than 30 mL per day, a contrast swallow can be made to demonstrate if leak is closed so that the patient can start with oral intake. If the fistula keeps on producing

>500 mL/day, repositioning of the covered stents may be necessary. If this is impossible or the fistula continues to leak, surgery is the best option.

If the leak is distal, the LSG can be converted to a gastric bypass (GB), while the distal part of the stomach with the leak is resected. If the leak is proximal and a part of the fundus left in place, a small resection and conversion to a GB is an option. If not enough fundus is left in place, the fistula can be covered with small bowel by a Roux-Y construction, or a Roux-Y reconstruction can be performed on the esophagus.

Enterocutaneous Fistula – After leakage subphrenic abscess formation is a regularly seen complication. Fistulas in the left upper abdominal quadrant or left thoracic wall sometimes arise spontaneously or after percutaneous drainage of an abscess. In essence, the treatment of fistulas is the same as in GI surgery. The general principles of management of enterocutaneous fistulae are control of sepsis, attention to nutrition, definition of the anatomy, protection of the skin around the drain, and planning for definitive management.

A CT scan of the abdomen with oral contrast is helpful to identify any undrained collections. Contrast swallow during the follow-up to monitor the progress of the fistula is helpful. If the leak is difficult to diagnose, a radio-opaque contrast injected into the drain as a tubogram can be made to see if any contrast will enter the gastrointestinal tract.

Internal Bleeding – Internal bleeding after LSG is in almost all cases in the first days after operation. If the patient is pale, has abdominal discomfort, and tachycardia, hemorrhage must be suspected. In the majority of cases, conservative management suffices; however, when an active bleeding is evident or hemodynamic instability, emergency surgery is needed. Most of the times, the bleeding is on the gastric staple line and is easily controlled by clips.

Gastroesophageal Dysmotility and Reflux – The number of patients that has postoperative gastroesophageal dysmotility and reflux and needed a specific treatment besides regular proton pump inhibitors (PPIs) was reported in one cohort study as 1.1 %. A combination of a dilated upper part of the sleeve with a relative narrowing of the midstomach, without complete obstruction, is common in most patients with a severe gastroesophageal dysmotility and reflux. The sleeve volume, the bougie size, and the starting point of the antral resection do not seem to have an effect in this complication. Operatively converting the gastric sleeve to a gastric bypass often dramatically improves motility.

Vertical Banded Gastroplasty (VBG)

The VBG was used for the first time in 1980 by Edward Mason (Fig. 10.12). It is a true restrictive procedure that entails the creation of a small gastric pouch with staples. The pouch stoma is controlled by a small Marlex band. The VBG has been a very popular bariatric procedure for years, because it provided good weight loss. However, the procedure is mostly abandoned because of a relatively high incidence of complications in the long term.

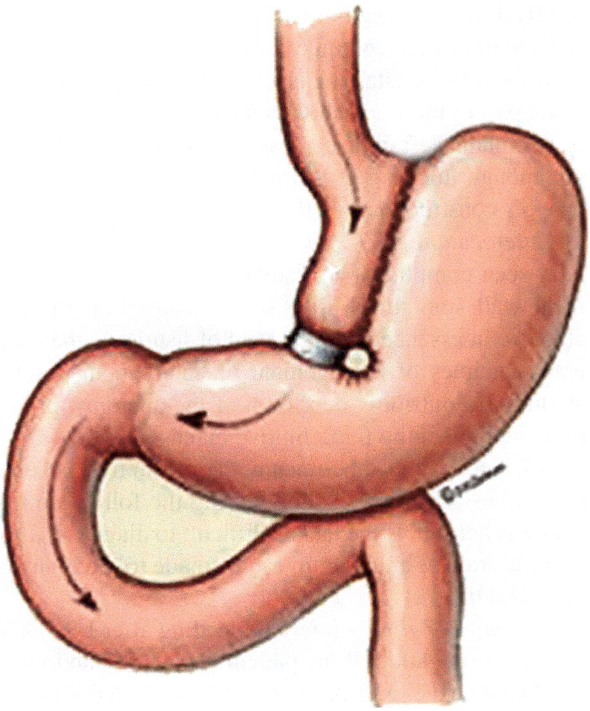

Fig. 10.12 Vertical banded gastroplasty

Staple line disruption and weight regain is reported in 30 % of patients. Staple line disruption enables the patient to increase their intake. On the other hand, obstruction, stenosis, or even erosion of the band leads to vomiting, pouch dilatation, reflux, extreme weight loss, and malnutrition. Although revisional surgery with ligation of the band is technically possible, this leads to significant weight regain in almost all cases.

Many failed VBGs are nowadays converted to other bariatric procedures among which RY gastric bypass and BPD are the most popular. Conversion after open VBG in the past to another bariatric procedure can be performed laparoscopically. However, due to dense scarring tissue especially around the band and adherence to the liver can make this a very challenging procedure.

Duodenal Switch (DS) and Biliopancreatic Diversion (BPD)

DS and BPD are bariatric procedures that have in common that they bypass a large portion of the small intestine, thus creating a true malabsorption. The common channel in DS and BPD ranges from 60 to 100 cm. Although both procedures give superior weight loss, even better than RYGB, they are not widespread because they are technically difficult and are associated with higher morbidity and mortality than other bariatric procedures. Perioperative complications are comparable to RYGB. However, the most important complications after DS and BPD are the nutritional deficits on the longer run.

Recognition of Complications and Timing of Surgery

Complications in morbidly obese patients happen regularly even in high-volume centers. However, they are very difficult to diagnose even for experienced physicians. For that reason every unusual event and every deviant postoperative course must raise a serious suspicion of a complication. Usually bariatric patients follow a fast-track postoperative course enabling them to be discharged after 2 or 3 days. In case of prolonged reconvalescence in a patient, a complication can be imminent. Several studies have demonstrated that overall morbidity and mortality in a bariatric center is influenced by both the experience of the surgeon and the experience of the hospital, in particular the nursing staff on the bariatric ward. Therefore, any change in the patient's vital signs, mental status, pain level, or location should prompt the nursing staff to alert the surgeon. Although diagnostic examinations can be helpful when a complication is suspected, they can easily lead to false-negative findings and a wrongly expectant attitude. Literature demonstrates that it often takes 2 to 3 days after initiation of symptoms to adequately treat a leakage of the gastrointestinal anastomosis. Probably the wisest approach to a suspected complication is early reoperation without delay. In that way deterioration, sepsis, and death can often be avoided. The method of reintervention depends on the complication present, the patient's condition, and the experience of the surgeon. For some complications, it suffices to perform percutaneous drainage or gastroscopic treatment, whereas other complications require immediate reoperation. Laparoscopic management of complications is often possible, especially when the primary procedure was also performed minimally invasive. However, paralytic ileus, severe peritonitis, and deep sepsis are relative contraindications for laparoscopy and may need open explorative laparotomy.

References

1. American Society for Metabolic and Bariatric Surgery. Fact sheet: metabolic & bariatric surgery; 2009. Available online at: www.asbs.org/Newsite07/media/asbspresskit.htm.
2. Kremen AJ, LInner LH, Nelson CH. An experimental evaluation of the nutritional importance of proximal and distal small intestine. Ann Surg. 1954;140:439–44.
3. Tordjman J, Guerre-Millo M, Clément K. Adipose tissue inflammation and liver pathology in human obesity. Diabetes Metab. 2008;34(6 Pt 2):658–63.
4. Jones D, Adair JD, Prachand VN, Friedman LS, Lipman TO, Pories S. Complications of bariatric surgery. Available online at: http://www.uptodate.com/contents/complications-of-bariatric-surgery.

5. Arterburn D, Livingston EH, Schifftner T, Kahwati LC, Henderson WG, Maciejewski ML. Predictors of long-term mortality after bariatric surgery performed in Veterans Affairs medical centers. Arch Surg. 2009;144(10):914–20.
6. Smith MD, Patterson E, Wahed AS, Belle SH, Bessler M, Courcoulas AP, Flum D, Halpin V, Mitchell JE, Pomp A, Pories WJ, Wolfe B. Relationship between surgeon volume and adverse outcomes after Roux-en-Y gastric bypass in Longitudinal Assessment of Bariatric Surgery (LABS) study. Surg Obes Relat Dis. 2010;6(4):463.
7. DeMaria EJ, Murr M, Byrne TK, Blackstone R, Grant JP, Budak A, Wolfe L. Validation of the obesity surgery mortality risk score in a multicenter study proves it stratifies mortality risk in patients undergoing gastric bypass for morbid obesity. Ann Surg. 2003;246(4):578–82.
8. Hamilton EC, Sims TL, Hamilton TT, Mullican MA, Jones DB, Provost DA. Clinical predictors of leak after laparoscopic Roux-en-Y gastric bypass for morbid obesity. Surg Endosc. 2003;17(5):679–84.
9. Eid I, Birch DW, Sharma AM, Sherman V, Karmali S. Complications associated with adjustable gastric banding for morbid obesity: a surgeon's guides. Can J Surg. 2011;54(1):61–6.
10. O'Brien PE, Dixon JB. Weight loss and early and late complications—the international experience. Am J Surg. 2002;184(6B):42S–5.
11. Abu-Abeid S, Szold A. Laparoscopic management of Lap-Band erosion. Obes Surg. 2001; 11:87–9.
12. Shi X, Karmali S, Sharma AM, Birch DW. A review of laparoscopic sleeve gastrectomy for morbid obesity. Obes Surg. 2010;20:1171–7.
13. Tan JT, Kayawasam S, Wijeratne T, Chandratna HS. Diagnosis and management of gastric leaks after sleeve gastrectomy for morbid obesity. Obes Surg. 2010;20:403–9.
14. Court I, Wilson A, Benotti P, Szomstein S, Rosenthal RJ. T-tube gastrostomy as a novel approach for distal staple line disruption after sleeve gastrectomy for morbid obesity: case report and review of the literature. Surgery. 2009;145(1):106–13.

Chapter 11
Prevention and Treatment of Major Complications After Liver Surgery (and Liver Transplantation)

Pascual Parrilla Paricio, Ricardo Robles Campos, and Francisco Sánchez Bueno

Keywords Liver surgery • Intraoperative/postoperative bleeding • Air embolism • Postoperative liver failure • Biliary complications • Liver transplantation

Liver Resection

In recent decades we have witnessed a significant reduction in morbidity and mortality after liver resection (LR) (less than 30 % morbidity and less than 5 % mortality) [1–6], which is related to several factors: better selection and preparation of patients for surgery; better knowledge of hepatic surgical anatomy; possibility of calculating, prior to surgery, the minimum liver remnant volume for maintaining liver function; better instruments for parenchyma transection aimed at reducing blood loss; and lastly liver transplantation, which has developed alongside liver surgery and facilitated the training of surgeons (Tables 11.1 and 11.2).

We shall analyze the most frequent and serious surgical complications.

Intraoperative and/or Postoperative Bleeding

This complication leads to a polytransfusion, which has been related to higher morbidity and mortality rates and may require prolonged hilar clamping and cause liver failure due to hepatic ischemia.

P.P. Paricio • R.R. Campos • F.S. Bueno, MD (✉)
Department of Surgery and Liver Transplantation Unit,
Virgen de la Arrixaca University Hospital,
Murcia, Spain
e-mail: sbuenof@um.es

M.A. Cuesta, H.J. Bonjer (eds.), *Treatment of Postoperative Complications after Digestive Surgery*, DOI 10.1007/978-1-4471-4354-3_11,

Table 11.1 Indications, surgical technique, and morbidity in our liver resection series ($n = 850$)

Parameters	No. of cases	%
Indications		
Benign lesions: hemangioma (25), FNH (9), IHL (7), others (20)	70	8.2
Colorectal liver metastases	562	66.2
Non-colorectal liver metastases	53	6.2
Malignant primary tumors: HCC (72), others non-CC (6)	78	9.2
Bile duct tumors: Klatskin (32), peripheral CC (26), gallbladder carcinoma (29)	87	10.2
Surgical technique[a]		
Extreme liver surgery (two IVC grafts and five left renal vein grafts)	7	0.8
Right trisectionectomy	24	2.8
Right hepatectomy	151	17.8
Left hepatectomy	100	11.8
Lateral sectionectomy	49	5.8
Segmentary and wedge resections	519	61
Central hepatectomy (12), resections of three segments (70), resections of two segments (178), resection of one segment (191), wedge resections (68)		
Morbidity		
Biliary complications	41	5
Infected waste collections	83	10
Postoperative bleeding	4	0.5
Postoperative liver failure	12	1.4
Mortality		
Total	13	1.52
Related to biliary complications	4	
Related to infected waste collections – sepsis	1	
Related to hemorrhage	3	
Related to other complications (no deaths due to postoperative liver failure)	5	

FNH focal nodular hyperplasia, *IHL* intrahepatic lithiasis, *IVC* inferior vena cava, *HCC* hepatocellular carcinoma, *CC* cholangiocarcinoma

[a]121 liver resections were performed by laparoscopic approach

Origin of Bleeding

Bleeding may be located at the portal pedicle, inferior vena cava (IVC), or surface of the parenchymal transection. Portal pedicle bleeding usually occurs during intra- or extraglissonian transection. Injury may also occur to the middle hepatic vein during the left extraglissonian approach. Bleeding of the IVC or hepatic veins (HVs) may cause bleeding and/or air embolism, the origin of which is the IVC itself, the caudate collaterals or an inferior right hepatic vein. Bleeding of a parenchymal origin may come from the hilar vessels or hepatic veins. This complication is more frequent in the case of anatomical anomalies such as portal trifurcation or when there are hepatic drainage branches from the right segments to the middle HV.

Favoring Factors

(1) Extended liver resections, especially when it is necessary to occlude the IVC or use a venovenous bypass or vascular grafts [7]; (2) atypical resections

Table 11.2 Indications, surgical technique, and morbidity in our liver transplant series ($n=884$)

Parameters	No. of cases	%
Indications		
1. Hepatocellular cirrhosis	473	53.5
2. Hepatocellular carcinoma with cirrhosis	126	14.2
3. Acute hepatic failure	49	5.5
4. Cholestatic diseases	47	5.3
5. Metabolic diseases	43	4.9
6. Retransplant	102	11.5
7. Others	44	5.1
Surgical technique		
1. Classic technique	156	17.6
2. Cava vein preservation (piggyback technique)	728	82.4
Morbidity		
1. Postoperative abdominal hemorrhage which requires surgical treatment	32	3.6
2. Arterial complications	18	2
Arterial thrombosis	15	1.7
Arterial stenosis	3	0.3
3. Venous complications	6	0.6
Cava vein and/or suprahepatic vein thrombosis	3	0.3
Portal vein thrombosis	2	0.2
Stenosis portal vein	1	0.1
4. Biliary complications	108	12.2
Early biliary leak	43	4.9
Biliary peritonitis after removal of Kehr tube which requires surgical treatment	31	3.5
Biliary stenosis	25	2.8
Biliary necrosis	9	1

(not following fissure planes); (3) resection of large tumors or tumors invading vascular pedicles; (4) *hepatic cirrhosis*, in which bleeding is favored by the hardness of the liver, previous coagulopathy, and portal hypertension; (5) patients receiving *chemotherapy* [8] prior to surgery, as they develop a fatty liver and considerable fibrosis, which means there is a greater risk of bleeding; (6) patients with *extrahepatic cholestasis*, as they have an impaired intestinal absorption of vitamin K and decreased prothrombin in peripheral blood [6, 9]; and (7) diseases with *hematological alterations* (Kasabach-Merritt syndrome in the case of hemangiomas).

Prevention

(1) We must preoperatively correct any hematological alterations with platelets, cryoprecipitates, fresh plasma, and parenteral vitamin K. (2) Patients with extrahepatic cholestasis will have improved liver functionality with percutaneous drainage of the liver lobe to be preserved. (3) To reduce intraoperative bleeding a central venous pressure of less than 5 mmHg must be maintained (in laparoscopic LR, due to the risk of air embolism, it is debated whether central venous pressure should be decreased or not). (4) Large-bore peripheral lines are necessary, together with a system of rapid fluid infusion and the venovenous bypass, in the event that it is

necessary to perform total vascular occlusion. (5) The surgical technique must be careful and follow the anatomical fissures under ultrasonographic guidance. Prior to parenchymal transection a vascular control – either total or selective (intra- or extra-glissonian) – should be made of the elements of the hepatic hilum depending on the surgical technique to be performed and the surgeon's experience. (6) In extreme liver surgery [7, 10] or major hepatectomies, besides controlling the hilum it is also advisable to control the infrahepatic IVC and suprahepatic IVC for possible total vascular occlusion; even the piggyback technique can be performed to completely dissect the IVC and thus avoid occlusion. (7) To reduce bleeding during parenchymal transection, numerous cutting and coagulation instruments have been designed, of which the most commonly used are the ultrasonic dissector, argon scalpel, hydrojet, harmonic scalpel, LigaSure, TissueLink, and bipolar forceps. These methods must be associated with ligations and sutures of the vascular and biliary elements, although finger fracture and kellyclasia are still very useful techniques. Recently a large series of LRs was published in which parenchymal transection was performed with vascular endostapler [11]. A number of hemostatic substances have also been developed for application to the surface of the liver to reduce bleeding, although results are contradictory regarding their use [12].

Treatment

Hilar bleeding is easy to control, as at the very start of the operation, a loop is passed round the pedicle and simple traction performs hemostasis. It is also useful to insert the index finger of the left hand through the Winslow hiatus to compress the hilum between two fingers and suture the lesion. IVC tears can be controlled by applying pressure with the fingers of the left hand inserted behind it and suturing the point of bleeding once the hemostasis has been identified. If the bleeding cannot be controlled, vascular occlusion of the IVC is performed and the injury repaired. HV tears are controlled with the hanging maneuver, with a loop passed initially between the right HV and middle HV, which surrounds the liver behind and in front of the dissected IVC. If it is not controlled with traction, manual compression is applied or vascular occlusion of the IVC. Parenchymal bleeding is controlled well with manual compression and suture of the injured vessels. Bleeding may occur postoperatively, diagnosed by a drop in hematocrit (HCT) or blood escaping through the drains or the existence of a hemoperitoneum. Alterations in coagulation must be corrected, and if the bleeding continues a re-laparotomy is necessary

Air Embolism

This is an uncommon complication that occurs following tears in veins close to the right auricle (IVC and HVs), in which there is negative pressure. Publications exist suggesting that the use of an argon scalpel and ultrasonic dissector might increase airflow into the HVs and favor embolism and also that laparoscopic surgery would increase the risk of air embolism due to the use of CO_2 at a pressure of more than 14 mmHg in the abdominal cavity [13], something which has not yet been demonstrated.

Perioperative Management

If this is detected, the field must be irrigated with physiological saline to prevent more air from entering and the orifice through which the air penetrates compressed, or occlusion should be performed with a vascular clamp and the tear sutured. The anesthetist must aspirate through the central line to try to extract as much air as possible, and the perfusion of fluids must be incremented to increase central venous pressure.

Postoperative Liver Failure

This is the main cause of postoperative mortality. Mild or moderate liver failure appears with mild jaundice, ascites, hypoproteinemia, and hypoalbuminemia. Serious cases are revealed by significant jaundice, hypoglycemia, encephalopathy, coagulopathy with a Quick of less than 30 %, kidney failure, respiratory failure, and even multisystemic failure. In 2011 *an International Study Group of Liver Surgery [*14] classifies LF in three grades: LF with abnormal laboratory parameters, but not requiring changes in the patient's management is grade A; deviation from the regular clinical course but without invasive measures is grade B; and deviation from the regular clinical course requiring invasive treatment is grade C.

Origin and Favoring Factors

(1) Child A *cirrhosis* when performing major LRs (≥3 segments) and Child B and C cirrhosis even if the LR is segmental [15, 16]. (2) *Extensive resections* or *extreme liver surgery* that requires a venovenous bypass or prolonged vascular occlusion in healthy livers, but especially if there is severe steatosis, cholestasis, or the patients have received neoadjuvant chemotherapy [7, 8]. (3) *Intra- and postoperative bleeding* which conditions hypotension and a secondary hepatic ischemia. (4) Very prolonged complete *hilar clamping* [17].

Prophylaxis

With hepatic cirrhosis there is no test to accurately predict the risk of LF. The Child-Pugh classification is the most commonly used functional test, with indocyanine green clearance used in oriental countries. In order to prevent LF, the Hospital Clínic in Barcelona [18] selects cirrhotic patients for liver resection who are Child A and have a portal pressure of less than 10 mmHg (measured by suprahepatic vein catheterization) and a TB of less than 1. In healthy livers it is important to perform a preoperative liver volumetry when a major LR is to be done, and if the remnant volume is insufficient (less than 25 % or less than 35 % if the patient has received chemotherapy or there is cholestasis or a fatty liver), a preoperative portal vein embolization is recommended or a two-stage resection combined with portal occlusion techniques [5, 19]. In the case of patients with cholestasis, oriental authors recommend percutaneous drainage of the lobe to be preserved, accompanied by portal vein embolization of the pathological lobe. This enables extended liver resections to be performed [20].

During the operation, we must avoid serious episodes of bleeding that condition hepatic ischemia; occlusion of the hepatic hilum must be for as short a time as possible and done intermittently; some authors recommend ischemic preconditioning and occlude the hilum for 10 min, which appears to adapt the hepatic cell to the ischemia and stimulate liver regeneration [21].

Treatment

This includes correction of the alterations in coagulation and metabolic acidosis, administration of liver-protecting parenteral nutrition to correct hypoproteinemia and hypoalbuminemia, and antibiotic treatment to prevent infectious complications that aggravate LF.

Biliary Complications

These are the most common and potentially serious complications and can appear postoperatively as fistulas and/or bile collections, as a diffuse bile peritonitis, or as a sepsis due to the existence of segments with poor bile drainage.

Biliary fistulas were recently classified in three grades [22]: grade A biliary fistula has little or no clinical impact on the patient, the fistula is controlled by drainage, the drainage volume decreases daily, and bile drainage lasts less than 1 week. Grade B biliary fistula causes a change in the patient's clinical situation and treatment, requiring additional radiological or endoscopic approaches, the hospital stay is lengthened, or it is a grade A fistula with more than 1-week hospital stay. Grade C biliary fistula requires laparotomy for treatment, and occasionally a clinical situation of sepsis or multisystemic failure occurs. Hospital stay is very prolonged and patients may have secondary complications (e.g., wall abscesses).

Favoring Factors

(1) Anatomical anomalies of the biliary tree, especially intrahepatically; (2) reresections in which a right hemihepatectomy was performed, as the liver is rotated and the hepatic hilum blocked; (3) presence of an HJ; (4) existence of poorly vascularized liver segments or bile duct; and (5) presence of biliary metallic prostheses.

Prevention

Prevention is implemented by performing a systematic intraoperative cholangiography (IOC) in the case of hemihepatectomies or extended LRs. When a hepatectomy is finished, the bile duct must also be explored by IOC or by injecting serum through the cystic duct to identify minor biliary leaks on the liver surface. Segments which have become ischemic during the liver resection should be excised.

Treatment

Injury to a principal hepatic duct must be treated with an HJ reconstruction. If a segment is left poorly drained, it must be excised to avoid secondary infectious complications, or the biliary radicle sutured if it is of little importance.

If it appears as a biliary fistula through the drain, which does not close conservatively, we must identify the origin by performing a cholangiography through the drain or an ERCP, which allows a papillotomy to be performed, and also insert a nasobiliary drain or an endoscopic plastic prosthesis. If endoscopic treatment fails, the next step is surgical treatment. If it appears as an infected perihepatic collection, detected by CT, a radiological drain must be inserted, and if a high volume of drainage is maintained, it should be treated as a biliary fistula.

Infected Collections

Favoring factors include liver resections with biliodigestive anastomoses, patients with previous chemotherapy, the application of intraoperative radiofrequency, and immunodepressed patients.

Perioperative Management

In the presence of fever, leukocytosis, increased CRP, and procalcitonin, we must indicate an emergency abdominal CT. If there are clinical data of sepsis or air inside the collection, the collection must be drained radiologically as an emergency procedure. On rare occasions these collections are not resolved with radiological treatment, and surgical treatment is necessary. In selected cases with less than 38 °C fever, no leukocytosis, and no hemodynamic repercussion, antibiotic treatment can be started under clinical, analytical, and serial CT guidance.

Liver Transplantation

Liver transplantation (LT) is an extremely complex technique associated with a high rate of surgical complications, notably – due to their frequency and prognostic impact – postoperative bleeding and vascular and biliary complications [23].

Postoperative Bleeding

The significance of postoperative bleeding is related to its frequency (0–10 %), severity (mortality 0–3 %), and to the fact that it conditions a shorter graft survival and longer hospital stay [1–6].

Predisposing Factors

1. *Recipient-Related [*24, 25]. Patients with severe hepatopathy present with severe coagulopathy prior to LT, which may condition a greater risk of postoperative bleeding, although this has not been corroborated by all authors. Portal hypertension increases the risk of bleeding due to the increase in number, size, and pressure of the venous capillaries and to thrombopenia secondary to hypersplenism. When previous abdominal surgery is also associated, the risk of bleeding is greater.

2. *Operation-Related.* A poor dissection that does not take hemostasis into account from the outset of the operation is going to condition an excessive consumption of hemoderivatives, which will aggravate the patient's previous coagulopathy. Moreover, there is an alteration in coagulation during LT, which starts in the hepatectomy phase, increases during the anhepatic phase, and worsens during reperfusion (fibrinolysis occurs in 20–30 % of LTs) [25].

   As far as surgical technique is concerned, for some authors [26] the classical technique involves a greater risk of bleeding than the piggyback procedure, as a wider retroperitoneal dissection is necessary to remove the recipient inferior vena cava. Moreover, the portal vein and IVC require clamping during the classical technique, which means greater hypertension in the splanchnic venous system and IVC territory. Placement of a venovenous bypass prevents this venous hypertension, but small doses of heparin added to the circuit may aggravate the coagulopathy.
3. *Organ Donation-Related.* The lack of donors has led to the need to use "suboptimal" livers. Suboptimal livers imply a greater incidence of primary graft dysfunction, which is associated with a higher risk of bleeding due to alterations in coagulation. Reduced transplants have a variable-sized cutting surface, which may be a focus of bleeding after revascularization.

Etiology

During the operation bleeding may start during the hepatectomy phase, generally related to technical difficulties. In these cases, once the liver has been removed, bleeding usually stops with careful hemostasis. *If the bleeding persists or starts during reperfusion,* it may be secondary to the existence of a severe fibrinolysis which would cause a diffuse hemorrhage [24, 25, 27].

If the bleeding starts in the immediate postoperative period and there is *good graft function*, the origin is usually the retroperitoneal surface freed during the hepatectomy, the vascular anastomoses, or the donor liver (lacerations, vesicular bed, non-ligated small vein branches, etc.). When there is *graft dysfunction*, coagulation alters seriously, with an increase in bleeding, which would further aggravate graft function due to hypoperfusion and associate a diffuse hemorrhage that would be difficult to cohibit.

Diagnosis

Here we should distinguish two situations:

1. *When the drains function correctly,* diagnosis is based on an increase in hemorrhagic drainage, which will be accompanied by hemodynamic instability, oliguria or anuria, and a decrease in hematocrit (HCT). If the drained blood is hot and red, it indicates the bleeding is recent; if there are doubts as to the characteristics of the bleeding, it would be useful to perform an HCT of the drained fluid, which might differentiate hemorrhage from bloodstained ascites.
2. *When the drains do not function*, diagnosis might be based on hemodynamic instability, transfusion needs, diuresis, and a decrease in HCT. It is also useful to measure the abdominal perimeter at the umbilical level as the patient will present with hemoperitoneum and a secondary abdominal distension. It is very useful in this situation to perform ultrasound and CT. Ultrasound is more feasible when the patient is unstable, as it can be performed at the patient's bedside.

Prevention

Preoperative correction of alterations in coagulation has not proved effective for reducing intraoperative bleeding. During the operation, we must monitor the factors involved in coagulation (Quick, APTT, platelets, PDF, etc.), and some authors also recommend performing a thromboelastogram [27]. Any alteration must be corrected using the corresponding substances such as coagulation factors, platelets, and antifibrinolytics. These alterations are usually corrected 1 or 2 h after reperfusion, while the surgeon is preparing the arterial and biliary anastomosis.

A correct surgical technique with special attention to hemostasis is fundamental. The hemorrhage from the retroperitoneum is better controlled by transfixion suture of the points of bleeding [26]. When the classical technique is performed, some authors report that the use of a venovenous bypass or an early portacaval shunt (internal bypass) may reduce blood loss during the hepatectomy by decreasing portal hypertension [39]. The piggyback technique is associated with a lower percentage of postoperative bleeding because it avoids removing the IVC and coming into conflict with the right suprarenal gland, as occurs with the classical technique. When a reduced transplant is used, a bleeding cutting surface must be coagulated.

Treatment

When bleeding causes hemodynamic instability, the patient must undergo reoperation as early as possible to prevent prolonged hypotension from causing irreversible damage to the graft. All the blood in the lower abdomen and all perihepatic clots must be eliminated. On some occasions, the bleeding is diffuse and the point of bleeding cannot be identified, which is usually associated with a primary or secondary graft dysfunction; on other occasions, the bleeding comes from a specific point (retroperitoneum, arterial anastomosis, donor liver, etc.) and is resolved. The vascular pedicles must be explored during the operation in order to rule out any complications that might cause a graft dysfunction and aggravate the bleeding.

Vascular Complications

They are common in the immediate postoperative period (first month) and carry high morbidity and mortality rates if diagnosed late.

Arterial Complications

The incidence of arterial complications (ACs) in most series [28–32] ranges from 7to 10 %, with thrombosis being the most frequent, especially in pediatric recipients

Etiology

In the early forms (first postoperative month) the most common causes are technical problems arising from differences in size and the poor quality of the vessels to be anastomosed, as well as the presence of arterial anomalies that require complex

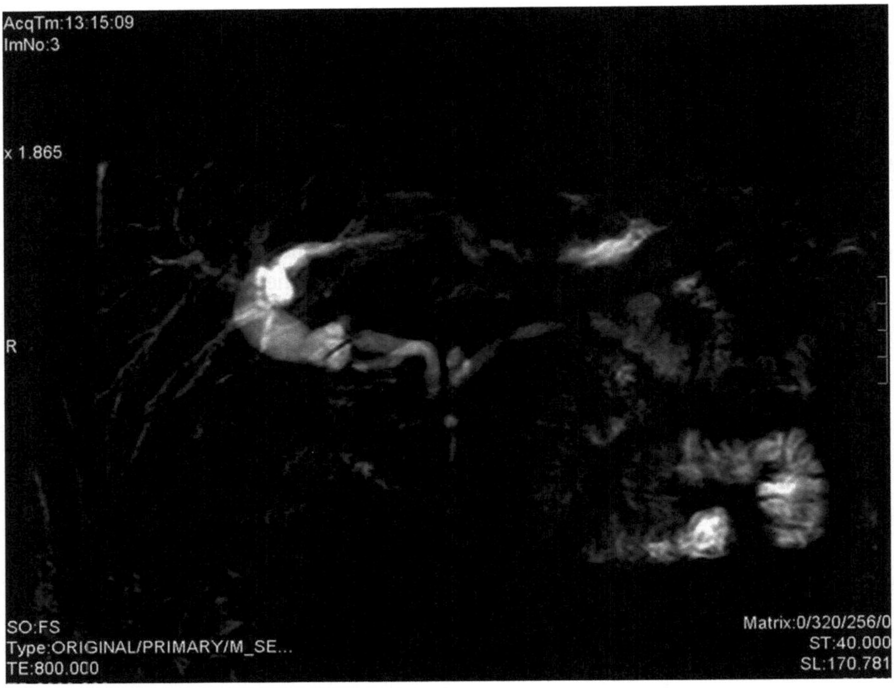

Fig. 11.1 Early thrombosis hepatic artery aortography showing the coeliac trunk, hepatic artery, and one centimeter from the gastroduodenal artery, at the level of the anastomosis, a thrombosis of the hepatic artery without arterial flow in the liver

arterial reconstructions in bench surgery or during the surgical intervention. Etiology in the late forms (after the first month) is more controversial and related to immunological factors (anticardiolipin antibodies), ABO incompatibility, cytomegalovirus infections, protein C deficiency, presence of multiple episodes of acute rejection, chronic graft rejection, etc.

Clinical Features

There is a close relation to the early or late appearance of thrombosis (Fig. 11.1) and to the fact that the bile duct is only irrigated by the hepatic artery. In the early forms there is usually a sharp, steady deterioration in liver function, especially in the coagulation parameters after normal graft functioning. This fulminant liver failure leads to patient death if an emergency retransplant is not performed. Conversely, the late forms have a predominance of biliary manifestations, in the form of a biliary fistula or biloma secondary to necrosis of the extrahepatic biliary tree or a progressive obstructive jaundice due to stenosis and/or cloacae of the intrahepatic biliary tree. Occasionally, even, there are no biliary manifestations, but only recurrent septic episodes that cause fever symptoms of an unknown origin or multiple liver abscesses. Lastly, asymptomatic forms have been described, without graft dysfunction, which have been detected on routine angiographic exploration. When we suspect an AC, we must perform an echo Doppler of the hepatic artery and if in doubt an arteriography of the coeliac trunk.

Treatment

The ideal procedure for early thrombosis is retransplantation, although good outcomes have been achieved with an early thrombectomy, which avoids retransplantation, if the liver damage is not irreversible [29–31].

If there is an arterial stenosis, the best treatment is retransplantation, although on occasions a percutaneous transluminal angioplasty using high-pressure inflatable balloon catheters may be effective [33]. The aim of these intraluminal maneuvers is to tear the fibrosis responsible for the stenosis, which means it is contraindicated during the first 2 weeks postoperatively. Other authors [34] advocate the placement of metallic prostheses in the stenosed area.

Prevention

The best prevention is a very meticulous surgical technique, and it is therefore fundamental to perform the anastomosis with a patch on the two artery ends. In our experience of 900 liver transplants, 85 % of the cases received an anastomosis between the donor coeliac trunk and the bifurcation of the recipient common hepatic artery and gastroduodenal artery. Some authors [33, 35] recommend the systematic measurement of arterial flow after reconstruction, but we agree with those who do not perform. If there are arterial anomalies that require complex reconstructions, it is preferable to perform arterial anastomosis, if possible, at the coeliac trunk, splenic artery, or supracoeliac aorta. Lastly, in high-risk patients (complex reconstructions, pediatric transplants, etc.) a thrombosis prophylaxis with administration of dextran and platelet antiaggregants (dipyridamole, aspirin, etc.) is recommended in the immediate postoperative period. In our experience only 1.6 % of our patients had an arterial thrombosis.

Venous Complications

Venous complications are infrequent and encountered in the portal vein and inferior vena cava. In most cases they are related to technical errors committed during the surgical operation; predisposing factors include the presence of previous portal vein thrombosis and the Budd-Chiari syndrome, which favor venous thrombosis, or anatomical anomalies in the venous structures of the donor and/or recipient (preduodenal portal vein, vena cava agenesis, etc.) [28].

Vena Cava Thrombosis

This occurs in 1–2 % of cases and is generally associated with a stenosis of the anastomosis.

Etiology

Technical errors are the main cause of vena cava thrombosis (VCT); one predisposing factor is the disproportion between the size of the graft and the recipient hepatic fossa. When the graft is bigger than the hepatic fossa, the suprahepatic anastomosis may be narrow, which leads to a slower blood flow and, secondarily, a VCT.

A reduced graft (segmental transplant) or small-sized graft and a large hepatic fossa can lead to torsion of the graft and, secondarily, a venous thrombosis, as may also occur in venous reconstruction following the piggyback technique, when there is poor orientation between the graft and the recipient suprahepatic veins.

Clinically it may appear as a Budd-Chiari syndrome or as an occlusive syndrome of the inferior vena cava depending on whether the thrombosis is located suprahepatically, which compromises drainage of the suprahepatic veins, or infrahepatically, which does not affect the hepatic veins. In a series of 1,112 orthotopic liver transplants with conservation of the inferior vena cava [36], a 2.5 % overall rate of intraoperative anastomosis-related complications was reported, particularly congestion of the graft due to malrotation of the suprahepatic veins, and a 1 % rate of early postoperative complications (first week), which began as an acute Budd-Chiari syndrome. These surgical complications are reduced drastically if a patch is used on the three recipient suprahepatic veins to perform anastomosis with the donor suprahepatic vena cava, instead of a patch with two veins (0.59 % vs 5 % for congestion of the graft and 0.28 % vs 1.6 % for acute Budd-Chiari, respectively).

The fundamental *exploratory techniques* to suspect this complication are Doppler ultrasound, angio-CT, and angio-NMR which assess the degree of permeability of the suprahepatic veins and inferior vena cava and the echogenicity of the hepatic parenchyma. Abdominal CT may reveal the degree of hepatic parenchyma destructuring.

Treatment

Therapeutic guidelines depend on the site of the thrombosis, either in the suprahepatic veins or in the infrahepatic cava. If thrombosis of the suprahepatic veins is detected early and there is no severe liver failure, a percutaneous transluminal angioplasty is performed associated with anticoagulant therapy (heparin and dicumarinics). If there are severe hepatic repercussions, the most effective therapeutic procedure is an emergency retransplant. If the thrombosis is in the infrahepatic cava, some authors favor immediate surgical reconstruction, whereas others advocate percutaneous transluminal angioplasty and/or local thrombolytic therapy with urokinase or streptokinase [37]. Patients undergoing transplantation for Budd-Chiari syndrome have demonstrated the usefulness of prophylaxis with anticoagulant treatment in the immediate postoperative period to avoid recurrence of posttransplant thrombosis of the vena cava.

Portal Vein Thrombosis

This occurs in 1–3 % of cases [28, 38].

Etiology

The most frequent causes are technical errors related to venous redundancy and torsion and/or stenosis, with risk factors including the presence of previous surgery on the portal vein or splanchnic axis (portacaval shunt, mesentericocaval shunt, splenorenal shunt, splenectomy, etc.) or a pre-transplant portal vein thrombosis that requires a thrombectomy during the surgical intervention.

Clinical Features

Depending on the time the thrombosis occurs, we can differentiate between early forms (during the first postoperative week) and late forms (after the first week). If the thrombosis is early, there is a predominance of symptoms and signs typical of a severe acute liver failure, with steady clinical deterioration which leads to patient death. With the late form clinical symptoms depend on the degree of existing porta-caval collateral circulation; it is generally not serious, with a predominance of upper gastrointestinal bleeding due to esophagogastric varices and ascites and rarely with severe deterioration of the liver function.

Diagnosis

Diagnosis is established with clinical data and an abdominal Doppler ultrasonography and confirmed by arteriography of the coeliac trunk and superior mesenteric artery. The most common radiological data are absence of portal vein flow and the existence of collateral circulation to the inferior vena cava.

Treatment

In the early forms the treatment of choice is thrombectomy of the splenoportal axis and reconstruction of the portal anastomosis, with or without the use of vein grafts, although some authors have suggested using intraportal thrombolytic therapy. If there is no success, the best is to perform an emergency retransplant if there is severe acute liver failure. As for the late forms, spontaneous resolution has been reported when portal vein recanalization occurs, and in some cases a distal splenorenal shunt has been performed if there are episodes of bleeding due to rupture of esophageal varices.

Biliary Complications

Biliary complications are still the Achilles' heel of liver transplantation due to the high rate of postoperative morbidity they imply [39–43]. Although some groups have an incidence of less than 10 % [4], most authors report figures of 10–34; it is higher in the case of living donor liver transplantation [44], related to the smaller caliber of the bile duct and greater risk of devascularization.

Prevention: Biliary Reconstruction Techniques

Most groups use end-to-end choledochocholedochostomy as the first-choice procedure and Roux-en-Y choledochojejunostomy in cases of sclerosing cholangitis, secondary biliary cirrhosis, retransplantation, or in situations in which there is a clear discordance in caliber between the donor and recipient choledochus. The appearance of complications is related to the diameter of the bile duct, vascularization of the ends, and the technical skill of the surgeon performing the anastomosis.

A controversial point is whether or not to leave a T tube [45]. Although randomized prospective studies are needed to compare the two techniques, the outcomes of the series published suggest that not leaving a T tube reduces fistulas and cholangitis at the expense of increasing the rate of stenosis of the anastomosis [46]. A T tube is probably only recommended when the bile duct is very thin.

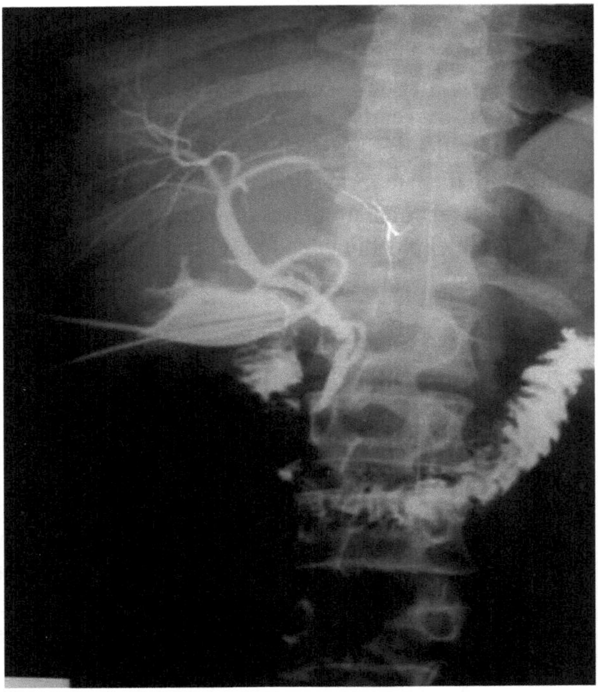

Fig. 11.2 Biliary fistula. Cholangiography through Kehr tube showing a biliary fistula at the level of the common bile duct – common bile duct anastomosis

The choledochocholedochal anastomosis is done in a single layer using absorbable 4 or 5/0 sutures, although some studies show no differences if the suture is continuous [47]. The choledochojejunal anastomosis is also done in a single layer using absorbable 4 or 5/0 sutures, and a multiperforated stent may or may not be left in the anastomosis. In cases in which a stent is left, it must be exteriorized after fixing to the jejunal loop using a Witzel tunnel technique. The T tube is removed between the 12th and 16th weeks and the hepaticojejunostomy stent between the 4th and 8th weeks.

Analysis of Biliary Complications

Early Biliary Fistula with a Permeable Hepatic Artery

In 90 % of cases the bile leak or fistula may originate in three different locations: (a) the biliary anastomosis, (b) the choledochotomy through which the long branch of the T tube is extracted, and (c) a necrosis of the intra- and/or extrahepatic bile duct secondary to a thrombosis of the hepatic artery. Less frequently it comes from the cystic duct or biliary radicles.

The most common scenario is that the bile leak is not very significant, originating at the anastomosis and collecting in the subhepatic space (biloma, Fig. 11.2). The factors that influence its origin most significantly are a defective surgical technique and deficient vascularization of the terminal portion of the choledochus. It is therefore recommended that the donor choledochus be as short as possible.

Clinically bilomas appear as a circumscribed peritonitis located in the upper hemiabdomen. Ultrasound will reveal the existence of a subhepatic collection. If a biliary fistula is suspected, a trans-Kehr cholangiography should be performed to confirm the fistula and locate its origin. Endoscopic retrograde cholangiography is used if a T tube has not been left and transparietohepatic cholangiography if a hepaticojejunostomy has been performed.

Most authors advocate treating any biloma conservatively at first, with drainage under ultrasonographic guidance, and may or may not associate decompression and drainage of the bile duct transparietohepatically with a nasobiliary catheter or an endoscopic papillotomy [48–50]. Surgery is indicated when the fistula persists after several days.

Biliary Peritonitis After T Tube Removal

Liver transplant patients undergo an immunosuppressive treatment with corticosteroids, which inhibit the formation of the fistulous tract between the choledochus and the exterior. As a result, when the T tube is removed 3 or 4 months after transplantation, the appearance of peritoneal reactions is not uncommon, due to a bile leak to the peritoneal cavity through the choledochotomy, such that up to 5–12 % of patients may require surgical treatment. This surgical treatment can be performed via laparoscopy due to the small amount of adhesions these patients have [51]. Lavage of the abdominal cavity and drainage of the subhepatic space is sufficient. It is also possible to implement an early fistula treatment with endoscopic placement of a transpapillary nasobiliary catheter, with or without radiological drainage, which thus avoids surgical treatment.

Stenosis of the Bile Duct

The most frequent cause is stenosis of the choledochocholedochal anastomosis or hepaticojejunostomy [52]. The clinical symptoms are an extrahepatic obstructive jaundice and ultrasound reveals dilatation of the intra- and extrahepatic bile duct above the anastomosis. Cholangioresonance is very useful for diagnostic confirmation. An endoscopic retrograde (Fig. 11.3) or trans-Kehr or transparietohepatic cholangiography can also be done. The latter is especially indicated in cases of hepaticojejunostomy stenosis.

Various authors have reported good results from treating anastomotic stenosis with one or several sessions of dilatations, occasionally associating placement of an endoprosthesis via the transparietohepatic or endoscopic retrograde approach [48, 53]. However, the long-term follow-up of this treatment has shown that more than 50 % of cases restenose within a year [54], which together with the

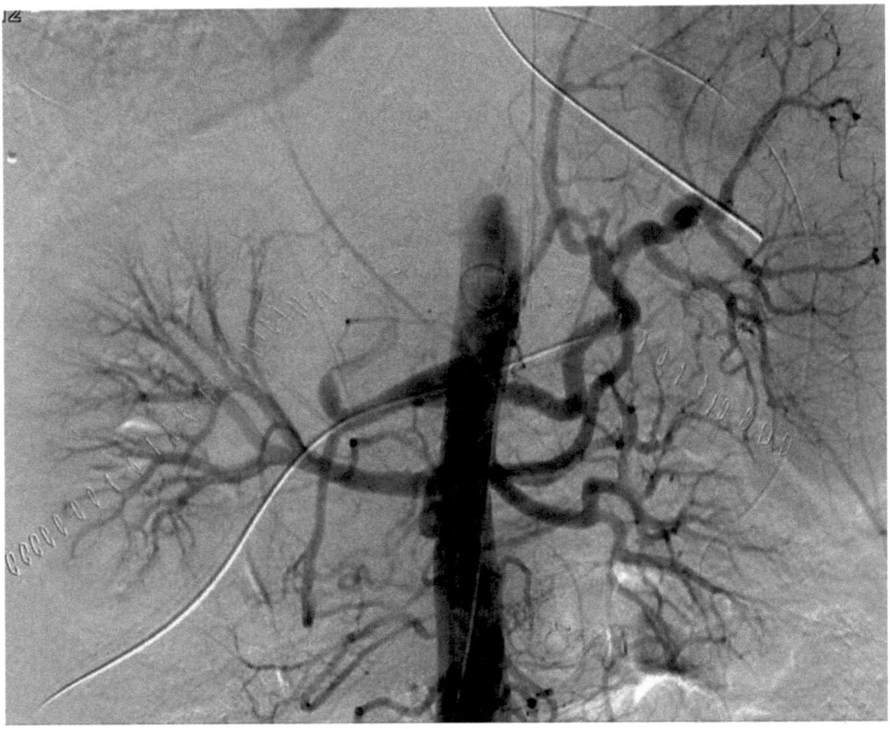

Fig. 11.3 Biliary stenosis at the place of anastomosis. MRCP cholangiography showing stenosis at the level of the biliary anastomosis

complications described for radiological or endoscopic manipulation of the bile duct (hemobilia, hemorrhage, cholangitis, pancreatitis, choledochal perforation, duodenal perforation, biliary fistula, and migration of the endoprosthesis) lead a number of groups to favor surgical treatment for stenosis by means of a hepaticojejunostomy.

Other causes of biliary obstruction include kinks or obstruction of the T tube or hepaticojejunostomy stent, those caused by biliary sludge or biliary lithiasis, and compressions of the bile duct by cystic mucoceles. Finally, when non-anastomotic single or multiple stenoses of the intra- and/or extrahepatic bile duct appear, an ischemic origin should be considered.

Biliary Complications Related to Thrombosis of the Hepatic Artery

Arterial thrombosis may appear clinically as a biliary complication, either as a biliary fistula or as a biliary stenosis. Therefore when a liver transplant patient reveals a postoperative biliary complication, we must always explore the hepatic artery using Doppler ultrasound and/or selective arteriography to rule out an ischemic origin. It is important to note that this type of biliary complication is extremely serious, as it is associated with a marked alteration in graft function and most cases will finally require liver retransplantation.

Biliary fistulas of an ischemic origin are due to a necrosis of the intra- and/or extrahepatic bile duct, leading to the formation of cavities or "cloacae" in the hepatic hilum and/or intrahepatic, which contain bile and which can be seen characteristically on cholangiography.

The gravity of this type of fistula, often associated with serious infections of the biliary cloacae, liver abscesses, and serious alterations in graft function, prompts a liver retransplant as the best therapeutic option, although in some cases with preserved liver function, it is possible to perform a hepaticojejunostomy or cloacojejunostomy associated with an arterial revascularization via thrombectomy or thrombolysis.

Biliary stenosis due to thrombosis of the hepatic artery usually appears between the first and third months after liver transplantation as symptoms of cholestasis, and it is typical to see a cholangiographic pattern with multiple stenosis and segmental dilatations of the intrahepatic biliary tree. Although this complication was initially described as secondary to arterial thrombosis, it occasionally appears without arterial thrombosis, related to a cold ischemia time of more than 12 h, with chronic ductopenic rejection or rejection due to incompatibility of the ABO system, which receives the name "ischemic-type biliary complication." Once Doppler or selective arteriography confirms the ischemic origin of the non-anastomotic stenosis, retransplantation is recommended as the most effective, definitive treatment.

References

1. Jarnagin WR, Gonen M, Fong Y, De Matteo RP, Ben-Porat L. Littles, et al. Improvement in perioperative outcome after hepatic resection. Análisis of 1803 consecutive cases over the past decade. Ann Surg. 2002;236(4):397–407.
2. Fan ST, Lo CM, Liu CL, Lam CM, Yuen NK, Yeung C, et al. Hepatectomy for hepatocellular carcinoma: toward zero hospital deaths. Ann Surg. 1999;229(3):322–30.
3. Bolton JS, Fuhrman GM. Survival after resection of multiple bilobar hepatic metastases from colorectal carcinoma. Ann Surg. 2000;231(5):743–51.
4. Nagasue N, Ono T, Yamanoi A, Kohno H, El-Assal ON, Tamura H, et al. Prognostic factors and survival after hepatic resection for hepatocellular carcinoma without cirrhosis. Br J Surg. 2001;88:515–22.
5. Morales MD, Robles R, Marín C, Capel A, Vázquez V, Reus M, et al. Cálculo del volumen hepático mediante TC espiral: utilidad en la planificación de la resección hepática en pacientes no cirróticos. Cir Esp. 2004;76:152–9.
6. Jarnagin N, Fong Y, De Matteo R, Gonen M, Burke E, Bodniewicz J, et al. Staging, resectability, and outcome in 225 patients with hilar cholangiocarcinoma. Ann Surg. 2001;234:507–19.
7. Azoulay D, Andreani P, Maggi U, Salloum C, Perdigao F, Sebagh M, et al. Combined liver resection and reconstruction of the supra-renal vena cava. The Paul Brousse experience. Ann Surg. 2006;244:80–8.
8. Adam R, Delvart V, Pascal G, Valeanu A, Castaing D, Azoulay D, et al. Rescue surgery for unresectable colorectal liver metastases downstaged by chemotherapy: a model to predict long-term survival. Ann Surg. 2004;240:644–58.

9. Liu CL, Fan ST, Lo CM, Tso WK, Lam CM, Wong J. Improved operative and survival outcomes of surgical treatment for hilar cholangiocarcinoma. Br J Surg. 2006;93:1488–94.
10. Ohwada S, Hamada K, Kawate S, Sunose Y, Tomizawa N, Yamada T, et al. Left renal vein graft for vascular reconstruction in abdominal malignancy. W J Surg. 2007;31(6):1215–20.
11. Kaneko H, Otsuda Y, Takagi S, Tsuchiya M, Tamura A, Shiba T. Hepatic resection using stapling devices. Am J Surg. 2004;187:280–4.
12. Figueras J, Lladó L, Miro M, Ramos E, Torras J, Fabregat J, et al. Application of fibrin glue sealant after hepatectomy does not seem justified: results of a randomized study of 300 patients. Ann Surg. 2007;245:536–42.
13. Ikegami T, Shimada M, Imura S, Nakamura T, Kawahito S, Morine Y, et al. Argon gas embolism in the application of laparoscopic microwave coagulation therapy. J Hepatol Biliary-Pancreatic Surg. 2009;16:394–8.
14. Rahbari NN, Garden OJ, Padbury R, Brooke-Smith M, Crawford M, Adam R, et al. Posthepatectomy liver failure: a definition and grading by the International Study Group of Liver Surgery (ISGLS). Surgery. 2011;149(5):713–24.
15. Tanaka K, Shimada H, Matsumoto C, Matsuo K, Nagano Y, Engo I, et al. Anatomic versus limited nonanatomic resection for solitary hepatocellular carcinoma. Surgery. 2008;143: 607–15.
16. Robles R, Marín C, Parrilla P. Complicaciones de La cirugía hepática. En: Cirugía AEC, manual de La Asociación Española de Cirujanos. Directores P. Parrilla y JI Landa. 2ª edición. Editorial Médica Panamericana; 2010. p. 671–676.
17. Figueras J, Lladó L, Ruiz D, Ramos E, Busquets J, Rafecas A, et al. Complete versus selective portal triad clamping for minor liver resections: a prospective randomized trial. Ann Surg. 2005;241(4):582–90.
18. Llovet JM, Fuster J, Bruix J. Barcelona-Clinic Liver Cancer Group: diagnosis, staging, and treatment of hepatocellular carcinoma. Liver Tranpl. 2004;10 suppl 1:S115–20.
19. Azoulay D, Castaing D, Smail A, Adam R, Cailliez V, Laurent A, et al. Resection of nonresectable liver metastases from colorectal cancer after percutaneous portal vein embolization. Ann Surg. 2000;231:480–6.
20. Baumgart J, Lang S, Lang H. A new method for induction of liver hypertrophy prior to right trisectionectomy: a report of three cases. HPB. 2011;13 suppl 2:72–3.
21. Scatton O, Zalinski S, Jegou D, Compagnon P, Lesurtel M, Belghiti J, et al. Randomized clinical trial of ischaemic preconditioning in major liver resection with intermittent Pringle manoeuvre. Br J Surg. 2011;98(9):1236–43.
22. Koch M, Garden OJ, Padbury R, Rahbari NN, Adam R, Capussotti L, et al. Bile leakage after hepatobiliary and pancreatic surgery: a definition and grading of severity by the International Study Group of Liver Surgery. Surgery. 2011;149(5):680–8.
23. Robles R, Ramírez P, Sánchez-Bueno F, Sansano T, Parrilla P. Hemorragia postoperatoria. En Trasplante Hepático, el postoperatorio inmediato, capítulo 17. Complicaciones quiúrgicas. Berenguer J and Parrilla P. Ed. Elsevier, Barcelona: Autores; 2008.
24. Ramos E, Dalmau A, Sabaté A, et al. Intraoperative red blood cell transfusion in liver transplantation: influence of patient outcome, prediction of requirements and measures to reduce them. Liver Transpl. 2003;9:1320–7.
25. Ickx BE, Van der Linden PJ, Melot C, et al. Comparison of the effects of aprotinin and tranexamic acid on blood loss and red blood cell transfusion requirements during the late stages of liver transplantation. Transfusion. 2006;46:595–605.
26. Tzakis A, Todo S, Starlz TE. Orthotopic liver transplantation with preservation of the inferior vena cava. Ann Surg. 1989;210:649–52.
27. Porte RJ, Molenaar IQ, Begliomini B, et al. Aprotinin and transfusion requirements in orthotopic liver transplantation: a multicentre randomised double-blind study. EMSALT study group. Lancet. 2000;355(9212):1303–9.
28. Sánchez-Bueno F, Robles R, Ramírez P, Parrilla P. Complicaciones vasculares del trasplante hepático. En Trasplante Hepático, el postoperatorio inmediato, capítulo 17. Complicaciones quiúrgicas. Berenguer J and Parrilla P. Ed. Elsevier, Barcelona: Autores; 2008.

29. Sanchez-Bueno F, Robles R, Ramirez P, Acosta F, Rodriguez JM, Lujan J. et al.- Hepatic artery complications after liver transplantation. Clin. Transplantation. 1994;8:399–404.
30. Silva MA, Jambulingam PS, Gunson BK, Mayer D, Buckels JA, Mirza DF. Bramhall SR.- Hepatic artery thrombosis following orthotopic liver transplantation: a 10-year experience from a single centre in the United Kingdom. Liver Transpl. 2006;12:146–51.
31. John P. Duffy, Johnny C Hong, Douglas G Farmer, Rafik M Ghobrial, Hasan Yersiz, Jonathan R Hiatt, Ronald W Busuttil.- Vascular complications of orthotopic liver transplantation: Experience in more than 4,200 patients. J Am Coll Surg. 2009;208:896–905.
32. Jain A, Costa G, Marsh W, Fontes P, Devera M, Mazariegos G. et al.- Thrombotic and non-thrombotic hepatic artery complications in adults and children following primary liver transplantation with long-term follow-up in 1000 consecutive patients. Transpl Int. 2006; 19:27–37.
33. Saad WE, Davies MG, Sahler L, Lee DE, Patel NC, Kitanosono T, et al. Hepatic artery stenosis in liver transplant recipients: primary treatment. With percutaneous transluminal angioplasty. J Vasc Intervent Radiol. 2005;16:795–805.
34. Ueno T, Jones G, Martin A, Ikegami T, Sanchez EQ, Chinnakotla S, et al. Clinical outcomes from hepatic artery stenting in liver transplantation. Liver Transpl. 2006;12:422–7.
35. MA Yi, LI Qiang, YE Zhi-Ming, ZHU Xiao-feng, HE Xiao-shunm. Use of arterial conduit for arterial revascularization during liver and multivisceral transplantation. Chin Med J. 2011;124:2986–2989.
36. Parrilla P, Sánchez-Bueno F, Figueras J, Jaurrieta E, Mir J, Margarit C, et al. Analysis of the complications of the piggy-back technique in 1.112 liver transplants. Transplantation. 1999;67:1214–7.
37. Parrilla P, Sanchez-Bueno F, Ramirez P, et al. Urokinasa locorregional en trombosis de la vena cava inferior. Postrasplante ortotópico de higado. Cir Esp. 1990;48:212–6.
38. Kishi Y, Sugawara Y. Late on set portal vein trombosis and its risk factors. Hepatogastroenterology. 2008;55:1008–9.
39. Ramírez P, Robles R, Sánchez-Bueno F, Parrilla P. Complicaciones biliares del trasplante hepático. En Trasplante Hepático, el postoperatorio inmediato, capítulo 17. Complicaciones quiúrgicas. Berenguer J and Parrilla P. Ed. Elsevier, Barcelona: Autores; 2008.
40. Bismuth H, Cataíng J, Gugenhein J, Traynor O, Ciardullo M. Roux-en-Y hepaticojejunostomy: a safe procedure for biliary anastomosis in liver transplantation. Transpl Proc. 1987;1:2413–5.
41. Starzl TE, Putnam CW, Hansbrough JF, Porter KA, Reid HA. Biliary complications after liver transplantation: with special reference to the biliary cash syndrome and techniques of secondary duct repair. Surgery. 1977;81:212–21.
42. Calne RY, McMaster P, Portman B. Observations on preservation, bile drainage and rejection in 64 human orthotopic liver allografts. Ann Surg. 1977;186:282–90.
43. Ramirez P, Parrilla P, Bueno FS, Robles R, Pons JA, Acosta F. Reoperation for biliary tract complications following orthotopic liver transplantation. Br J Surg. 1993;80:1426–8.
44. Yazumi S, Chiba T. Biliary complication after a right-lobe living donor liver transplant. J Gastroenterol. 2005;40(9):861–5.
45. Riediger C, Muller MW, Michalski CW, Huser N, Schuster T, Kleeff J, Friess H. T-tube or no T-tube in the reconstruction of the biliary tract during orthotopic liver transplantation: systematic review and metaanalysis. Liver Transpl. 2010;16:705–17.
46. Bawa SM, Mathew A, Kríshnan H, Minford E, et al. Biliary reconstruction with or without an internal biliary stent in orthotopic liver transplantation: a prospective randomised trial. Transpl Int. 1998;11(Supp 1):S245–5247.
47. Castaldo ET, Pinson CW, Feurer ID, Wright JK, Gorden DL, Kelly BS, Chari RS. Continuous versus interrupted suture for end-to-end biliary anastomosis during liver transplantation gives equal results. Liver Transpl. 2007;13:234–8.
48. Kuo PC, Lewis WD, Stokes K, Pleskow D, Simpson MA, Jenkins RL. A comparison of operation, endoscopic retrograde cholangiopancreatography and percutaneous transhepatic cholangiography in biliary complications after hepatic transplantation. J Am Coll Surg. 1994; 179:177–81.

49. Ostroff JW, Roberts JP, Gordon RL, Ring EJ, Ascher NL. The management of t tube leaks in orthotopic liver transplant recipients with endoscopically placed nasobiliary catheters. Transplantation. 1990;49(5):922924.
50. Liao JZ, Zhao Q, Qin H, Li RX, Hou W, Li PY, Liu NZ, Li DM. Endoscopic diagnosis and treatment of biliary leak in patients following liver transplantation: a prospective clinical study. Hepatobiliary Pancreat Dis Int. 2007;6:29–33.
51. Robles R, Parrilla P, Luján J, et al. Laparoscopic treatment of biliary peritonitis after T tube removal in patients undergoing orthotopic liver transplantation. Br J Surg. 1997;82:1244.
52. Akamatsu N, Sugawara Y, Hashimoto D. Biliary reconstruction, its complications and management of biliary complications after adult liver transplantation: a systematic review of the incidence, risk factors and outcome. Transplant Int. 2011;24:379–92.
53. Nishida S, Nakamura N, Kadono J, Komokata T, Sakata R, Madariaga JR, Tzakis AG. Intrahepatic biliary strictures after liver transplantation. J Hepatobiliary Pancreat Surg. 2006;13:511–6.
54. Alazmi WM, Fogel EL, Watkins JL, McHenry L, Tector JA, Fridell J, Mosler P, Sherman S, Lehman GA. Recurrence rate of anastomotic biliary strictures in patients who have had previous successful endoscopic therapy for anastomotic narrowing after orthotopic liver transplantation. Endoscopy. 2006;38:571–4.

Chapter 12
Prevention and Treatment of Major Complications After Cholecystectomy

Klaske A.C. Booij, Dirk J. Gouma, Thomas M. van Gulik, and Olivier R.C. Busch

Keywords Cholecystectomy • Laparoscopic cholecystectomy • Vasculo-biliary injury • Peroperatively diagnosed injury • BDI • Quality of life • Litigation claims

Introduction

Annually, over 19.000 patients undergo a cholecystectomy in the Netherlands, of which approximately 16.500 are performed laparoscopically [1]. The complication rate after laparoscopic cholecystectomy (LC) is 2–12 % and the mortality rate about 0.2 % [2, 3]. General complications include wound infection, intra-abdominal abscess formation, and postoperative bleeding from the cystic artery which occurs in about 0.05 % and usually presents within a few hours after surgery [4]. Laparoscopy-induced "access injuries" are visceral and vascular injuries that are mostly related to the puncture technique. Although the incidence of these complications is low, ranging from 0 to 0.05 % for the open technique versus 0.044 to 0.07 % for the closed technique [5], the overall mortality rate is high, ranging from 13 to 21 % [6, 7]. The most specific and devastating complication after cholecystectomy is bile duct injury (BDI). This complication is, especially in combination with vascular injury, accompanied by substantial morbidity, mortality, and a decrease in the life expectancy and long-term quality of life [2, 8, 9]. The incidence reported in literature is dependent on its definition, study design, and study population and ranges from 0.16 to 1.5 % after LC versus 0.0 to 0.9 % after open cholecystectomy (OC) [2, 10]. After the introduction of LC, initially there seemed to be

K.A.C. Booij • D.J. Gouma • T.M. van Gulik • O.R.C. Busch, MD, PhD (✉)
Department of Surgery, Academic Medical Center,
University of Amsterdam, Amsterdam, The Netherlands
e-mail: d.j.gouma@amc.uva.nl; o.r.busch@amc.uva.nl

M.A. Cuesta, H.J. Bonjer (eds.), *Treatment of Postoperative Complications after Digestive Surgery*, DOI 10.1007/978-1-4471-4354-3_12,

an increase in the number of BDI. Go et al. [2] evaluated the incidence of BDI after the introduction of LC in the Netherlands in 1990 until 1992 by using a written questionnaire which was sent to all 138 Dutch surgical institutions and reported an incidence of BDI of 0.86 %. Gouma et al. [11] studied the incidence of BDI in 1991 using a questionnaire to all Dutch surgical departments to analyze the number of surgical reconstructions for BDI and therefore the true incidence of severe BDI and reported an incidence of 1.09 % after LC and 0.51 % BDI after OC. The higher incidence of BDI after LC in those days was mostly related to technical difficulties, unfamiliarity with the procedure, and the "learning curve" effect. A Cochrane systematic review from Keus et al. [12] in 2006 suggests that the incidence of BDI has been stabilized since they found no difference in complications after LC or OC, with BDI occurring in 0.2 % in both groups. Nevertheless, annually 40–45 patients are still referred to the Academic Medical Center, without any sign of decrease in recent years [13]. This suggests a higher incidence of BDI in the Netherlands than reported in the literature [13]. As stated before, initially inexperience probably contributed to the high incidence of BDI, but other factors such as anatomical variation and techniques without using the critical view of safety (CVS) of Strasberg [14] as the standard of care seem to be responsible for the current incidence of BDI. Furthermore, there appears to be a lack of knowledge of escape techniques in difficult cholecystectomies to prevent BDI. Buddingh et al. [15] recently conducted a nationwide survey in which 97.6 % of Dutch surgeons reported to use the technique of CVS. Hereby the incidence of BDI in the Netherlands might decline in the future.

Even though the incidence of BDI may not be high and the results of treatment are excellent, especially when performed in a multidisciplinary team in a tertiary referral center [16, 17], the consequences of this injury have a negative impact on the life expectancy [9] and the quality of life (QoL) [18]. Therefore a thorough knowledge of the possibilities for prevention, early diagnosis, and treatment of this complication are mandatory for every surgeon and surgical resident performing cholecystectomies, either performed open or laparoscopically.

Prevention of BDI

The key issue in the management of BDI and other complications is prevention. Prevention of BDI is only possible with the thorough knowledge of pre- and intraoperative risk factors for BDI. Furthermore, the surgeon should be familiar with various escape techniques in difficult cases.

Risk Factors for BDI

Informed consent, in which the risk of BDI and its possible consequences are mentioned, should be obtained and registered in all cases, particularly in the presence of preoperative risk factors.

Risk factors and measures to prevent and recognize BDI are outlined in many publications [19–22]. Adverse outcome after LC is particularly associated with male gender, comorbidity, complexity and urgency of surgery, and conversion [23, 24]. Local risk factors are acute cholecystitis, aberrant anatomy, severe local fibrosis due to previous inflammation [10, 25], and bleeding in the Calot's triangle disturbing the operative view. Other risk factors are misuse of cautery, technical problems, and misidentification of the anatomy [21, 26]. Injuries due to misidentification usually occur when the surgeon interprets the common bile duct or an aberrant right hepatic duct for the cystic duct [21]. Way et al. [22] suggested that errors leading to laparoscopic bile duct injuries result principally from visual perceptual illusion, not from errors in skills, knowledge, or judgment. Lillemoe [20] stated that the concept of human error should not be used as an "excuse" for surgeons to avoid responsibility for complications. Knowledge of the anatomy and the mechanism of injury, an appropriate level of suspicion, the standard use of the CVS technique, and probably the use of an intraoperative cholangiogram (IOC) will prevent misperception errors that may occur during cholecystectomy.

Especially in the presence of risk factors, adequate expertise in the operating room should be ensured [21], and familiarity with escape techniques should be present. In the case of acute cholecystitis, there is a higher conversion rate and a longer duration of surgery when operated by a surgeon without laparoscopic expertise [27]. In the presence of acute cholecystitis, the operation should therefore be upgraded to an advanced laparoscopic procedure [21]. Obviously, this will have consequences for on call shifts. In 2009 the Dutch Association on Endoscopic Surgery has already stated that surgeons who only incidentally operate laparoscopically are not allowed to perform laparoscopic procedures without supervision. Recently the Dutch Society of General Surgery has confirmed this by formulating specific agreements and certifications concerning this problem. During shifts, a surgeon on call should not perform procedures that he or she is not familiar with, i.e., that are not regularly performed during daytime shifts, without consulting or help from an experienced surgeon. For on call shifts certain procedures, such as small bowel obstruction due to adhesions, appendicitis, and rupture of a spleen, can still be performed by the general surgeon. For other acute procedures such as gastric, pancreatic, colon, and rectal resections and also cholecystectomy, specific expertise is mandatory. Thereby these procedures will be exclusively performed by experienced surgeons. A clear shift schedule should be available and well known by surgeons on call within a hospital or region. In some cases consultation of or even referral to a tertiary center may be the best option.

Critical View of Safety

Already in 1995 Strasberg described the guidelines for a critical view of safety (CVS) [28]. This technique is generally adopted by the Dutch Society of Surgery in the guidelines on gallstone disease and best practice of cholecystectomy in 2007 [10] and introduced as the standard of care in all training programs. The objective

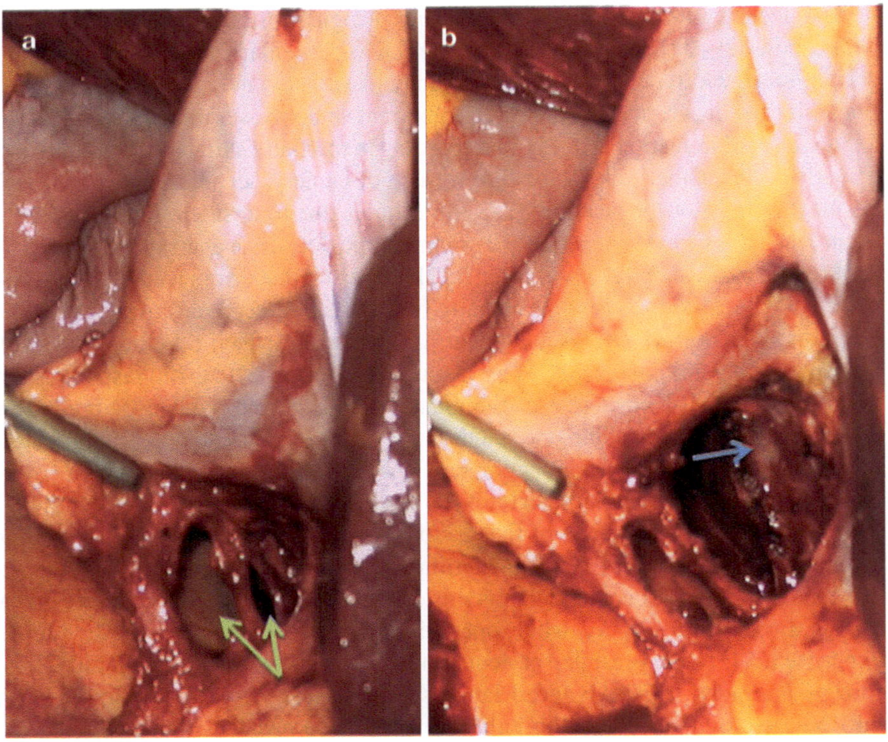

Fig. 12.1 Difference between two "windows" and CVS. (**a**) After dissection, two windows are created, one between the cystic duct and cystic artery and one between the artery and the liver bed (*arrows*). Because the cystic plate is not fully cleared of tissue, CVS has not been reached. (**b**) Here the cystic plate (*white, arrow*) is clearly identified and hence CVS is reached. (Published with permission of Elsevier. *J Am Coll Surg* [29])

of this technique is to conclusively identify the cystic duct (CD) and cystic artery (CA) before they are clipped and cut. Calot's triangle cannot always be clearly identified due to retraction of the gallbladder against the liver. The principle of CVS is therefore to fully unfold Calot's triangle. First traction on the fundus and infundibulum of the gallbladder is applied in cranial and ventrocaudal direction, respectively. The peritoneal envelope is then opened bilaterally up to the liver bed. Using blunt meticulous dissection with limited and cautious use of cautery, the gallbladder is dissected for at least one third of its length out of the liver bed to ensure that no other structures besides the CA and CD are present between the gallbladder and the liver. Mobilization of the infundibulum is the essence of CVS. Hereby a two-window view is created between respectively the CD and CA and between the CA and liver bed (see Fig. 12.1a and b [29]). Thereby a definitive 360° identification of the cystic duct and cystic artery is achieved. CVS is captured photographically or by video and recorded together with the operation report [29]. Only after CVS is definitively reached, the cystic duct and artery can be clipped and divided safely.

Escape Techniques

If mobilization of the infundibulum is not possible and therefore CVS cannot be reached, the Dutch guidelines on gallstone disease and best practice on laparoscopic cholecystectomy propagate conversion to OC [10]. However, this advice is not sufficient because conversion is not a solution for the situation per se. The main question is whether conversion will give a better overview on the anatomy and thereby make the operation easier or is it better to change the operation strategy to other escape procedures. In the current laparoscopic era, surgical residents have little experience with OC [30]. Nevertheless, as stated before, this procedure is used in those cases when LC cannot be performed at all. Paradoxically, there is progressively less experience with the technique that is necessary for the most challenging cases [30]. Recently, psychological factors were described that play a role in the decision making of either continuing a difficult procedure laparoscopically or to convert to OC [31]. As mentioned before, the underestimation of the risk of visual misperception and therefore misinterpretation of the anatomical relationships seems to be crucial in the occurrence of BDI. This means that despite conversion and persisting indistinct visualization, local dissection is continued. A stopping rule, such as using a different operative strategy or consulting a surgeon that is experienced in OC and different escape techniques in those cases when CVS cannot be reached, may be much more important than conversion per se.

In the preoperative planning of cholecystectomy, the presence of preoperative risk factors for difficult cholecystectomy and conversion such as acute cholecystitis should be considered in choosing the right surgical team. Another option is to plan a primary open procedure [23]. In that way, patients with a suspected difficult cholecystectomy according to preoperative risk factors play an important role in the surgical training of young residents with the open procedure and alternative techniques. Recently primary percutaneous gallbladder drainage has been shown to be a safe and successful treatment option in high-risk patients less eligible for surgery [32].

Several techniques are suggested to prevent BDI [21, 33, 34]. The infundibular technique, which depends on observing the cystic duct flare as it becomes the infundibulum, can be misleading especially in case of acute inflammation [21]. This technique should therefore not be used for the identification of the ducts. Another error trap is the fundus-down cholecystectomy in the case of severe inflammation, the failure to perceive the presence of an aberrant right hepatic duct on cholangiography, and injury to the CBD in the case of a "parallel union" of the cystic duct [26]. Loss of the dissection plane between the liver and gallbladder might even lead to injury of the right portal vein.

An alternative strategy is the antegrade technique, also called the fundus-first technique, where the gallbladder is dissected from the liver bed starting at the fundus. This technique is used for difficult procedures and is a frequently used technique in OC. It can also be used laparoscopically and will, in the hands of an experienced surgeon, reduce the chance of BDI in the same manner [35].

An additional technique that may be used instead is leaving the infundibulum in situ. This principle is used in the method of Terblanche, or subtotal cholecystectomy, which can be performed open or laparoscopically [30, 36, 37]. Excision of the gallbladder is performed using cautery at the gallbladder-liver bed junction leaving a small rim of the posterior gallbladder wall. After that, the residual gallbladder mucosa must be destructed with electrocoagulation to prevent mucus production [36].

Another option, for example, in case of severe local inflammation, is to terminate the procedure and convert to percutaneous gallbladder drainage with delayed cholecystectomy or referral to a tertiary center.

It is unclear if intraoperative cholangiography (IOC), in difficult cases, can truly reduce the risk of BDI [10]. Flum et al. [9] and more recently Buddingh et al. [38] showed a lower rate of major BDI after implementation of routine IOC compared to selective use of cholangiography. This may partly be related to the fact that the interpretation of IOC might be difficult in inexperienced hands and should be learned adequately. When IOC is not frequently used, misinterpretation in the presence of injury has been described [21, 22], in particular with segmental lesions. If bile leakage occurs during dissection, cholangiography should be performed by inserting a catheter in the lesion.

Diagnosis of BDI

Inadequate management of BDI may lead to severe deterioration with biliary peritonitis, sepsis, multiple organ failure, and even death. Therefore, early recognition is of utmost importance. Early symptoms are abdominal pain, anorexia, nausea, vomiting, and ileus. As a matter of fact, in any patient who fails to recover within 24–48 h after LC or has persistent abdominal complaints after LC, BDI should be considered. Jaundice is usually a symptom that occurs in a later postoperative phase after several days. There seems to be no relation between the severity of the injury and the presenting symptoms [4].

In general there are three different groups of patients that can be identified according to the moment of recognition of the BDI, all with different symptoms and a different treatment strategy.

In the first group of patients, the injury is detected during initial operation, usually by biliary leakage and sometimes by intraoperative cholangiography. This appears to be only the case in 15–30 % of the patients [4, 13].

In the second group there is a delayed identification of BDI in the direct postoperative period (34 % of cases [13]). However, the time interval between LC and diagnosis of the BDI varies widely with a median interval of 7 days and the mean interval of approximately 4 weeks [13]. These patients are frequently discharged on the second postoperative day and readmitted a few days later with a biloma, biliary peritonitis, obstructive jaundice, or sepsis due to abdominal leakage of infected bile.

In the last group of patients, there is a long symptom-free interval of several months up to more than a year after the initial injury. The cause is usually an ischemic stricture of the CBD, presenting with obstructive jaundice rather than cholangitis. A few patients present with intermittent obstruction and cholangitis, due to a spontaneous enteric fistula [4].

The type of diagnostic procedure to be performed is dependent on the presenting symptoms. In the case of sepsis, the first diagnostic procedure should be ultrasound or CT scanning for the detection of fluid collections. The next step is visualization of the biliary tree by endoscopic retrograde cholangiopancreatography (ERCP), magnetic resonance cholangiopancreatography (MRCP), percutaneous transhepatic cholangiography (PTC), or sometimes drainography to establish the diagnosis and classify the injury. In the case of jaundice without sepsis, visualizing the biliary tree should be the first step. The diversity in the types of injury demands a multidisciplinary approach in which treatment options are discussed in a team of surgeons, gastroenterologists, and radiologists, all familiar with these patients [13]. Interpretation of completeness of the biliary tree before any intervention is undertaken is of utmost importance to exclude segmental injury and anatomical variation (see Fig. 12.2).

Classification of BDI

Before proceeding with the actual treatment of BDI, the type of injury should first be classified or staged. Several classifications of BDI exist. The oldest one is the Bismuth classification [39] which classifies the injury in terms of the level of the lesion in the biliary tree. The classification of McMahon [40] classifies the injury into major and minor injuries, and the Strasberg classification [28] classifies the injury in terms of level and severity. In 1996 the Amsterdam classification was developed which links the type of injury directly to the further clinical management of BDI and is in our opinion therefore of practical use [41]. Type A injury (see Fig. 12.3) involves cystic duct leakage. Type B injury (see Fig. 12.4) is bile duct leakage. Type C injury (see Fig. 12.5) is a bile duct stricture. Type D injury (see Fig. 12.6) is a bile duct transection [41].

Vasculo-biliary Injury

Unfortunately, it is not uncommon that a BDI is combined with a vascular injury. The most common type of vasculo-biliary injury (VBI), also called the "classical injury," is injury to the right hepatic artery (RHA) and common bile duct (CBD), with an incidence around 25 % of all the BDIs [14]. The cause of the misidentification is frequently a combination of adverse operative conditions and the use of suboptimal identification techniques, such as the infundibular technique [42]. In the operative report, the division of a so-called second cystic duct or accessory duct may

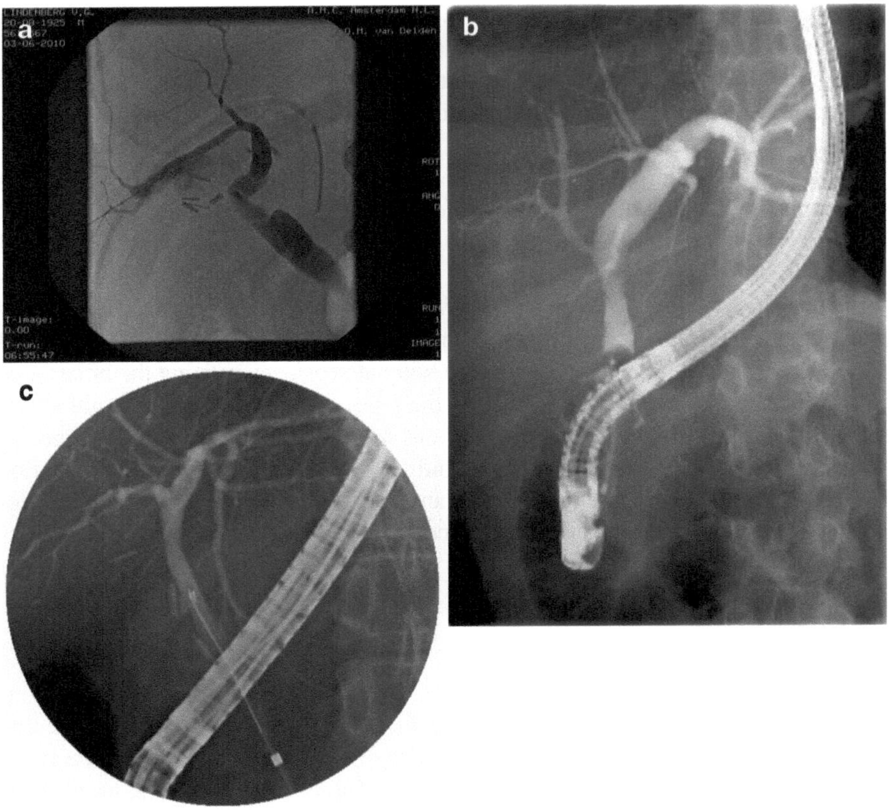

Fig. 12.2 Segmental injury. (**a**) Cholangiogram. Leakage from the RHD near an operation clip. (**b**) ERCP. Occlusion RHD. (**c**) ERCP. Occlusion of the anterior segment of the RHD due to an operation clip (later confirmed by MRCP)

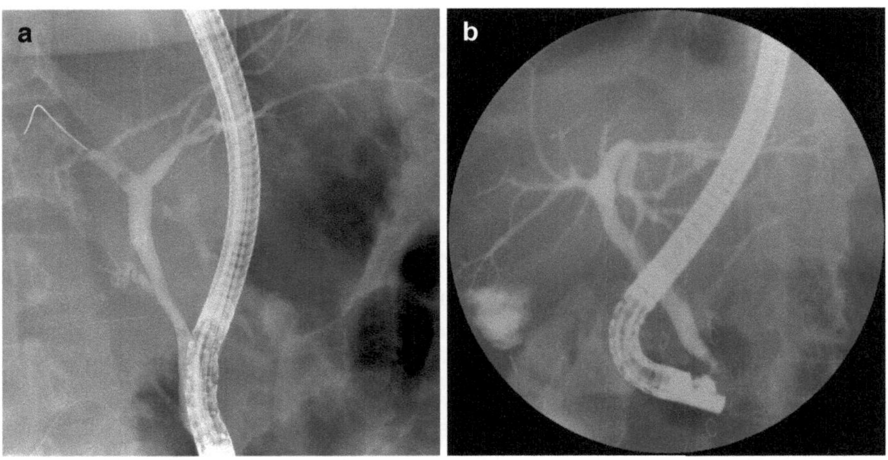

Fig. 12.3 Type A injury. (**a**) ERCP. Leakage from the cystic stump near the operation clips (*red arrow*). The tip of a PTC drain is shown (*black arrow*). (**b**) ERCP. Leakage from a duct of Luschka (*arrow*)

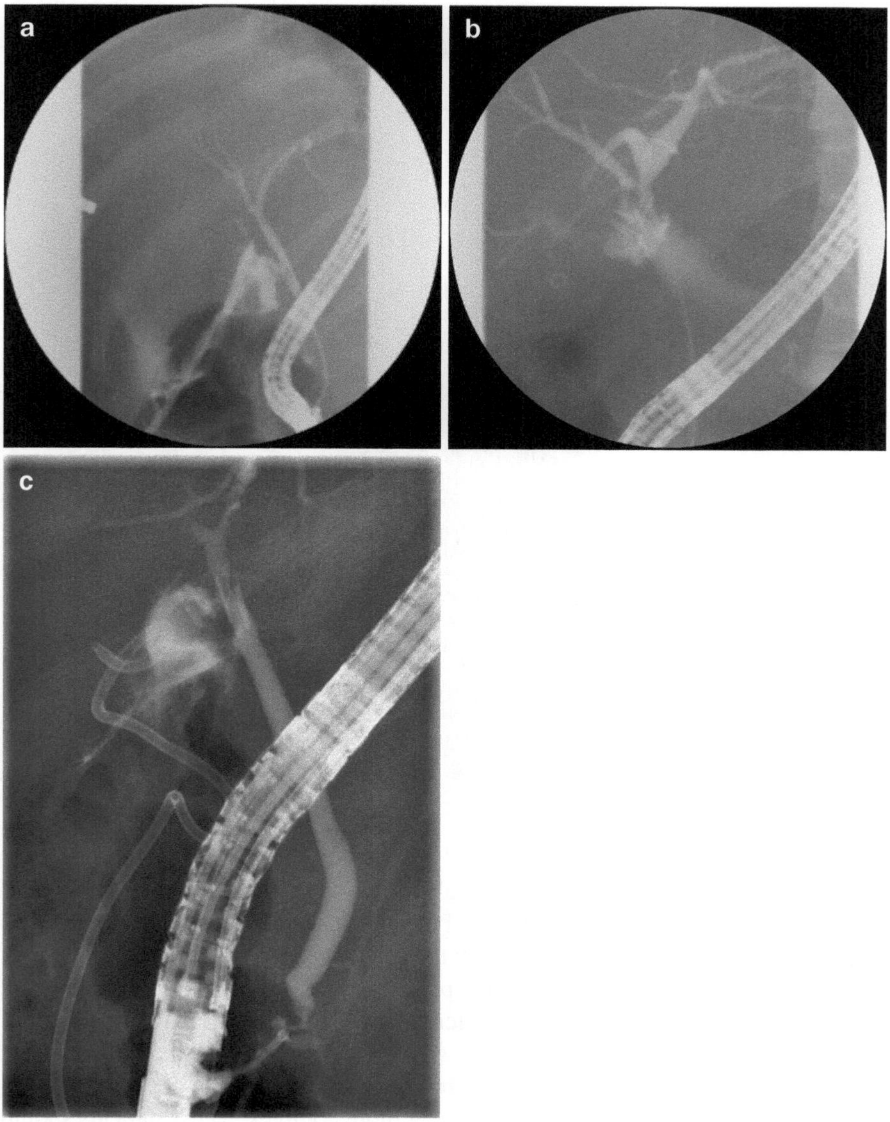

Fig. 12.4 Type B injury. (**a**) ERCP. Leakage of the CBD (*red arrow*). Part of the right hepatic system is missing (*black arrow*). MRCP showed aberrant anatomy with the posterior segment of the RHD originating from the LHD (not shown). (**b** and **c**) ERCP shows diffuse leakage of the CBD around multiple operation clips (*arrows*)

undeserved be described. The cause of this may be the tendency to persist in the anatomic frame of reference. This seems to be caused by the complexity of the human brain in which strongly held assumptions, i.e., being convinced of operating in the correct anatomical plane, cause that peroperative complications are attributed to behavioral factors, e.g., an "accessory duct," instead of leading to corrective feedback, i.e., considering the anatomical plane may not be correctly chosen [14, 22, 33].

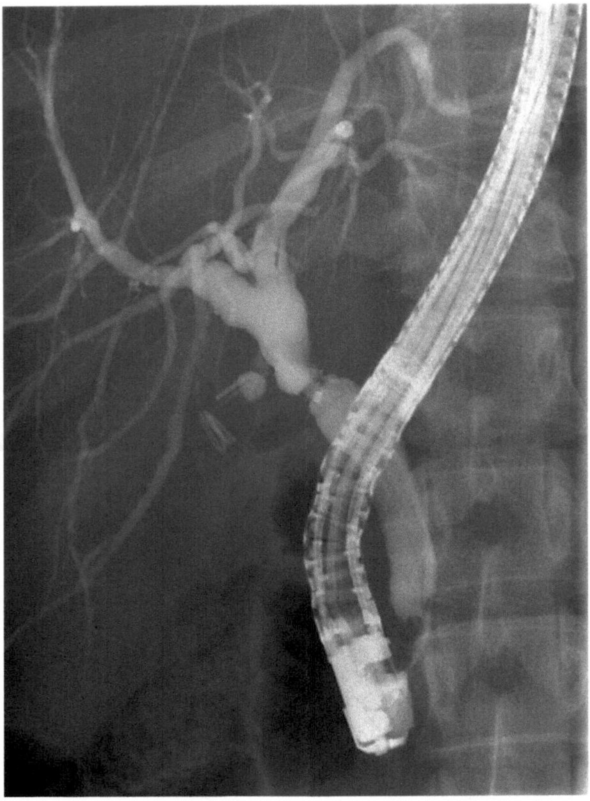

Fig. 12.5 Type C injury ERCP. Stenosis of the proximal CBD, approximately 1 cm below the bifurcation of the left and right hepatic duct (*red arrow*). The biliary tree is intact

Clinically, isolated RHA injury is rarely noticed due to compensatory collateral flow, but in combination with BDI part of the collateral blood supply is damaged as well. Therefore in combination with BDI the actual injury tends to be more complex and higher up in the biliary tree than the primary observed injury [14]. This process may also be responsible for stenosis after early biliary reconstruction due to ischemia of the bile duct [14]. Repair of the artery is rarely possible and the benefit of such a reconstruction is not proven [14]. Injuries to the portal vein or proper or common hepatic artery are uncommon but much more complex. These patients should immediately be referred to a tertiary center and considered to have vascular reconstruction or partial hepatectomy [14].

Treatment of BDI

As mentioned earlier, the treatment of BDI requires a multidisciplinary approach by surgeons, gastroenterologists, and interventional radiologists, all experienced in this field [13]. BDI can only be treated adequately after a thorough classification of the type of injury. In discussing the treatment of BDI, we routinely use the Amsterdam classification and consider the timing of diagnosis as well [10, 41].

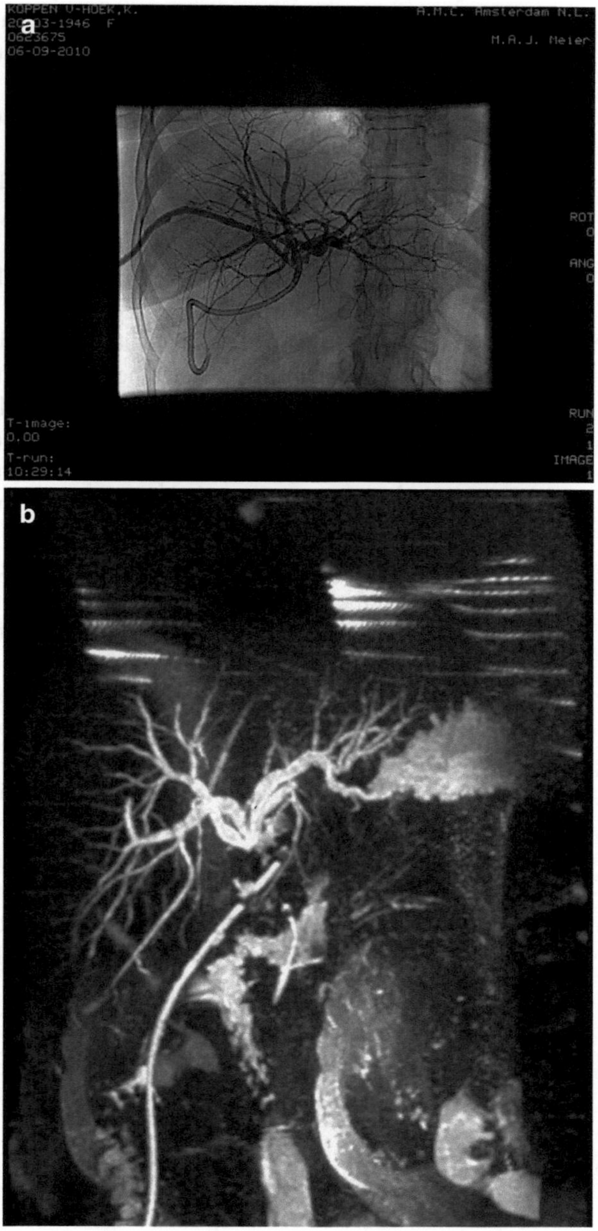

Fig. 12.6 Type D injury. (**a**) Cholangiogram via PTC drain (*black arrow*). The *red arrow* shows the bifurcation. Below the bifurcation the CBD is missing. Above this level, the biliary tree is intact. (**b**) MRCP. The *red arrow* shows a subhepatic drain. The red line shows the part of the CBD that is missing. The biliary tree is intact

Peroperatively Diagnosed Injury

In a study by de Reuver et al. [13], BDI was detected peroperatively in 21 % of the patients. In 17 % of the patients, a repair procedure was performed directly during the initial operation. However, it is known that patients in whom a repair procedure is performed during the initial cholecystectomy by the same surgeon who caused the BDI have a significantly worse prognosis than patients who were referred to a tertiary center [9, 13]. When the choice for a direct repair of the injury still is made, the presence of an experienced surgical team is mandatory. If there is not enough experience present, the patient should be referred to a tertiary center or a surgeon from the referral center should visit the concerned hospital to perform a repair procedure.

Type A injuries can usually be secured primarily. The same is true for type B injuries, which can be closed over a T-drain. However, in both types of injury, care must be taken not to worsen the injury by occluding the CBD or one of the vascular structures. If sufficient surgical experience is lacking, a bailout technique is external drainage and subsequent referral to a tertiary center.

In type D lesions, peroperative classification of the injury is usually difficult. In these cases IOC may be helpful. As stated before, expertise in interpreting IOC is of great importance to avoid misinterpretation of the cholangiogram. In the presence of an experienced surgeon and when there are no signs of tissue loss, an end-to-end anastomosis using a T-drain can usually safely be constructed. After this type of reconstruction, there is a 68 % chance of stricture formation [43]. However, de Reuver et al. [43] showed that this complication can be adequately managed by endoscopic stenting or percutaneous drainage with a success rate of 66 % in these patients [43]. When the stricture is resistant to dilatation, reconstructive surgery by performing a hepaticojejunostomy (HJ) can still be performed with a relatively low morbidity [43]. However, when there is tissue loss of the CBD in the first place, hepaticojejunostomy should be performed, but especially for this procedure, adequate experience is mandatory, since this is the last resort operation. HJ in the acute setting without dilatation of the bile ducts is a difficult procedure, and one should be very careful not to further extend the injury into the intrahepatic ducts or subsequently damage the arterial supply [43]. In most cases there will not be enough experience present during the initial operation, and therefore the options are either to place a subhepatic drain and refer the patient to a tertiary center or let an experienced surgeon from the tertiary center perform a direct reconstruction in the referring hospital. The results of an early repair are actually good if performed by an experienced surgeon.

Postoperatively Diagnosed Injury

When BDI is diagnosed postoperatively, at first sepsis should be controlled using fluid resuscitation, antibiotics, and percutaneous drainage of fluid collections. When the patient is treated in a hospital without sufficient experience in the treatment of BDI, the patient should be referred. Appropriate classification with visualization of the entire biliary tree is mandatory before the type of treatment can be determined. In the presence of local expertise in performing an ERCP, type A injuries can be directly treated by endoscopic stenting with an overall success of 97 % [44]. Even in type B and C injuries, when sepsis has subsided, the patients can be treated early by endoscopic dilatation and or stenting. In type B injuries the success rate is 89 %, and stent-related complications occur in 3.8 % of the patients [44]. For type C injuries, the success rate of stenting is 74 %, with stent-related complications occurring in 33 % of the patients during a median duration of stenting of 11 months (range 1–69 months). Most complications were mild (19 % stent migration, 14 % stent occlusion) and managed by stent exchange. For type D injuries, hepaticojejunostomy should be constructed after sepsis is adequately treated and the patient is recovered from this period. The preferred timing of this procedure seems to be after about 6 weeks to 3 months after the initial procedure to prevent progressive ischemia and thereby postoperative leakage and stricture formation [14, 45]. Of the 500 patients referred to our tertiary center, 151 patients (30.2 %) underwent reconstructive surgery for BDI [45]. Surgery-related complications occurred in 29 patients (19 %). Severe complications include anastomotic leakage that occurred in 6 patients (4 %) and postoperative bleeding in 1 patient (1 %). Five patients with anastomotic leakage were successfully treated with a temporary percutaneous transhepatic stent. There was no hospital mortality. After a mean interval of 46 months (median 24, range 8–120) after surgical reconstruction, anastomotic strictures were diagnosed in 10 % of the patients. In 20 % of these patients, surgical reconstruction had to be performed, and most (80 %) of these patients could be adequately treated by percutaneous transhepatic dilatation. Independent negative predictive factors for outcome are extended injury in the biliary tree, secondary referral, and repair in the acute phase after the injury. Similar results after reconstruction have been published by others [46, 47]. Recently, it has been reported that the results of an early repair are as good when performed in the absence of sepsis and by an experienced team [48, 49].

Quality of Life and Litigation Claims

Although results after treatment of BDI in referral centers are fairly good, during follow-up of these patients, 62 % reported suffering from symptoms that are linked to the injury (De Reuver, unpublished data). Tiredness was reported by the majority of the patients (69 %), while more specific symptoms for BDI, such as fullness (59 %), periodical fever (22 %), and jaundice (9 %), were reported less frequently (De Reuver, unpublished data). These symptoms are in striking contrast with the functional outcome after treatment since the success rate of the nonoperative treatment of type A, B, and C injuries is 97 %, 89 %, and 74 %, respectively, and the success rate after surgical reconstruction in terms of strictures is 90 % [44]. The long-term QoL of patients after the treatment of BDI seems to be impaired [16, 17, 50], independent on the type of injury and type of treatment [16, 17]. The phenomenon of bias by response shift may also be responsible for the reported poor QoL, meaning that the patients do not accept a decline in daily health status after a surgical procedure that is perceived as relatively minor and was tremendously complicated [51].

The 10-year survival of BDI patients is 88 %, which is not significantly worse compared to the age-matched general population. The hazard of death is two times as high in male patients and when the repair procedure was performed during the initial cholecystectomy [13]. Flum et al. [9] showed an 11 % death increase in patients who underwent a repair procedure by the same surgeon who performed the initial cholecystectomy. Furthermore, they reported a mortality rate after BDI almost three times as high compared to patients who underwent cholecystectomy without an injury [9].

The number of claim procedures in BDI patients in the Netherlands treated in a tertiary center is only 19 %. Factors associated with starting a claim procedure are younger age, severity of injury, employment, and the use of social securities. A complete transection of the CBD is an independent predictive factor for starting a claim procedure [52]. Most patients feel that they had not been taken seriously at the time of the first postoperative symptoms which has led to a delay in diagnosis of the injury. They were disappointed by the reluctance of the primary surgeon to admit to a procedural error and to give full information on the severity of the injury [51]. It has been suggested that settlement and liability payment can lead to a reduction of complaints related to QoL in patients after BDI.

Summary

The most devastating complication after cholecystectomy is BDI, with a reported incidence of 0–1.5 %. The key issue in the management of BDI is prevention. Prevention is only adequate with the awareness of pre- and intraoperative risk factors, the use of CVS, experience in performing cholecystectomy, and knowledge of the different escape strategies in the case of a difficult cholecystectomy. BDI can be diagnosed either peroperatively or in the direct or late postoperative phase. In case BDI occurs, the severity of the injury should be classified thoroughly before a proper treatment can be chosen. The treatment of BDI should be performed by a multidisciplinary team and only if sufficient experience in dealing with this complication is present. If not, the patients should be referred to a tertiary center. Even after an objectively excellent outcome of treatment, the reported QoL is still reduced.

References

1. Prismant. Utrecht, the Netherlands: National Medical Registration; 2005–2009.
2. Go PM, Schol F, Gouma DJ. Laparoscopic cholecystectomy in the Netherlands. Br J Surg. 1993;80:1180–3.
3. Deziel DJ, Millikan KW, Economou SG, Doolas A, Ko ST, Airan MC. Am J Surg. 1993;165:9–14.
4. Van Erpecum KJ, Bergman JJGHM, Gouma DJ, Terpstra OT. Gallstone disease. In: Van Lanschot JJB, Gouma DJ, Jansen PLM, Jones EA, Pinedo HM, Schouten WR, Tytgat GNJ, editors. Integrated medical and surgical gastroenterology. Houten: Bohn Stafleu van Loghum; 2004. p. p146–66.

5. Larobina M, Nottle P. Surg Laparosc Endosc Percutan Tech. 2005;15:119–23.
6. Chandler JG, Corson SL, Way LW. Three spectra of laparoscopic entry access injuries. J Am Coll Surg. 2001;192:478–91.
7. Bhoyrul S, Vierra M, Nezhat R, et al. Trocar injuries in laparoscopic surgery. J Am Coll Surg. 2001;192:677–83.
8. Gouma DJ, Rauws EA, Keulemans YC, Bergman JJ, Huibregtse K, Obertop H. Galwegletsel na laparoscopische cholecystectomie. Ned Tijdschr Geneeskd. 1999;143:606–11.
9. Flum DR, Cheadle A, Prela C, Dellinger EP, Chan L. Bile duct injury during cholecystectomy and survival in medicare beneficiaries. JAMA. 2003;290:2168–73.
10. Nederlandse Vereniging voor Heelkunde. Evidence based richtlijn. Onderzoek en behandeling van galstenen; 2007.
11. Gouma DJ, Go PM. Bile duct injury during laparoscopic and conventional cholecystectomy. J Am Coll Surg. 1994;178:229–33.
12. Keus F, de Jong J, Gooszen HG, Laarhoven CJHM. Laparoscopic versus open cholecystectomy for patients with symptomatic cholecystolithiasis. Cochrane Database Syst Rev. 2006(4):CD006231. DOI: 10.1002/14651858.CD006231.
13. De Reuver PR, Rauws EA, Bruno MJ, Lameris JS, Busch OR, van Gulik TM, Gouma DJ. Survival in bile duct injury patients after laparoscopic cholecystectomy. A multidisciplinary approach by gastroenterologists and surgeons. Surgery. 2007;142:1–9.
14. Strasberg SM, Helton WS. An analytical review of vasculobiliary injury in laparoscopic and open cholecystectomy. HPB. 2011;13:1–14.
15. Buddingh KT, Hofker HS, Ten Cate Hoedemaker HO, van Dam GM, Ploeg RJ, Nieuwenhuijs VB. World J Surg. 2011;35:1235–41. discussion 1242–3.
16. Boerma D, Rauws EA, Keulemans YC, Bergman JJ, Obertop H, Huibregtse K, Gouma DJ. Impaired quality of life 5 years after bile duct injury during laparoscopic cholecystectomy: a prospective analysis. Ann Surg. 2001;234:750–7.
17. De Reuver PR, Sprangers MA, Gouma DJ. Quality of life in bile duct injury patients. Ann Surg. 2007;246:161–3.
18. De Reuver PR, Sprangers MA, Rauws EA, Lameris JS, Busch OR, van Gulik TM, Gouma DJ. Impact of bile duct injury after laparoscopic cholecystectomy on quality of life: a longitudinal study after multidisciplinary treatment. Endoscopy. 2008;40:637–43.
19. Chapman WC, Abecassis M, Jarnagin W, Mulvihill S, Strasberg SM. Bile duct injuries 12 years after the introduction of laparoscopic cholecystectomy. J Gastrointest Surg. 2003;7:412–6.
20. Lillemoe KD, Yeo CJ, Talamini MA, Wang BH, Pitt HA, Gadacz TR. Selective cholangiography. Current role in laparoscopic cholecystectomy. Ann Surg. 1992;215:669–74.
21. Strasberg SM. Avoidance of biliary injury during laparoscopic cholecystectomy. J Hepatobiliary Pancreat Surg. 2002;9:543–7.
22. Way LW, Stewart L, Gantert W, Liu K, Lee CM, Whang K, Hunter JG. Causes and prevention of laparoscopic bile duct injuries: analysis of 252 cases from a human factors and cognitive psychology perspective. Ann Surg. 2003;237:460–9.
23. Giger UF, Michel JM, Opitz I. Th Inderbitzin D, Kocher T, Krahenbuhl L; Swiss Association of Laparoscopic and Thoracoscopic Surgery (SALTS) Study Group. Risk factors for perioperative complications in patients undergoing laparoscopic cholecystectomy: analysis of 22,953 consecutive cases from the Swiss Association of Laparoscopic and Thoracoscopic Surgery database. J Am Coll Surg. 2006;203:723–8.
24. Kanakala V, Borowski DW, Pellen MG, Dronamraju SS, Woodcock SA, Seymour K, Attwood SE, Horgan LF. Risk factors in laparoscopic cholecystectomy: a multivariate analysis. Int J Surg. 2011;9:318–23.
25. Georgiades CP, Mavromatis TN, Kourlaba GC, Kapiris SA, Bairamides EG, Spyrou AM, Kokkinos CN, Spyratou CS, Ieronymou MI, Diamantopoulos GI. Is Inflammation a significant predictor of bile duct injury during laparoscopic cholecystectomy? Surg Endosc. 2008;22:1959–64.

26. Strasberg SM. Error traps and vasculo-biliary injury in laparoscopic and open cholecystectomy. J Hepatobiliary Pancreat Surg. 2008;15:284–92.
27. Kortram K, Reinders JS, van Ramshorst B, Wiezer MJ, Go PM, Boerma D. Laparoscopic cholecystectomy for acute cholecystitis should be performed by a laparoscopic surgeon. Surg Endosc. 2010;24:2206–9.
28. Strasberg SM, Hertl M, Soper NJ. Analysis of the problem of biliary injury during laparoscopic cholecystectomy. J Am Coll Surg. 1995;180:101–25.
29. Strasberg SM, Brunt LM. Rationale and use of the critical view of safety in laparoscopic cholecystectomy. J Am Coll Surg. 2010;211:132–8.
30. Visser BC, Parks RW, Garden OJ. Open cholecystectomy in the laparoscopic era. Am J Surg. 2008;195:108–14.
31. Dekker SW, Hugh TB. Laparoscopic bile duct injury: understanding the psychology and heuristics of the error. ANZ J Surg. 2008;78:1109–14.
32. Kortram K, de Vries Reilingh TS, Wiezer MJ, van Ramshorst B, Boerma D. Percutaneous drainage for acute calculous cholecystitis. Surg Endosc. 2011. [Epub ahead of print].
33. Hugh TB. New strategies to prevent laparoscopic bile duct injury-surgeons can learn from pilots. Surgery. 2002;132:826–35.
34. Wijsmuller AR, Leegwater M, Tseng L, Smaal HJ, Kleinrensink GJ, Lange JF. Optimizing the critical view of safety in laparoscopic cholecystectomy by clipping and transecting the cystic artery before the cystic duct. Br J Surg. 2007;94:473–4.
35. Huang SM, Hsiao KM, Pan H, Yao CC, Lai TJ, Chen LY, Wu CW, Lui WY. Overcoming the difficulties in laparoscopic management of contracted gallbladders with gallstones: possible role of fundus-down approach. Surg Endosc. 2011;25:284–91.
36. Michalowski K, Bornman PC, Krige JE, Gallagher PJ, Terblanche J. Laparoscopic subtotal cholecystectomy in patients with complicated acute cholecystitis or fibrosis. Br J Surg. 1998;85:904–6.
37. Philips JA, Lawes DA, Cook AJ, Arulampalam TH, Zaborsky A, Menzies D, Motson RW. The use of laparoscopic subtotal cholecystectomy for complicated cholelithiasis. Surg Endosc. 2008;22:1697–700.
38. Buddingh KT, Weersma RK, Savenije RA, van Dam GM, Nieuwenhuijs VB. Lower rate of major bile duct injury and increased intraoperative management of common bile duct stones after implementation of routine intraoperative cholangiography. J Am Coll Surg. 2011;213:267–74.
39. Bismuth H, Lazorthes F. 83rd Congress of the French Surgical Society (Paris, 21–24 September 1981). Second report. Operative injuries of the common biliary duct. J Chir (Paris). 1981; 118:601–9.
40. McMahon AJ, Fullarton G, Baxter JN, O'Dwyer PJ. Bile duct injury and bile leakage in laparoscopic cholecystectomy. Br J Surg. 1995;82:307–13.
41. Bergman JJ, van den Brink GR, Rauws EA, de Wit L, Obertop H, Huibregtse K, Tytgat GN, Gouma DJ. Treatment of bile duct lesions after laparoscopic cholecystectomy. Gut. 1996;38:141–7.
42. Strasberg SM, Eagon CJ, Drebin JA. The 'hidden cystic duct' syndrome and the infundibular technique of laparoscopic cholecystectomy-the danger of the false infundibulum. J Am Coll Surg. 2000;191:661–7.
43. De Reuver PR, Busch OR, Rauws EA, Lameris JS, van Gulik TM, Gouma DJ. Long-term results of a primary end-to-end anastomosis in peroperative detected bile duct injury. J Gastrointest Surg. 2007;11:296–302.
44. De Reuver PR, Rauws EA, Vermeulen M, Dijkgraaf MG, Gouma DJ, Bruno MJ. Endoscopic treatment of post-surgical bile duct injuries: long term outcome and predictors of success. Gut. 2007;56:1599–605.
45. De Reuver PR, Grossmann I, Busch OR, Obertop H, van Gulik TM, Gouma DJ. Ann Surg. 2007;245:763–70.
46. Stewart L, Way LW. Bile duct injuries during laparoscopic cholecystectomy. Factors that influence the results of treatment. Arch Surg. 1995;130:1123–8.

47. Lillemoe KD, Melton GB, Cameron JL, Pitt HA, Campbell KA, Talamini MA, Sauter PA, Coleman J, Yeo CJ. Postoperative bile duct strictures: management and outcome in the 1990s. Ann Surg. 2000;232:430–41.
48. Perera MT, Silva MA, Hegab B, Muralidharan V, Bramhall SR, Mayer AD, Buckels JA, Mirza DF. Specialist early and immediate repair of post-laparoscopic cholecystectomy bile duct injuries is associated with an improved long-term outcome. Ann Surg. 2011;253:553–60.
49. Kapoor VK. Bile duct injury repair: when? what? who? J Hepatobiliary Pancreat Surg. 2007;14:476–9.
50. Moore DE, Feurer ID, Holzman MD, Wudel LJ, Strickland C, Gorden DL, Chari R, Wright JK, Pinson CW. Long-term detrimental effect of bile duct injury on health-related quality of life. Arch Surg. 2004;139:476–81.
51. Gouma DJ, Obertop H. Br J Surg. 2002;89:385–6.
52. De Reuver PR, Rauws EA, Lameris JS, Sprangers MA, Gouma DJ. Claims for damages as a result of bile-duct injury during (laparoscopic) cholecystectomy. Ned Tijdschr Geneeskd. 2007;151:1732–6.

Chapter 13
Prevention and Treatment of Major Complications After Surgery of Klatskin Tumors

Geert Kazemier and Miguel A. Cuesta

Keywords Postoperative complications • Klatskin tumors • Cholangiocarcinomas • Liver resection • Postoperative bleeding • Bile leakage

Cholangiocarcinomas are rare in the Western world, but they are highly lethal because most are locally advanced at presentation. Currently, the term cholangiocarcinoma is used to describe bile duct cancers arising in the intrahepatic, perihilar, or extrahepatic biliary tree, excluding gallbladder or ampulla Vateri carcinomas. Tumors involving the perihilar region or hepatic duct bifurcation are often referred to as Klatskin tumors [1].

Symptoms and Differential Diagnosis

Cholangiocarcinomas usually become only symptomatic when the tumor obstructs the proper hepatic duct, causing painless jaundice. Painless jaundice is often accompanied by anorexia, weight loss, and abdominal discomfort or pain. The differential diagnosis includes primary sclerosing cholangitis (PSC), choledocholithiasis, benign (iatrogenic) biliary strictures, or compression of the common bile duct by pancreatic carcinoma, chronic pancreatitis, or metastatic cancers involving perihilar lymph nodes. Up to one-third of patients with symptoms and imaging suggestive of a cholangiocarcinoma will have either a benign disease or another malignancy that obstructs the biliary system [2]. Biochemical liver tests

G. Kazemier (✉) • M.A. Cuesta, MD (✉)
Department of Surgery, VU University Medical Center, Amsterdam, The Netherlands
e-mail: ma.cuesta@vumc.nl

M.A. Cuesta, H.J. Bonjer (eds.), *Treatment of Postoperative Complications after Digestive Surgery*, DOI 10.1007/978-1-4471-4354-3_13,

are of little use in differentiating since all these conditions can be associated with cholestasis, reflected in elevated serum levels of bilirubin and alkaline phosphatase.

Diagnostic Tools

Due to its localization, manner of growth, and pathological characteristics, treating patients with Klatskin tumors can be challenging. In those patients, the actual tumor mass is typically unimpressive, and upstream bile ducts may not be dilated in cholangiocarcinomas with underlying PSC or cirrhosis. Preoperative evaluation includes ultrasound, contrast-enhanced triple-phased helical CT scan, magnetic resonance cholangiopancreatography (MRCP), and endoscopic retrograde cholangiopancreatography (ERCP) or percutaneous transhepatic cholangiography (PTC) ([3], Fig. 13.1). Both ERCP and PTC can be used to obtain brush cytology of the tumor. Unfortunately, the diagnostic yield of brush cytology has only a limited sensitivity. Tumor markers such as CEA, CA 19–9, or a combination of both can also be useful to confirm the diagnosis, but positive predictive value has been shown to be low. Despite all these diagnostic modalities and even more advanced imaging techniques, such as intraductal ultrasound, positron emission tomography (PET scan), or staging laparoscopy, true resectability can be determined only by operative evaluation in a large proportion of patients, and up to 50 % are surgically not curable during surgery [4].

Preoperative Approach and Prevention of Postoperative Complications

The only potentially curative option for patients suffering from Klatskin tumors is complete resection. The growth characteristics along the ducts, and in the hepatic parenchyma, mandate liver resection in order to get free resection margins and gain a better prognosis in the majority of cases. This requires extensive preoperative measures in many of these patients, such as biliary decompression, preoperative assessment of quality and volume of the remnant liver segments, and possible induction of preoperative hypertrophy of that remnant in case of concerns about insufficient postoperative residual liver volume.

Whether biliary decompression prior to surgery should be carried out in patients with hilar cholangiocarcinoma who present with obstructive jaundice is under debate. Placement of stents, either endoscopically or percutaneously, induces complications, and stents might hinder preoperative imaging, particularly MRI/MRCP, and even hamper intraoperative palpation in determining the actual tumor extent. On the other hand, liver dysfunction due to cholestasis can develop with unrelieved

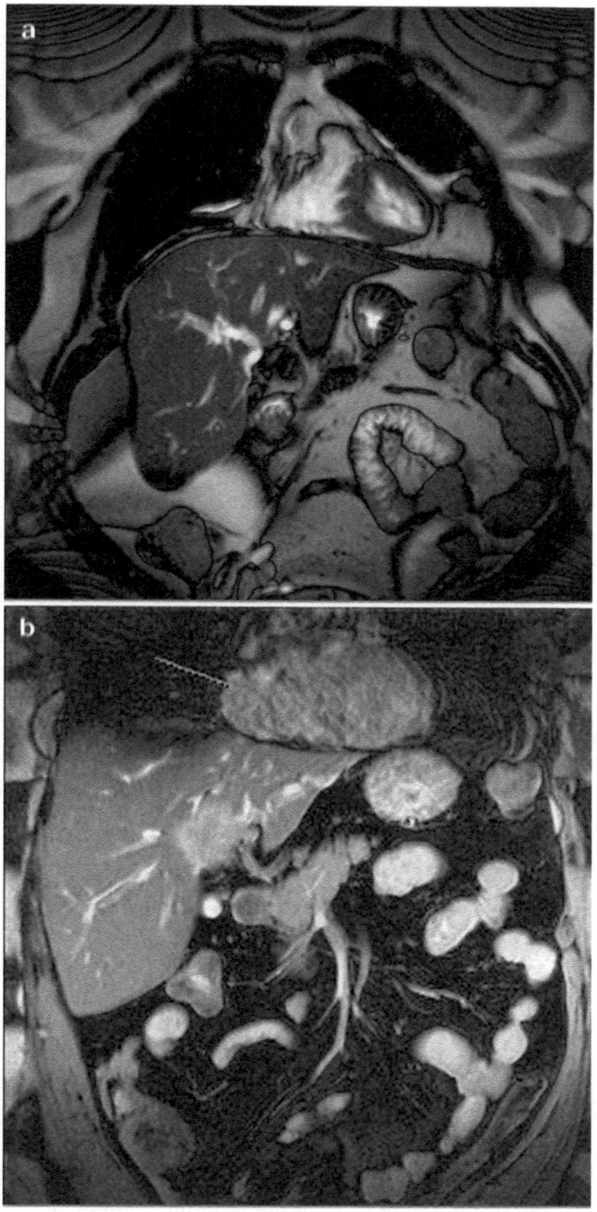

Fig. 13.1 (**a**) MRI of a Klatskin tumor, Bismuth-Corlette type 3b. (**b**) MRI, mass cholangiocarcinoma, type 3b (*green line*) is the line of liver resection

bile duct obstruction, and liver dysfunction is a known risk factor for increased postoperative morbidity and mortality following major liver resections [5, 6]. From a more practical point of view, preoperative stenting can be mandatory to alleviate jaundice and its sequelae such as pruritus during the frequently long preoperative period. A meta-analysis aiming at unraveling the effect of preoperative biliary drainage in jaundiced patients with hilar cholangiocarcinoma showed no difference in postoperative mortality or length of hospital stay with and without preoperative biliary decompression [7]. Whether to perform preoperative biliary drainage endoscopically or percutaneously is also controversial. Many surgeons prefer the percutaneous route as this allows for use of the same percutaneous stent after the biliary reconstruction to guide through the anastomosis.

Histologically negative resection margins are critical to postoperative cancer-free survival. Liver resections of 70 % or more are often necessary to achieve this. Preoperative portal vein embolization (PVE) of the portal vein branches supplying that segments of the liver that have to be removed has been shown to result in hypertrophy of the expected liver remnant. PVE is often used in patients with Klatskin tumors who have a predicted postoperative liver remnant volume of less than 30 %; patients with less than 30 % residual liver tumor are prone to postoperative (sub)acute liver failure. It can be done during a separate operation by suture ligation of that portal vein branches, but transhepatic, endovascular techniques have been shown to be more successful at achieving the wanted hypertrophy. This has been attributed to the fact that with the latter technique, portal vein thrombosis is often more complete because more thrombogenic agents can be used [8–12].

Besides the volume of the expected liver remnant, assessing the quality of liver tissue of the residual liver segment is pivotal. Percutaneous biopsy of this expected residual liver remnant to rule out severe fibrosis or cirrhosis is recommended. To perform this safely and without intra-abdominal biliary spill, adequate biliary decompression of the expected liver remnant is crucial before the procedure.

Classification of Klatskin Tumors and Consequences for Types of Resections

Cholangiocarcinomas arising in the perihilar region have been classified according to the degree of involvement of the hepatic ducts, the Bismuth-Corlette classification ([13], Fig. 13.2). To predict resectability and type of resection, a stenosis in the hepatic ducts suspected for cholangiocarcinoma can be classified according to the Bismuth-Corlette classification. Type I are tumors localized in the common hepatic duct without involvement of the hepatic duct bifurcation. Type II are tumors involving the hepatic duct bifurcation without segmental duct involvement excluding the caudate lobe. Type III a and b are tumors involving the hepatic duct bifurcation and the right or the left hepatic duct, respectively. Type IV concerns tumors involving the bifurcation and both ducts right and left or segmental duct in both liver halves (Fig. 13.1).

For type I lesions, the procedure is en bloc resection of the extrahepatic bile ducts and gallbladder with tumor-free bile duct margins and a regional lymphadenectomy followed by Roux-en-Y hepaticojejunostomy. In addition to the above operation,

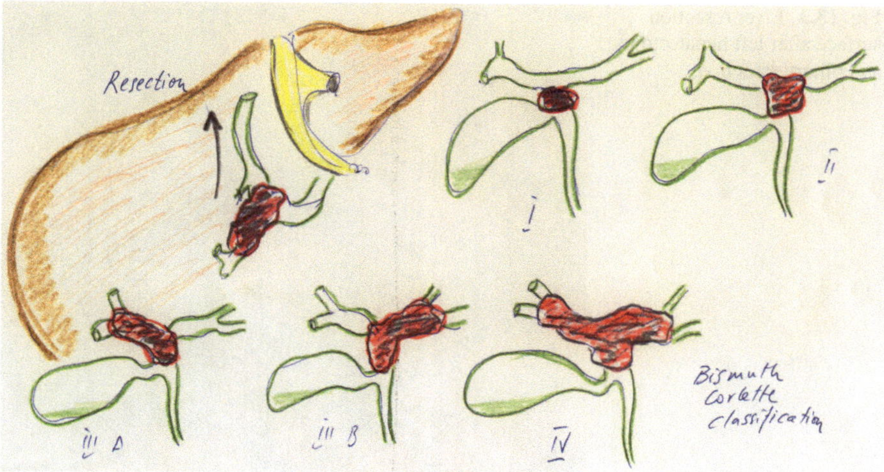

Fig. 13.2 Bismuth-Corlette classification of cholangiocarcinoma

type II tumors require en bloc resection of the caudate lobe because the segmental bile duct of this segment typically enters the left and/or right hepatic duct at the site of the bifurcation. In addition to the above operations, type III and IV tumors require (extended) right or left hepatectomy to ensure tumor-free margins. In case of portal vein involvement, more advanced techniques such as extended liver resection combined with portal vein resection and reconstruction to achieve negative margins have been shown to result in acceptable survival. Additional pancreaticoduodenectomy is sometimes necessary, particularly in patients with type I and II Klatskin tumors to ensure a radical resection.

Pathological staging is done according to the TNM classification. The clinical staging of Jarnagin and Blumgart defining radial as well as longitudinal extension of Klatskin tumors has also been shown to be useful [14]. This classification entails three elements: (a) location and extent of ductal involvement, (b) presence or absence of portal vein invasion, and (c) presence or absence of hepatic lobe atrophy. According to Jarnagin et al., criteria for unresectability include patient factors, local factors, and distant disease, factors which have been demonstrated to correlate correctly with radical resectability. There are different pathological types and different growth patterns having the potential for causing vascular encasement and lymphatic metastasis, and this makes radical surgical resection more difficult.

Surgery

In patients with Klatskin tumors, as mentioned earlier, true resectability is ultimately determined at surgery. In the absence of retropancreatic and paratruncal nodal metastases, liver or more distant metastases, invasion of the main hepatic

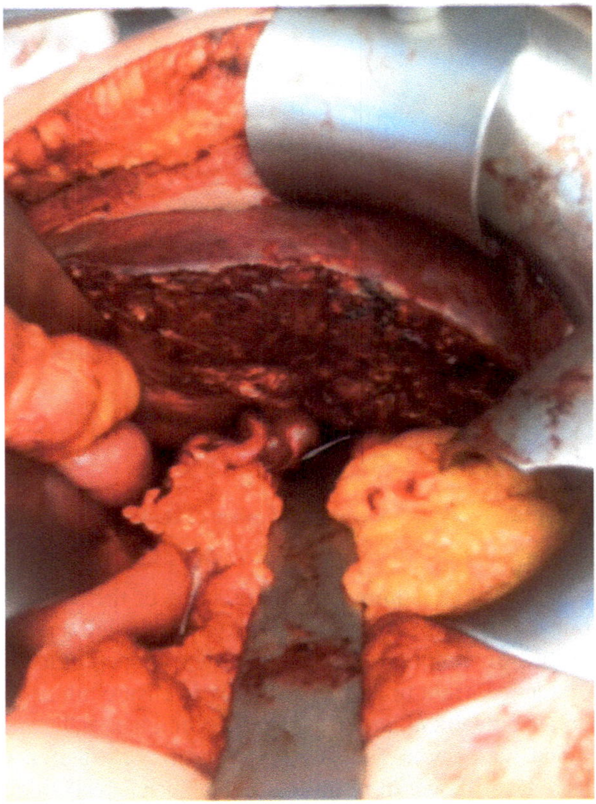

Fig. 13.3 Liver resection surface after left hepatectomy and biliary resection

artery, and of extrahepatic adjacent organ invasion, resection of Klatskin tumors should be attempted. During surgery, after general abdominal inspection to exclude distance metastases, the perihilar tumor can be locally assessed by palpation. Intraoperative ultrasonography can be useful to determine the exact resection plane. Once the resection plan is made, liver parenchyma dissection is performed, and the bile duct(s) is cut at the presumed tumor-free site(s); fresh frozen section pathology of the bile duct(s) is performed in many centers. Often dysplasia, sometimes even severe, is noted at these sites. Only in case of overt adenocarcinoma, however, an attempt should be made to further extend the resection if possible. Another strategy is to perform the most radical resection believed necessary and possible depending on the preoperative imaging and intraoperative findings, to reconstruct the bile duct(s) and to wait for the definitive pathology report (Figs. 13.3 and 13.4). There are few data regarding the benefits of lymphadenectomy for perihilar cholangiocarcinoma. Lymph node involvement however is a prognostic factor. Selective portal lymphadenectomy is often recommended. PTC drains placed preoperatively can be placed through the anastomosis or anastomoses, but one should be aware of seeding of tumor when these drains were passed through the tumor preoperatively. Despite all preoperative measures and often extensive resections, cure is still possible in

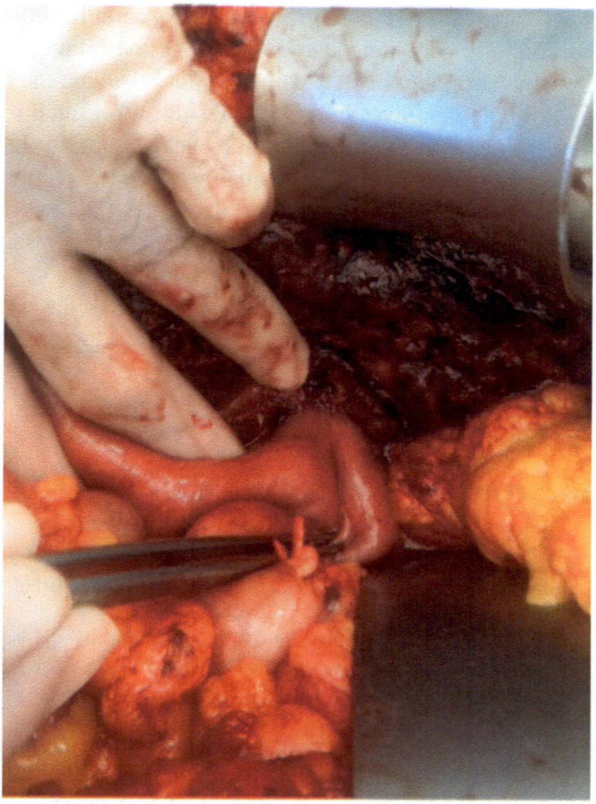

Fig. 13.4 Hepaticojejunostomy

fewer than 50 % of patients, and in the majority of cases, long-term disease control is rarely achieved [15, 16]. Within some clinical protocols, liver transplantation has been shown to have great potential as treatment for non-resectable Klatskin tumors. It is however too early to recommend this as standard of care [17].

Complications and Mortality

Treating patients with Klatskin tumor is challenging. Large series describe considerable postoperative morbidity (up to 76 %) and mortality (up to 19 %) [4, 18, 19]. Morbidity includes infectious complications including cholangitis, liver abscesses, intra-abdominal abscesses, and wound infection. The majority can be treated non-surgically, but percutaneously or with wound drainage.

Direct postoperative bleedings are rare but require re-exploration in the majority of cases. Bleeding later postoperatively as a result of septic complications is mostly arterial and resulting from biliary leak and biliary fistula. This should be treated by angiography and coiling if possible.

Biliary leak is a common postoperative complication. The majority can be treated successfully percutaneously by draining the biloma first and diverting the biliary flow by placement of PTC catheter after resolving the first septic period.

Postoperative liver failure as a result of too small residual liver capacity can be very difficult to treat, and its associated mortality has been associated with the extent of the resection and the quality of the liver remnant. In case of acute postoperative liver failure in the first few days after operation, accompanied by high serum transaminases, torsion of the liver remnant and its vasculature should be considered as it mandates prompt surgical intervention.

Because of the significant perioperative risk for complications, complex nature of operative management and rarity of this tumor, patients are better served by referral to tertiary centers.

References

1. Klatskin G. Adenocarcinoma of the hepatic duct at its bifurcation within the porta hepatis. An unusual tumor with distinctive clinical and pathological features. Am J Med. 1965;38:241–56.
2. Wetter LA, Ring EJ, Pellegrini CA, et al. Differential diagnosis of sclerosing cholangiocarcinomas of the common hepatic duct (klatskin tumors). Am J Surg. 1991;161:57–62.
3. Manfredi R, Barbaro B, Masselli G, et al. Magnetic resonance imaging of cholangiocarcinoma. Semin Liver Dis. 2004;24:155–64.
4. Ito F, Cho Clifford S, Rikkers Layton F, et al. Hilar cholangiocarcinoma: current management. Ann Surg. 2009;250:210–8.
5. Nimura Y, Kamiya J, Kondo S, et al. Aggressive preoperative management and extended surgery for hilar cholangiocarcinoma: Nagoya experience. J Hepatobiliary Pancreat Surg. 2000;7:155–62.
6. Cherqui D, Benoist S, Malassagne B, et al. Major liver resection for carcinoma in jaundiced patients without preoperative biliary drainage. Arch Surg. 2000;135:302–8.
7. Van Gulick TM, Kloek JJ, Ruys AT, et al. Multidisciplinary management of hilar cholangiocarcinoma (Klatskin tumour): extended resection is associated with improved survival. Eur J Surg Oncol. 2011;37:65–71.
8. Figueras J, Llado L, Valls C, et al. Changing strategies in diagnosis and management of hilar cholangiocarcinoma. Liver Transpl. 2000;6:786–94.
9. Qiu YD, Bai JL, Xu FG, Ding YT. Effect of preoperative biliary drainage on malignant obstructive jaundice: a meta-analysis. World J Gastroenterol. 2011;17:391–6.
10. Seyama Y, Kubota K, Sano K, et al. Long term outcome of extended hemihepatectomy for hilar bile duct cancer with no mortality and high survival rate. Ann Surg. 2003;238:73–83.
11. Abdalla EK, Barnett CC, Doherty D, et al. Extended hepatectomy in patients with hepatobiliary malignancies with and without preoperative portal vein embolization. Arch Surg. 2002;137:675–80.
12. Nagino M, Kamiya J, Nishio H, et al. Two hundred forty consecutive portal vein embolizations before extended hepatectomy for biliary cancer: surgical outcome and long term follow-up. Ann Surg. 2006;243:364–72.
13. Bismuth H, Corlette MB. Intrahepatic cholangioenteric anastomosis in carcinoma of the hilus of the liver. Surg Gynecol Obstet. 1975;140:170–8.
14. Jarnagin WR, Fong Y, De Matteo RP, et al. Staging, resectability, and outcome in 225 patients with hilar cholangiocarcinoma. Ann Surg. 2001;234:507–17.

15. Kondo S, Hirano S, Ambo Y, et al. Forty consecutive resections of hilar cholangiocarcinoma with no postoperative mortality and no positive ductal margins: results of a prospective study. Ann Surg. 2004;240:95–101.
16. Seyama Y, Makuuchi M. Current surgical treatment for bile duct cancer. World J Gastroenterol. 2007;13:1505–15.
17. Robles R, Parrilla P, Ramirez P, et al. Liver transplantation increases R0 resection and survival of patients with a non-disseminated unresectable Klatskin tumour. Cir Esp. 2010;87:82–8.
18. Su CH, Tsay SH, Wu CC, et al. Factors influencing postoperative morbidity, mortality, and survival after resection for hilar cholangiocarcinoma. Ann Surg. 1996;223:384–94.
19. Gerhards MF, van Gulik TM, de Wit LT, et al. Evaluation of morbidity and mortality after resection for hilar cholangiocarcinoma- a single center experience. Surgery. 2000;127:395–404.

Chapter 14
Prevention and Treatment of Major Complications After Duodeno-pancreatic Head Surgery

Johanna A.M.G. Tol, Thomas M. van Gulik, Olivier R.C. Busch, and Dirk J. Gouma

Keywords Duodeno pancreatic head surgery • Biliary anastomosis • Whipple procedure • Postoperative bleeding • Pancreatic leakage • Biliary leakage • Angiography

Pancreatic carcinoma is the fourth most deadly cancer in the United States and was responsible for 36.800 deaths in 2010. The incidence is 11/100,000 per year, and in about 80 %, the cancer is located in the pancreas' head. Together with ampullary carcinoma, distal common bile duct carcinoma, and duodenal carcinoma, they are referred to as periampullary carcinomas [1, 2].

When diagnosed the overall 5-year survival rate is around 5 %. While prognosis is poor and survival low, surgical resection remains the only potential curative procedure for periampullary carcinomas. After radical resection the 5-year survival is currently 20–25 % and up to 50 % is found in ampullary tumors [3]. However in 80 % of patients with pancreatic cancer, curative procedure is infeasible, because of local vascular ingrowth or metastatic disease [4]. For patients with a resectable lesion partial pancreatoduodenectomy is the procedure of choice as introduced by Kausch and Whipple, currently modified for a pylorus-preserving pancreatoduodenectomy (PPPD) [5].

In the early years mortality rates of 10–40 % have been reported, but after increasing experience and improved perioperative care, mortality rate reduced to less than 5 % in high-volume centers [6, 7]. With improved results pancreatoduodenectomy (PD) is now widely accepted as treatment of choice for malignant tumors and even used for some benign lesions such as chronic pancreatitis with radiological signs of a mass in the pancreatic head region.

J.A.M.G. Tol • T.M. van Gulik • O.R.C. Busch, MD, PhD • D.J. Gouma, MD (✉)
Department of Surgery, Academic Medical Center,
University of Amsterdam, Amsterdam, The Netherlands
e-mail: o.r.busch@amc.uva.nl; d.j.gouma@amc.uva.nl

M.A. Cuesta, H.J. Bonjer (eds.), *Treatment of Postoperative Complications after Digestive Surgery*, DOI 10.1007/978-1-4471-4354-3_14,

Unfortunately, the procedure is still accompanied by substantial morbidity rates ranging from 40 to 60 % [8–11]. The enormous difference in morbidity is partly due to a wide variety of definitions of complications used in the past. Fortunately the most common complications such as pancreatic anastomotic leakage, hemorrhage, and delayed gastric emptying now have been defined by the International Study Group of Pancreatic Surgery (ISGPS) [12–14]. A more general classification of surgical complication was introduced by Clavien in 2004 in which complications are graded following the invasiveness of their therapeutic interventions [15].

In this chapter we will discuss the diagnoses, grading, and management of the most important complications such as postpancreatectomy hemorrhage, anastomotic leakage, delayed gastric emptying, and chylous leakage as well as prevention and risk factors.

Complications

Anastomotic Leakage

Pancreatic Anastomosis

Incidence and Definition

Leakage of the pancreatic anastomosis is a key determinant in postoperative outcome and the most important complication after pancreatic surgery. It is associated with other complications such as intra-abdominal abscesses, sepsis, bleeding, and delayed gastric emptying that prolong hospital stay and are responsible for up to 88 % of postoperative mortality [9]. Due to a wide range in definitions, highly variable incidence rates between 2 and 30 % are reported in studies on pancreatic anastomotic leakage [16, 17]. The different definitions prevent a validated comparison of incidence and outcomes in different clinical trials. The International Study Group for Pancreatic Fistula (ISGPF) therefore developed a grading system for an objective and universally accepted definition of postoperative pancreatic fistula (POPF). It represents a "failure of healing/sealing of a pancreatic-enteric anastomosis, or it may represent a parenchymal leak not directly related to an anastomosis such as one originating from the raw pancreatic surface" [12].

Diagnosis and Grading

M. Trede reported many years ago the early clinical signs of POPF being abdominal tenderness, a slightly drier tongue, a rise in temperature and pulse, dyspnea, oliguria, and barely perceptible agitation [10]. These simple clinical changes are still the first step in early recognition of this complication. Pancreatic anastomosis leakage is generally recognized between the third and seventh POD (postoperative day).

When POPF is suspected, intra-abdominal drain effluent is tested on amylase contents. Amylase contents higher than three times the upper normal serum value

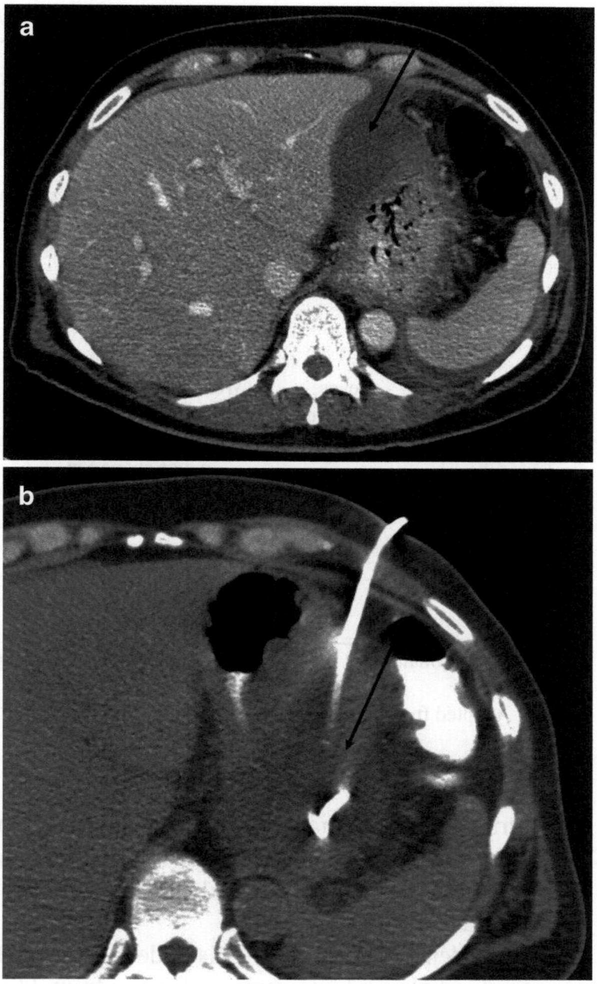

Fig. 14.1 (**a**) CT scan image of a patient after pancreatoduodenectomy who developed an intra-abdominal collection (*arrow*) due to leakage of the pancreaticojejunostomy. (**b**) CT-guided percutaneous drainage (*arrow*) to manage leakage of the pancreaticojejunostomy

associated with the symptoms mentioned above set the diagnosis POPF. Most patients generally will have a thorax X-ray examination because of the dyspnea showing pleural effusion due to the intra-abdominal collections. Computed tomography (CT) will confirm the diagnosis and identify the presence of intra-abdominal collections, see Fig. 14.1a.

Since the definition mentioned above will include clinically well patients with minor complaints, POPF is graded based on its clinical impact and therapeutic consequences following the ISGPF definition (Table 14.1) [12, 18].

Management and Outcome

Depending on the severity of POPF conservative management is adequate in up to 90 % of all patients and includes maintenance of perioperatively placed abdominal drains, supportive intravenous fluid and antibiotics, abstention of oral feeding,

Table 14.1 ISGPF definition postpancreatectomy pancreatic fistula

Grade A	Transient fistula	No clinical impact	No peripancreatic collections on CT scan; little/no change in management	Clinically well; no sepsis; no prolongation of hospital stay; slow removal of operatively placed drains
Grade B		Clinical impact	Peripancreatic drains in place or repositioned to drain collections; change in management is required	Clinically fairly well; degree of infection requiring specific treatment; prolongation of hospital stay; patients often discharged with drains in situ and observed in outpatient setting
Grade C		Severe clinical impact	Worrisome peripancreatic collections that require percutaneous drains; major change in management usually in ICU setting; possible re-surgery to salvage a difficult situation (completion pancreatectomy, etc.)	Clinically unwell; associated sepsis requiring aggressive antibiotics, octreotide, and other intensive care support; major prolongation of hospital stay; associated complications; and possibility of mortality

ISGPF International Study Group on Pancreatic Fistula, *CT* computed tomography, *ICU* intensive care unit
Source: Adapted from Shrikhande et al. [12, 18]

and nutritional support preferably by enteral feeding tube. Radiological intervention such as percutaneous drainage (Fig. 14.1b) is performed when conservative measures are unsuccessful and intra-abdominal collections or abscesses are found indicating a grade B POPF.

The incidence rate of grade B is widely variable, 13–63 %, and so is the frequency of radiological interventions ranging from 7 % up to 17 % in patients with POPF [19–21].

In the case of repeated unsuccessful percutaneous drainage or complications seen in POPF grade C such as sepsis, surgical intervention is almost mandatory. Like grade B POPF, the incidence rate of grade C and its subsequent surgical treatment is variable, ranging from 5.5 % up to 66 % of patients who undergo surgery [22]. The minimal approach during relaparotomy is extensive lavage and drainage. For a total dehiscent anastomosis, a more radical approach is needed. The anastomosis is discontinued, the jejunostomy closed by a stapler, and the pancreatic remnant can be closed and left behind with drainage of the pancreatic duct to create a controlled fistula, or even removed, a so called salvage pancreatectomy. This measure is under debate since definitive endocrine insufficiency is inevitable. More recently some advocate performing a new anastomosis into the stomach, a pancreaticogastrostomy.

In a study conducted in our institute surgical drainage was performed in 20 % of all patients with severe pancreatic leakage and completion pancreatectomy was

Table 14.2 Factors considered influencing the incidence of POPF

Disease and pancreas-related factors	Histopathological diagnosis, pancreatic texture, pancreatic duct size
Surgeon and hospital-related factors	Surgeon volume, hospital volume, hospital resources
Perioperative treatments	Preoperative biliary drainage, neoadjuvant treatment, prophylactic somatostatin or its analogs, perioperative nutritional support
Operative factors	Type of procedure, anastomotic technique, use of fibrin sealants, pancreatic duct stenting, intraoperative blood loss, perioperative transfusions, operative time, use of intraperitoneal drains
Patient-related factors	Age, gender, obesity, cardiovascular diseases, diabetes mellitus

POPF postoperative pancreatic fistula
Source: Adapted from Ramacciato et al. [23]

performed in 22 %. This study also showed a significant reduction in the overall relaparotomy rate of 16.1–7.7 % ($P=0.005$) in the period 1992–2002, despite a stable leakage rate, which has been further reduced during the past 10 years, indicating improvement of the nonsurgical management [22].

Radiological interventions have gained a more prominent role in the management of complications in most recent studies. These minimal-invasive techniques will shorten hospital stay and lower mortality rates and hospital costs by preventing extensive surgical procedures.

Risk Factors and Prevention

Many factors influence the incidence of POPF after PD as depicted in Table 14.2 [23]. Some factors are more significant than others. Generally accepted to be the most important risk factors are disease and pancreas-related factors as well as surgeons' experience and hospital volume.

Yeo et al. reported the strongest predictors of POPF being ampullary or duodenal disease and surgical volume [24]. Others reported additional risk factors in their multivariate analyses: coronary artery disease (OR 3.7; 95 % CI 1.2–12.1), a soft gland (OR 10.0; 95 % CI 2.1–47.6), and pancreatic duct diameter ≤3 mm (RR 2.5; 95 % CI 1.05–9.5). Similar predictive factors were found in our study: pancreatic duct size ≤2 mm ($P=0.002$), operating time ≥285 min ($P=0.031$), and ampullary adenocarcinoma ($P=0.035$) [22, 25].

Several surgical techniques have been described in order to find the optimal reconstruction after PD and prevent high rates of POPF. Two randomized controlled trials (RCT) compared the two most common techniques: pancreaticojejunostomy (PJ) versus pancreaticogastrostomy (PG). However, no superiority of either PJ or PG was reported [24, 26].

New techniques different from the conventional anastomotic techniques have been described in two other RCTs. A significant decrease in clinically relevant POPF from 18 % to 4 % was reported after comparing pancreaticogastrostomy with gastric partition versus conventional PJ, in favor of the PG with gastric partition ($P=0.01$) [27]. A new pancreaticojejunostomy binding technique compared with conventional PJ reported leakage rates in 0 % versus 7.2 %, respectively (OR 1.08; 95 % CI 1.02–1.14; $P=0.014$) [28].

The most optimal technique for the PJ reconstruction is still under debate ranging from end-to-side, duct-to-mucosa, to invagination, but only two randomized trials were performed. One study showed fewer POPF cases after the invagination technique compared with the duct-to-mucosa PJ (12 % vs. 24 %, $P=0.04$), though another study revealed no significant differences in POPF rates in patients with soft pancreatic texture when duct-to-mucosa was compared to end-to-side PJ. Another ongoing debate is one- or two-layer reconstruction with continuous or interrupted sutures, but no differences are reported. The experience of the surgeon with one of these techniques is the most important determinant [29].

Procedures to avoid a pancreatic anastomosis and thereby avoiding POPF have also been described. Occlusion of pancreatic duct after PD showed no difference in postoperative complications [30]. Total pancreatectomy will of course avoid anastomotic leakage but is associated with endocrine pancreatic insufficiency.

Drainage of the pancreatic duct as a preventive measure was studied in three RCTs. They compared drainage versus no drainage after PD. Internal pancreatic duct drainage did not reduce the POPF rate; however two studies reported a significantly lower rate after external drainage (26 % vs. 42 %, $P=0.034$; 6.7 % vs. 20 %, $P=0.032$) [20, 25, 31]. The role of fibrin glue was also evaluated but no decrease in POPF rates was reported [32].

Pharmacological intervention is another major preventive measure. Lai et al. reviewed 11 RCTs in which 6 showed a decreased postoperative complication rate after the use of perioperative somatostatin, but the other 5 did not. Two studies reported significantly less POPF cases in the somatostatin group ($P<0.05$). Though, due to the contradictory outcomes, the use of somatostatin remains controversial [9].

In conclusion, many different aspects to prevent leakage have been analyzed, and so far none have been proven superior in meta-analyses or large RCTs. The surgeon's experience in performing the anastomosis might be the most important factor, but new techniques/modifications as pancreaticogastrostomy with gastric partition, the invagination procedure, as well as stenting of the anastomosis are promising, but more research is necessary to prove superiority of any of those procedures.

Biliary Anastomosis

Incidence and Definition

Leakage of the hepaticojejunostomy is reported between 0.4 and 10 % of the patients after pancreatic surgery. It can initiate a biliary peritonitis and is associated with concomitant complications such as intra-abdominal abscesses, bleeding, and wound infection. This prolongs hospital stay and decreases quality of life. Unlike pancreatic leakage, it is a rare complication with very low mortality rates ranging from 1 to 3 % [33].

Table 14.3 Proposal of the ISGLS for grading bile leakage after hepatobiliary and pancreatic surgery

Grade A	Bile leakage requiring no or little change in patients' clinical management
Grade B	Bile leakage requiring a change in patients clinical management (e.g., additional diagnostic or interventional procedures) but manageable without relaparotomy *or* a grade A bile leakage lasting for >1 week
Grade C	Bile leakage requiring relaparotomy

ISGLS International Study Group of Liver Surgery
Source: Adapted from Koch et al. [34]

The International Study Group of Liver Surgery (ISGLS) recently developed a uniform definition and grading system of biliary leakage. It is defined as bile-stained fluid in the abdominal drain or biliary collections in the abdominal cavity in need for radiological or surgical intervention. Bilirubin concentration of the drained fluid is at least three times the serum bilirubin concentration [34].

Diagnosis and Grading

Biliary leakage is suspected when bile-stained fluid is present in the abdominal drain. Other anastomotic leakages have to be ruled out and ultrasonography and CT can detect any intra-abdominal perihepatic collections. Diagnostic aspiration of the collection will establish the diagnosis of biliary leakage. Magnetic resonance cholangiopancreatography (MRCP) can be used to detect the location of the leak.

In patients with biliary leakage, typical laboratory abnormalities are seen: isolated hyperbilirubinemia with normal Gamma-glutamyl transpeptidase and alkaline phosphatase due to the lack of obstruction.

The clinical characteristics and grading parameters are summarized in Table 14.3 [34].

Management and Outcome

Maintenance of preoperatively placed drains is the first step in managing biliary leakage. However in the case of an insufficiently drained leakage, percutaneous transhepatic biliary drainage (Fig. 14.2) is the treatment of choice and is performed in nearly 70 % of patients. A catheter is placed into the biliary system and preferably through the anastomosis into the jejunal loop which facilitates external and internal drainage.

This procedure changed the aggressive management of early relaparotomy in which the leakage was drained externally and abdominal lavage was performed. Anastomotic repair was performed when necessary but is currently avoided by the percutaneous approach. Surgical management is now only performed in less than 20 % of patients after drainage is unsuccessful or patients' clinical status asks for an immediate aggressive approach seen in grade C.

Prevention and Risk Factors

In a multivariate analysis, we found three independent predictors of biliary leakage: obesity BMI ≥ 35 (OR 11.32, 95 % CI 1.71–75, $P = 0.012$), no preoperative endoscopic biliary drainage (OR 2.43, 95 % CI 1.03–5.78, $P = 0.044$), and segmental anastomosis (OR 13.56, 95 % CI 4.23–43.49, $P < 0.001$) [33].

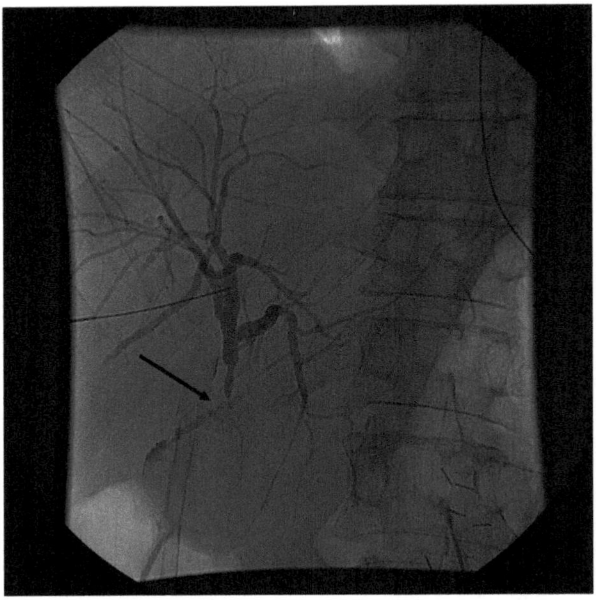

Fig. 14.2 Patient presenting with bile leakage after pancreatoduodenectomy. Cholangiogram reveals leakage of the hepaticojejunostomy (*arrow*). Percutaneous transhepatic biliary drainage is performed to manage the leakage

Preventing leakage of the hepaticojejunostomy can be achieved by placing a stent in the common bile duct during operation providing the bile to leak through the stent into the jejunum or drained externally.

Enteric Anastomosis

Incidence and Definition

Enteric anastomotic leak is very rarely seen after pancreatic surgery. Only one article solely describes duodenojejunostomy (DJ) or gastrojejunostomy (GJ) leakage after PPPD or standard PD, respectively [35]. The clinical symptoms might be the same as leakage of the PJ or HJ. Most large studies do not report DJ or GJ leak separately, simply because the complication did not occur, or in a low incidence rate ranging from 0.4 % to 1.2 %. The incidence is comparable with rates reported in other upper gastrointestinal operations. DJ or GJ leakage was defined as radiographic or visual evidence of the anastomotic defect [30, 35].

Diagnosis and Grading

DJ or GJ leakage can present within the first 10 days after surgery with one or more of the following clinical signs: an acute abdomen, fever, or enterocutaneous fistula or loss of bowel contents via the abdominal drain. Laboratory results will often reveal a leukocytosis. Radiological signs that indicate anastomotic failure will reveal free air on X-ray and fluid collections on CT (Fig. 14.3).

DJ or GJ leakage has been graded in a study previously mentioned according to the Clavien complication grading system [15].

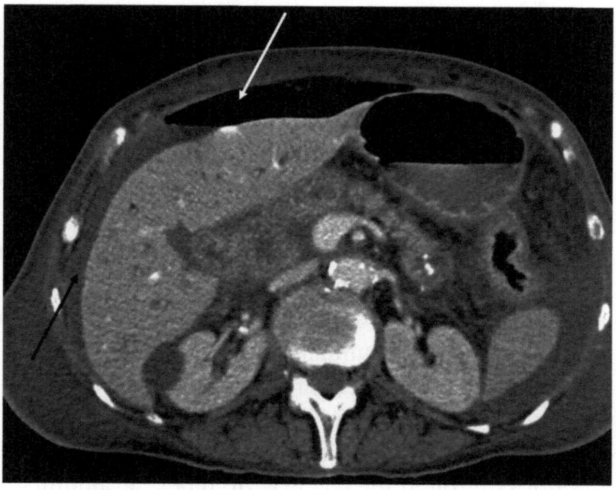

Fig. 14.3 CT scan image of a patient after pylorus-preserving pancreatoduodenectomy presenting with abdominal pain and fever revealing intra-abdominal free air (*white arrow*) and collections (*black arrow*) suggestive for leakage of the duodenojejunostomy

Management and Outcome

DJ or GJ leakage is a potentially fatal complication, it can prolong hospital stay with up to 25 days and surgical management is often required. In a study mentioned above, 12 out of 13 patients underwent relaparotomy. In >80 % of these patients, a distal gastrectomy had to be performed followed by new reconstruction. Only one patient was treated radiological with percutaneous drainage. Mortality rate reported in this study was substantial (38 %) [35].

Prevention and Risk Factors

Due to the low incidence, multivariate models of risk factors are unavailable. Furthermore the causes of these complications are unknown, but impaired perfusion of the anastomosis and a poorly vascularized duodenal stump might be causative factors in particular for the pylorus-preserving pancreatoduodenectomy.

Postpancreatectomy Hemorrhage

Incidence and Definition

Postoperative hemorrhage is another serious complication after pancreatic resection with incidence rates varying from 2 to 20 % and mortality rates exceeding 50 % [36]. The variability in incidence and mortality is partly caused by the many different definitions that are being used. Furthermore, substantial differences are seen in onset, cause, bleeding site, intensity, and clinical impairment of postoperative hemorrhage.

To enable a comparison between different surgical techniques in pancreatic surgery and the consequential incidence rate of postoperative hemorrhage and its mortality, one widely accepted definition is needed. The International Study Group of Pancreatic Surgery (ISGPS) developed a definition and proposed the term postpancreatectomy hemorrhage (PPH) [13]. They classified postoperative bleeding based on three criteria: time of onset, early PPH occurring within 24 h postoperatively and late PPH >24 h; location, intraluminal or extraluminal; and severity and impact, mild PPH with a similar clinical impairment and severe PPH with sequential blood transfusions and radiological and/or surgical interventions.

Since the introduction of the ISGPS hemorrhage classification, a number of studies validated the scoring system which is currently generally accepted [36, 37].

Diagnosis and Grading

Patients who develop PPH may present with hypotension, tachycardia, decreasing hemoglobin concentration, clinical deterioration, or blood loss through the gastrointestinal tract or abdominal drains depending on the site of the bleeding: intraluminal or extraluminal.

Intraluminal bleedings are seen near the anastomotic site, vessels in that area, the surface of the pancreas, or near a gastric ulcus. They generally present with blood loss through the gastrointestinal tract being hematemesis, melaena, and blood loss through the nasogastric tube. Intraluminal bleeding will usually manifest as an early hemorrhage. Consensus has been reached considering the cause of early hemorrhage which is likely due to technical failures during the index operation. In the case of intraluminal hemorrhage, endoscopy can be very useful since diagnosing and managing an anastomotic bleeding can be performed simultaneously. Angiography can be used to embolize bleeding from vessels. A recent analysis showed that angiography was performed in over 50 % of patients with PPH after pancreatic surgery and 18 % was subjected to an endoscopy. Both procedures were initially performed to detect the bleeding site [38]. All diagnostic interventions were performed provided that the patient was in a stable hemodynamic condition.

Extraluminal bleedings are seen in the abdominal cavity and may be evident by blood loss through the abdominal drain. The bleedings are caused by vascular erosion, anastomotic ulceration, arterial pseudoaneurysm, or disrupted suture line caused by POPF, biliary leakage, or intra-abdominal infections and generally present as late PPH. When PPH is suspected, ultrasonography and CT can detect intra-abdominal collections (hematoma as well as abscesses) seen in 70–80 % in late PPH. Furthermore, both procedures can detect pseudoaneurysms. The diagnosis is confirmed by angiography [39].

Blood loss through abdominal drains or nasogastric tubes is called a sentinel bleed and can be seen hours or even days before massive hemorrhage. Jagad et al. reviewed several studies and showed that in 30–100 %, a sentinel bleed resulted in PPH hours or days later [36]. A study performed in our institute reported that in 78 % of patients, a sentinel bleed was detected prior to late PPH and 74 % of patients with late PPH had septic complications [39].

When PPH is diagnosed, the clinical grading system proposed by the ISGPS classification, summarized in Table 14.4, can be used to state the severity of the hemorrhage [13].

Management and Outcome

Severe PPH asks for immediate treatment through either radiological intervention, e.g., angiography with embolization (Figs. 14.4a and b, 14.5a and b) or

Table 14.4 Proposal of the ISGPS for grading PPH after pancreatic surgery [13]

Grade A	Results in a temporary and marginal variation of the standard postoperative course
Grade B	Additional diagnostics and interventions are required leading to therapeutic consequences such as blood transfusion, intensive care necessity or even relaparotomy, or embolization
Grade C	A life-threatening situation in which surgical and radiological interventions are mandatory

ISGPS International Study Group, *PPH* postpancreatectomy hemorrhage

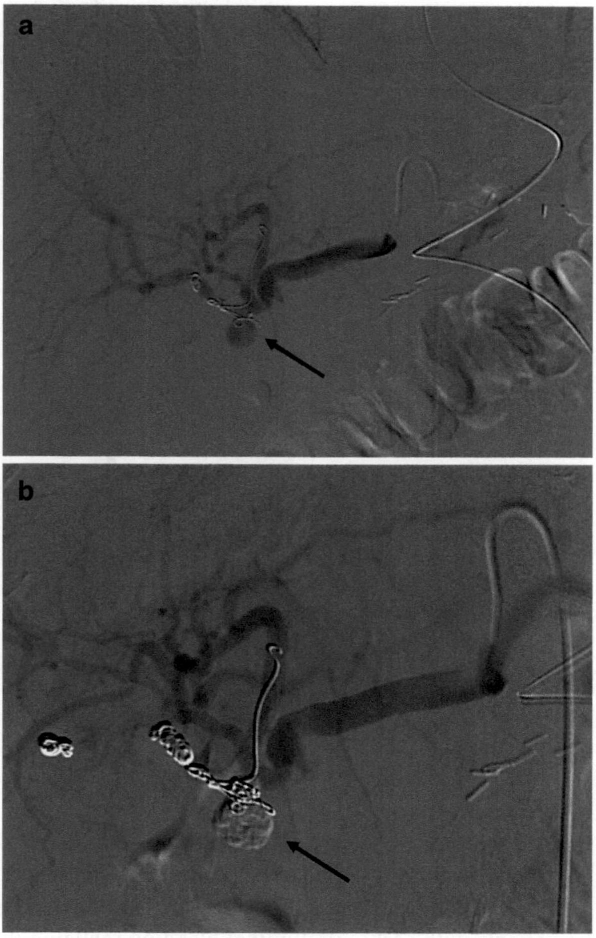

Fig. 14.4 Patient presenting with severe melaena after pancreatoduodenectomy was performed. Angiography of the arteria hepatica communis reveals a pseudoaneurysm shown in (**a**) (arrow) which is treated by means of coiling shown in (**b**) (*arrow*)

endoscopy with clips or sclerotherapy, or surgical intervention when the patients' condition is deteriorating rapidly or radiological interventions are unsuccessful or infeasible.

In a recent study on PPH, 38 % of patients underwent primary surgery, 57 % underwent primary radiological intervention, and 5 % were treated conservatively.

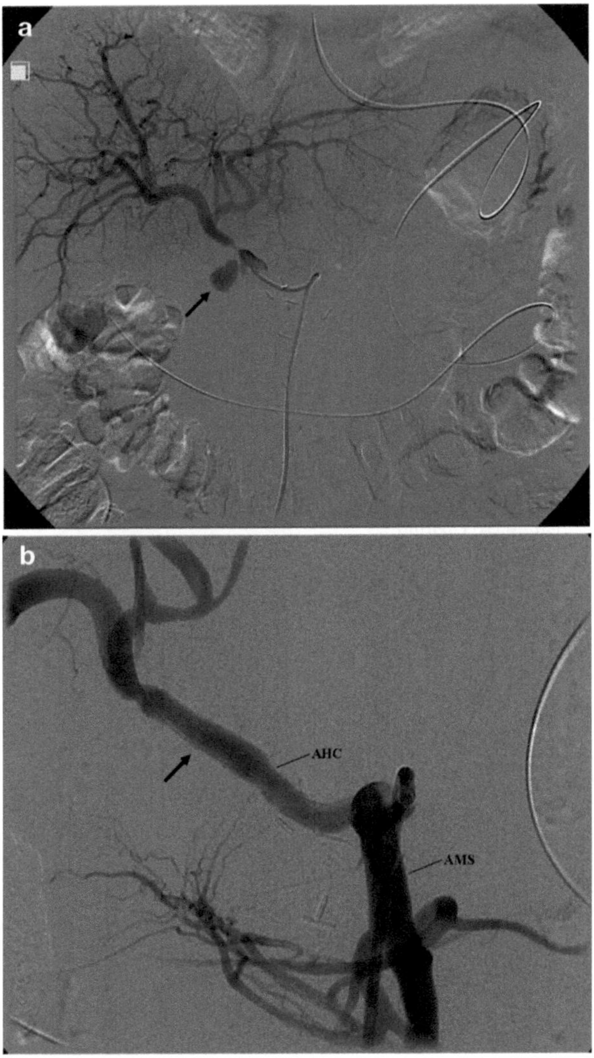

Fig. 14.5 Patient presenting with hematemesis after pancreatoduodenectomy was performed. Angiography reveals an aberrant arteria hepatica communis (AHC) originating from the arteria mesenterica superior (AMS) and a pseudoaneurysm of the arteria gastroduodenalis shown in (**a**) (*arrow*). A covered stent is placed in the arteria hepatica communis to manage the pseudoaneurysm shown in (**b**) (*arrow*)

More than half of the radiological interventions (54 %) were unsuccessful and a rescue laparotomy still had to be performed. The success rate of radiological coiling in terms of hemostasis was 80 % [38]. In this study endoscopic intervention was used in patients with early intraluminal bleeding realizing that a PJ bleeding generally is outside the reach of endoscopy but can also be managed by interventional angiography. Intraluminal bleeding can disrupt the anastomosis, causing a "false" extraluminal bleed since blood is then seen in the abdominal cavity. Early extraluminal PPH (within 24 h after surgery) is generally managed immediately with relaparotomy.

Management of late PPH is different since it is often caused by pseudoaneurysms due to POPF or intra-abdominal infections. An earlier study conducted at the AMC showed that 69 % of patients with late PPH underwent primary surgery and

Table 14.5 Therapeutic interventions in delayed massive hemorrhage [39]

Therapeutic intervention	Patients with late PPH (n = 23)
Conservative	2/5
Embolization	2/2
Surgical hemostasis	14/16
Anastomotic resection and reconstruction	2/3
Vessel ligation	8/8
Completion pancreatectomy	4/4
Exploration	0/1

PPH postpancreatectomy hemorrhage (no. successful/no. performed)

only 9 % were managed by radiological embolization. In half of all the surgical procedures, a vessel ligation was performed. Completion pancreatectomy was performed because of persistent anastomotic leakage (Table 14.5) [39].

More recently embolization is performed in the majority of patients.

A meta-analysis regarding the management of late PPH after PD showed 20 small case series with 163 patients in which 47.2 % of patients underwent primary surgery, 44.8 % underwent primary radiological intervention, and 8 % were treated conservatively. No significant differences were found regarding the morbidity or mortality between relaparotomy and radiological intervention. Though late hemorrhage is often already associated with other complications, in particular leakage and sepsis, as mentioned earlier, this combination is associated with a poor prognosis [40].

The pathophysiology of early PPH makes its management less complicated with better outcomes compared to late PPH. Identifying the importance of a sentinel bleed and an adequate aggressive approach towards the patients' clinical status will dictate the appropriate treatment. More research is needed to offer any standardized rules in the management of PPH.

Prevention and Risk Factors

The two most important predictive factors in PPH are sentinel bleed and pancreatic fistula [39]. A multivariate analysis reported three significant risk factors being pancreatic leakage (OR 3.5; 95 % CI 1.8–6.1), gastrojejunostomy leakage (OR 9.2; 95 % CI 1.5–56), and intra-abdominal abscess (OR 7.8; CI 4.2–14) [41]. Others suggest extended lymph node dissection being a risk factor [36]. PPH can be minimized by optimal preoperative preparation of the patient, exact attention to details during surgery, and close observation of the patient postoperatively.

Delayed Gastric Emptying

Incidence and Definition

The most common complication after pancreatoduodenectomy is delayed gastric emptying (DGE). Although DGE is not associated with a high mortality, it does have a severe impact on the postoperative course, hospital stay, and quality of life. It is most often found in patients with intra-abdominal complications. Although the

Table 14.6 Proposal of the ISGPS for grading DGE after pancreatic surgery

DGE grade	NGT required	Unable to tolerate solid oral intake by POD	Vomiting/gastric distension	Use of prokinetics
A	4–7 days or reinsertion > POD 3	7	±	±
B	8–14 days or reinsertion > POD 7	14	+	+
C	>14 days or reinsertion > POD 14	21	+	+

ISGPS International Study Group of Pancreatic Surgery, *DGE* delayed gastric emptying, *NGT* nasogastric tube, *POD* postoperative day
Source: Adapted from Wente et al. [14]

pathogenesis of primary DGE, without intra-abdominal complications, still remains unclear disruption of the neural connections, ischemic injury to the muscle mechanism and low levels of circulating motilin are thought to be involved.

Due to the lack of a generally accepted definition, the reported incidence rates vary widely from 5 to 57 % [42]. More recently, the International Study Group of Pancreatic Surgery (ISGPS) developed an objective and generally applicable definition with different grades [14]. The definition takes several aspects into account:

- Duration of nasogastric tube (NGT) and/or need for reinsertion of NGT
- Ability to tolerate solid oral intake
- Severity
- Therapeutic consequences

Diagnosis and Grading

The different grades of DGE describe its severity and clinical impact (Table 14.6) [14].

DGE is an early complication seen after pancreatic surgery. Patients are unable to tolerate solid oral intake by POD 7 and NGT is required for 4 days or more. When DGE arises, the underlying cause and in particular intra-abdominal collections due to leakage have to be excluded and generally a CT scan is performed. Diagnostic procedures to assess the gastric emptying are not routinely used but scintigraphy is considered the most accurate method for measurement of DGE [43].

Management and Outcome

The required intervention depends on the severity of DGE. Grade A will have no interventional consequences, but in grade C DGE adequate management aimed at the cause is necessary. When DGE is caused by intra-abdominal complications, managing these complications will subsequently manage DGE.

Standard treatment of DGE is mainly supportive by maintenance of perioperatively placed nasogastric tube and nutritional support preferably by the enteral route despite the fact that enteral infusion can potentially impair gastric emptying. A randomized trial was conducted in our institute to assess the effect of cyclic versus continuous enteral feeding on DGE. Cyclic enteral feeding after PPPD was associated with a shorter period of enteral nutrition, faster return to a normal diet ($P=0.04$), and a shorter hospital stay ($P=0.04$) [44].

Massive production of the NGT might lead to electrolyte and body fluid disturbances, and in these circumstances parental supplementation is mandatory.

Therapeutic measures have been sought to minimize the incidence of DGE. The reduction in circulating motilin levels after PD is thought to be causing DGE. Motilin agonists, erythromycin, have been administered in order to improve gastric emptying. DGE was reported in 14.3 % of patients who were administered erythromycin versus 57.1 % of patients who did not received erythromycin ($P<0.04$) [42].

Prevention and Risk Factors

Since the causes of DGE are unclear and likely to be multifactorial, it is difficult to take preventive measures. Various surgical techniques have been appointed to decrease the incidence of DGE.

Extended research has been conducted on the outcomes of standard PD versus pylorus-preserving PD (PPPD). A recently published RCT revealed that standard PD significantly reduces the incidence of DGE compared with PPPD ($P=0.02$) [45]. However three systematic reviews failed to report this. They did report perioperative differences, PPPD was a faster procedure (95 % CI −105.70 to −30.83; $P=0.0004$) with less intraoperative blood loss (95 % CI −0.96 to −0.56; $P<0.00001$) [46–48].

Two meta-analyses compared standard PD with extended lymphadenectomy PD and revealed slightly higher DGE rates in the extended group [49, 50]. The largest RCT reported DGE in 6 % in the PD group and in 16 % in the extended PD group ($P=0.006$) [51]. Explanation for this difference might be that more complex operations, with increased operation time and more blood loss, have a higher chance of DGE.

A more recently published study on DGE analyzed the effect of antecolic versus retrocolic reconstruction of the enterojejunostomy. DGE was seen in 30.9 % and no differences were found between the two techniques (antecolic 34 % vs. retrocolic 28 %, $P=0.6$). Age was the only significant predictive factor found after multivariate analysis ($P=0.02$) [52]. Another RCT did however show a significant difference. DGE was reported in 5 % in the antecolic group and in 50 % in the retrocolic group ($P=0.0014$), but the study population was very limited (n=40) [53]. Currently an RCT is being conducted in our own institute regarding DGE after retrocolic versus antecolic reconstruction of the duodenojejunostomy (registration number NTR1697).

The influence of prophylactic octreotide on DGE was analyzed in an RCT but failed to show an effect. They did however identify preoperative biliary drainage as an independent risk factor (OR 3.8; 95 % CI 0.98-14.9; $P=0.054$) [54].

Chylous Leakage

Incidence and Definition

Chylous leakage is caused by injury to the lymphatic system. The cisterna chyli, a saccular dilatation which contains ascending lymphatic trunks, is located on the

Table 14.7 Proposed grading system for isolated chylous leakage after pancreatoduodenectomy

Criteria	Grade A	Grade B	Grade C
Clinical conditions	Well	Often well	Ill appearing
Signs of infection	No	No	Yes
Ultrasound/CT (if obtained)	Negative	Negative/positive	Positive
Duration of CA production	< 7 days	7–14 days	>14 days
Dietary measure	Yes/no	Yes	Yes
Persistent drainage	No	Usually yes	Yes
Surgical intervention	No	No	Yes/no
Prolongation of hospital stay	No	Yes	Yes
Readmission	No	No	Yes/no

CT computed tomography, *CA* chylous ascites
Source: Adapted from Gaag et al. [57]

same level as the pancreas and injury to the cisterna chyli or its tributaries can occur during pancreatic dissection from the back site.

Chylous leakage is a rare complication; thus little is known about its incidence and management. Recent studies report a wide variation and incidence rates of 1.8, 5, 6.7, and 11 % [55–57]. In the absence of a uniform definition, our center proposed a grading system and a clear definition of chylous leakage. Chylous leakage was defined as a drain output of ≥275 mL with milky appearance and triglyceride level higher then 1.2 mmol/L in the absence of anastomotic leakage [57].

Diagnosis and Grading

Chylous leakage is usually seen on POD 1 or 2. It can appear as painless abdominal distension and respiratory embarrassment and can cause weight loss and fatigue. The appearance of the drain output and its high levels of triglycerides are sufficient to set the diagnosis. In some cases, CT can be helpful and some authors report more invasive diagnostic measures such as lymphangiography and lymphoscintigraphy [58]. However these techniques are very rarely used in daily practice.

Chylous leakage is graded in order to predict the severity and clinical impact (Table 14.7) [57].

Management and Outcome

In general, dietary therapy is the most frequently used conservative management. Enteral feeding with high protein and low fat with low or median-chain triglycerides is the treatment of choice. When enteral intake is impossible, total parenteral nutrition (TPN) is given. TPN is also given as an addition to enteral feeding when enteral feeding alone is insufficient [57]. The combination of dietary measures and somatostatin has been reported to be beneficial as well [55]. Paracentesis is performed when conservative measures alone are not adequate and is reported to be sufficient in up to 100 % [57]. Like the invasive diagnostic procedures, rigorous therapeutic measures for chylous leakage such as relaparotomy or a peritoneovenous shunt to close the leakage of the cisterna chyli are rarely performed [56].

Prevention and Risk Factors

Several factors were associated with a higher risk of chylous leakage. In a multivariate analysis, an increasing number of lymph nodes harvested (OR 1.07; 95 % CI 1.02–1.13; $P=0.007$) and vascular resection at the time of surgery (OR 8.25; 95 % CI 1.99–34.6; $P=0.004$) were two prognostic factors. Chronic pancreatitis was another independent-associated factor (OR 2.52; 95 % CI 1.19–5.32; $P=0.016$) [56, 57].

Summary

Pancreatic surgery is associated with a high incidence of complications. The most severe combination of complications responsible for high mortality rates is anastomotic leakage and hemorrhage. Clinical observation and an adequate approach are important in the postoperative management. This postoperative management has shifted over the last decade, and a nonoperative management is seen more often in which radiological intervention plays an important role.

References

1. Jemal A, Siegel R, Xu J, Ward E. Cancer statistics, 2010. CA Cancer J Clin. 2010; 60(5):277–300.
2. Sharma C, Eltawil KM, Renfrew PD, Walsh MJ, Molinari M. Advances in diagnosis, treatment and palliation of pancreatic carcinoma: 1990–2010. World J Gastroenterol. 2011;17(7): 867–97.
3. Riall TS, Cameron JL, Lillemoe KD, Campbell KA, Sauter PK, Coleman J, et al. Pancreaticoduodenectomy with or without distal gastrectomy and extended retroperitoneal lymphadenectomy for periampullary adenocarcinoma–part 3: update on 5-year survival. J Gastrointest Surg. 2005;9(9):1191–204.
4. Kuhlmann KF, de Castro SM, Wesseling JG, ten Kate FJ, Offerhaus GJ, Busch OR, et al. Surgical treatment of pancreatic adenocarcinoma; actual survival and prognostic factors in 343 patients. Eur J Cancer. 2004;40(4):549–58.
5. Whipple AO, Parsons WB, Mullins CRTREATMENTOFCARCINOMAOFTHE AMPULLAOFVATER. Ann Surg. 1935;102(4):763–79.
6. van Heek NT, Kuhlmann KF, Scholten RJ, de Castro SM, Busch OR, van Gulik TM, et al. Hospital volume and mortality after pancreatic resection: a systematic review and an evaluation of intervention in the Netherlands. Ann Surg. 2005;242(6):781–8.
7. Finks JF, Osborne NH, Birkmeyer JD. Trends in hospital volume and operative mortality for high-risk surgery. N Engl J Med. 2011;364(22):2128–37.
8. DeOliveira ML, Winter JM, Schafer M, Cunningham SC, Cameron JL, Yeo CJ, et al. Assessment of complications after pancreatic surgery: A novel grading system applied to 633 patients undergoing pancreaticoduodenectomy. Ann Surg. 2006;244(6):931–7.
9. Lai EC, Lau SH, Lau WY. Measures to prevent pancreatic fistula after pancreatoduodenectomy: a comprehensive review. Arch Surg. 2009;144(11):1074–80.
10. Trede M, Schwall G. The complications of pancreatectomy. Ann Surg. 1988;207(1):39–47.
11. Gouma DJ, van Geenen RC, van Gulik TM, de Haan RJ, de Wit LT, Busch OR, et al. Rates of complications and death after pancreaticoduodenectomy: risk factors and the impact of hospital volume. Ann Surg. 2000;232(6):786–95.

12. Bassi C, Dervenis C, Butturini G, Fingerhut A, Yeo C, Izbicki J, et al. Postoperative pancreatic fistula: an international study group (ISGPF) definition. Surgery. 2005;138(1):8–13.
13. Wente MN, Veit JA, Bassi C, Dervenis C, Fingerhut A, Gouma DJ, et al. Postpancreatectomy hemorrhage (PPH): an International Study Group of Pancreatic Surgery (ISGPS) definition. Surgery. 2007;142(1):20–5.
14. Wente MN, Bassi C, Dervenis C, Fingerhut A, Gouma DJ, Izbicki JR, et al. Delayed gastric emptying (DGE) after pancreatic surgery: a suggested definition by the International Study Group of Pancreatic Surgery (ISGPS). Surgery. 2007;142(5):761–8.
15. Dindo D, Demartines N, Clavien PA. Classification of surgical complications: a new proposal with evaluation in a cohort of 6336 patients and results of a survey. Ann Surg. 2004;240(2):205–13.
16. McKay A, Mackenzie S, Sutherland FR, Bathe OF, Doig C, Dort J, et al. Meta-analysis of pancreaticojejunostomy versus pancreaticogastrostomy reconstruction after pancreaticoduodenectomy. Br J Surg. 2006;93(8):929–36.
17. Wente MN, Shrikhande SV, Muller MW, Diener MK, Seiler CM, Friess H, et al. Pancreaticojejunostomy versus pancreaticogastrostomy: systematic review and meta-analysis. Am J Surg. 2007;193(2):171–83.
18. Shrikhande SV, D'Souza MA. Pancreatic fistula after pancreatectomy: evolving definitions, preventive strategies and modern management. World J Gastroenterol. 2008;14(38):5789–96.
19. Berger AC, Howard TJ, Kennedy EP, Sauter PK, Bower-Cherry M, Dutkevitch S, et al. Does type of pancreaticojejunostomy after pancreaticoduodenectomy decrease rate of pancreatic fistula? A randomized, prospective, dual-institution trial. J Am Coll Surg. 2009;208(5):738–47.
20. Pessaux P, Sauvanet A, Mariette C, Paye F, Muscari F, Cunha AS, et al. External Pancreatic Duct Stent Decreases Pancreatic Fistula Rate After Pancreaticoduodenectomy: Prospective Multicenter Randomized Trial. Ann Surg. 2011;253(5):879–85.
21. Prenzel KL, Holscher AH, Grabolle I, Fetzner U, Kleinert R, Gutschow CA, et al. Impact of duct-to-mucosa pancreaticojejunostomy with external drainage of the pancreatic duct after pancreaticoduodenectomy. J Surg Res. 2011;171:558–62.
22. de Castro SM, Busch OR, van Gulik TM, Obertop H, Gouma DJ. Incidence and management of pancreatic leakage after pancreatoduodenectomy. Br J Surg. 2005;92(9):1117–23.
23. Ramacciato G, Mercantini P, Petrucciani N, Nigri GR, Kazemi A, Muroni M, et al. Risk factors of pancreatic fistula after pancreaticoduodenectomy: a collective review. Am Surg. 2011;77(3):257–69.
24. Yeo CJ, Cameron JL, Maher MM, Sauter PK, Zahurak ML, Talamini MA, et al. A prospective randomized trial of pancreaticogastrostomy versus pancreaticojejunostomy after pancreaticoduodenectomy. Ann Surg. 1995;222(4):580–8.
25. Poon RT, Fan ST, Lo CM, Ng KK, Yuen WK, Yeung C, et al. External drainage of pancreatic duct with a stent to reduce leakage rate of pancreaticojejunostomy after pancreaticoduodenectomy: a prospective randomized trial. Ann Surg. 2007;246(3):425–33.
26. Duffas JP, Suc B, Msika S, Fourtanier G, Muscari F, Hay JM, et al. A controlled randomized multicenter trial of pancreatogastrostomy or pancreatojejunostomy after pancreatoduodenectomy. Am J Surg. 2005;189(6):720–9.
27. Fernandez-Cruz L, Cosa R, Blanco L, Lopez-Boado MA, Astudillo E. Pancreatogastrostomy with gastric partition after pylorus-preserving pancreatoduodenectomy versus conventional pancreatojejunostomy: a prospective randomized study. Ann Surg. 2008;248(6):930–8.
28. Peng SY, Wang JW, Lau WY, Cai XJ, Mou YP, Liu YB, et al. Conventional versus binding pancreaticojejunostomy after pancreaticoduodenectomy: a prospective randomized trial. Ann Surg. 2007;245(5):692–8.
29. Bassi C, Falconi M, Molinari E, Mantovani W, Butturini G, Gumbs AA, et al. Duct-to-mucosa versus end-to-side pancreaticojejunostomy reconstruction after pancreaticoduodenectomy: results of a prospective randomized trial. Surgery. 2003;134(5):766–71.

30. Tran K, Van Eijck C, Di Carlo V, Hop WC, Zerbi A, Balzano G, et al. Occlusion of the pancreatic duct versus pancreaticojejunostomy: a prospective randomized trial. Ann Surg. 2002;236(4):422–8.
31. Winter JM, Cameron JL, Campbell KA, Chang DC, Riall TS, Schulick RD, et al. Does pancreatic duct stenting decrease the rate of pancreatic fistula following pancreaticoduodenectomy? Results of a prospective randomized trial. J Gastrointest Surg. 2006;10(9):1280–90.
32. Lillemoe KD, Cameron JL, Kim MP, Campbell KA, Sauter PK, Coleman JA, et al. Does fibrin glue sealant decrease the rate of pancreatic fistula after pancreaticoduodenectomy? Results of a prospective randomized trial. J Gastrointest Surg. 2004;8(7):766–72.
33. de Castro SM, Kuhlmann KF, Busch OR, van Delden OM, Lameris JS, van Gulik TM, et al. Incidence and management of biliary leakage after hepaticojejunostomy. J Gastrointest Surg. 2005;9(8):1163–71.
34. Koch M, Garden OJ, Padbury R, Rahbari NN, Adam R, Capussotti L, et al. Bile leakage after hepatobiliary and pancreatic surgery: A definition and grading of severity by the International Study Group of Liver Surgery. Surgery. 2011;149(5):680–8.
35. Winter JM, Cameron JL, Yeo CJ, Lillemoe KD, Campbell KA, Schulick RD. Duodenojejunostomy leaks after pancreaticoduodenectomy. J Gastrointest Surg. 2008;12(2): 263–9.
36. Jagad RB, Koshariya M, Kawamoto J, Chude GS, Neeraj RV, Lygidakis NJ. Postoperative hemorrhage after major pancreatobiliary surgery: an update. Hepatogastroenterology. 2008;55(82–83):729–37.
37. Puppala S, Patel J, McPherson S, Nicholson A, Kessel D. Hemorrhagic complications after Whipple surgery: imaging and radiologic intervention. AJR Am J Roentgenol. 2011;196(1):192–7.
38. Yekebas EF, Wolfram L, Cataldegirmen G, Habermann CR, Bogoevski D, Koenig AM, et al. Postpancreatectomy hemorrhage: diagnosis and treatment: an analysis in 1669 consecutive pancreatic resections. Ann Surg. 2007;246(2):269–80.
39. de Castro SM, Kuhlmann KF, Busch OR, van Delden OM, Lameris JS, van Gulik TM, et al. Delayed massive hemorrhage after pancreatic and biliary surgery: embolization or surgery? Ann Surg. 2005;241(1):85–91.
40. Limongelli P, Khorsandi SE, Pai M, Jackson JE, Tait P, Tierris J, et al. Management of delayed postoperative hemorrhage after pancreaticoduodenectomy: a meta-analysis. Arch Surg. 2008;143(10):1001–7.
41. Wei HK, Wang SE, Shyr YM, Tseng HS, Tsai WC, Chen TH, et al. Risk factors for post-pancreaticoduodenectomy bleeding and finding an innovative approach to treatment. Dig Surg. 2009;26(4):297–305.
42. Yeo CJ, Barry MK, Sauter PK, Sostre S, Lillemoe KD, Pitt HA, et al. Erythromycin accelerates gastric emptying after pancreaticoduodenectomy. A prospective, randomized, placebo-controlled trial. Ann Surg. 1993;218(3):229–37.
43. Abell TL, Camilleri M, Donohoe K, Hasler WL, Lin HC, Maurer AH, et al. Consensus recommendations for gastric emptying scintigraphy: a joint report of the American Neurogastroenterology and Motility Society and the Society of Nuclear Medicine. Am J Gastroenterol. 2008;103(3):753–63.
44. van Berge Henegouwen MI, Akkermans LM, van Gulik TM, Masclee AA, Moojen TM, Obertop H, et al. Prospective, randomized trial on the effect of cyclic versus continuous enteral nutrition on postoperative gastric function after pylorus-preserving pancreatoduodenectomy. Ann Surg. 1997;226(6):677–85.
45. Kawai M, Tani M, Hirono S, Miyazawa M, Shimizu A, Uchiyama K, et al. Pylorus ring resection reduces delayed gastric emptying in patients undergoing pancreatoduodenectomy: a prospective, randomized, controlled trial of pylorus-resecting versus pylorus-preserving pancreatoduodenectomy. Ann Surg. 2011;253(3):495–501.
46. Diener MK, Knaebel HP, Heukaufer C, Antes G, Buchler MW, Seiler CM. A systematic review and meta-analysis of pylorus-preserving versus classical pancreaticoduodenectomy for

surgical treatment of periampullary and pancreatic carcinoma. Ann Surg. 2007;245(2):187–200.

47. Diener MK, Fitzmaurice C, Schwarzer G, Seiler CM, Antes G, Knaebel HP, et al. Pylorus-preserving pancreaticoduodenectomy (pp Whipple) versus pancreaticoduodenectomy (classic Whipple) for surgical treatment of periampullary and pancreatic carcinoma. Cochrane Database Syst Rev. 2011;5, CD006053.
48. Karanicolas PJ, Davies E, Kunz R, Briel M, Koka HP, Payne DM, et al. The pylorus: take it or leave it? Systematic review and meta-analysis of pylorus-preserving versus standard whipple pancreaticoduodenectomy for pancreatic or periampullary cancer. Ann Surg Oncol. 2007;14(6):1825–34.
49. Iqbal N, Lovegrove RE, Tilney HS, Abraham AT, Bhattacharya S, Tekkis PP, et al. A comparison of pancreaticoduodenectomy with extended pancreaticoduodenectomy: a meta-analysis of 1909 patients. Eur J Surg Oncol. 2009;35(1):79–86.
50. Michalski CW, Kleeff J, Wente MN, Diener MK, Buchler MW, Friess H. Systematic review and meta-analysis of standard and extended lymphadenectomy in pancreaticoduodenectomy for pancreatic cancer. Br J Surg. 2007;94(3):265–73.
51. Yeo CJ, Cameron JL, Lillemoe KD, Sohn TA, Campbell KA, Sauter PK, et al. Pancreaticoduodenectomy with or without distal gastrectomy and extended retroperitoneal lymphadenectomy for periampullary adenocarcinoma, part 2: randomized controlled trial evaluating survival, morbidity, and mortality. Ann Surg. 2002;236(3):355–66.
52. Gangavatiker R, Pal S, Javed A, Dash NR, Sahni P, Chattopadhyay TK. Effect of antecolic or retrocolic reconstruction of the gastro/duodenojejunostomy on delayed gastric emptying after pancreaticoduodenectomy: a randomized controlled trial. J Gastrointest Surg. 2011;15(5):843–52.
53. Tani M, Terasawa H, Kawai M, Ina S, Hirono S, Uchiyama K, et al. Improvement of delayed gastric emptying in pylorus-preserving pancreaticoduodenectomy: results of a prospective, randomized, controlled trial. Ann Surg. 2006;243(3):316–20.
54. Kollmar O, Moussavian MR, Richter S, de Roi P, Maurer CA, Schilling MK. Prophylactic octreotide and delayed gastric emptying after pancreaticoduodenectomy: results of a prospective randomized double-blinded placebo-controlled trial. Eur J Surg Oncol. 2008;34(8):868–75.
55. Aoki H, Takakura N, Shiozaki S, Matsukawa H. Milk-based test as a preventive method for chylous ascites following pancreatic resection. Dig Surg. 2010;27(5):427–32.
56. Assumpcao L, Cameron JL, Wolfgang CL, Edil B, Choti MA, Herman JM, et al. Incidence and management of chyle leaks following pancreatic resection: a high volume single-center institutional experience. J Gastrointest Surg. 2008;12(11):1915–23.
57. van der Gaag NA, Verhaar AC, Haverkort EB, Busch OR, van Gulik TM, Gouma DJ. Chylous ascites after pancreaticoduodenectomy: introduction of a grading system. J Am Coll Surg. 2008;207(5):751–7.
58. D'Hondt M, Foubert K, Penninckx F, Aerts R. Lymphangiography as a Treatment Method for Chylous Ascites Following Pancreaticoduodenectomy. Cancer: J Gastrointest; 2010.

Chapter 15
Treatment of Major Complications of Acute Pancreatitis

Hein Gooszen

Keywords Acute pancreatitis • Infected necrosis • Obstructive jaundice • Mechanical ileus • Infection • Intervention • (Peri)pancreatic necrosis • Perioperative care

Introduction

Acute pancreatitis is a relatively common disease with increasing incidence in the Western world. The cause for this increase is not fully clear but may be related to the increase in incidence of gallstone disease. It is the second most common gastrointestinal disorder requiring acute hospitalization in the United States, with annual costs exceeding $2 billion [1, 2]. Approximately 20 % of patients develop severe acute pancreatitis, defined by organ failure or necrotizing pancreatitis [3]. Severe pancreatitis is associated with a mortality of 15–30 % whereas the mortality of mild pancreatitis is only 0–1 % [4]. Organ failure is the most important determinant for mortality in acute pancreatitis, mainly occurring in the early phase of the disease, where the clinical course is dominated by the severity of the systemic inflammatory response syndrome (SIRS) [4].

At this early stage, there is essentially no place for surgical intervention, other than to treat abdominal compartment syndrome, persistent life-threatening bleeding in spite of attempted coiling, and (nonocclusive) small bowel ischemia.

Sterile pancreatic necrosis and sterile peripancreatic collections can be treated conservatively. Although the natural course of untreated (peri)pancreatic necrosis is unknown, there is accumulating data to suggest that spontaneous resolution by resorption, liquefaction, or perforation to the digestive tract can occur (Figs. 15.1 and 15.2).

H. Gooszen, MD
Department of Operating Room/Evidence Based Surgery,
Radboud University Nijmegen Medical Centre, Nijmegen, The Netherlands
e-mail: h.gooszen@ok.umcn.nl

M.A. Cuesta, H.J. Bonjer (eds.), *Treatment of Postoperative Complications after Digestive Surgery*, DOI 10.1007/978-1-4471-4354-3_15,

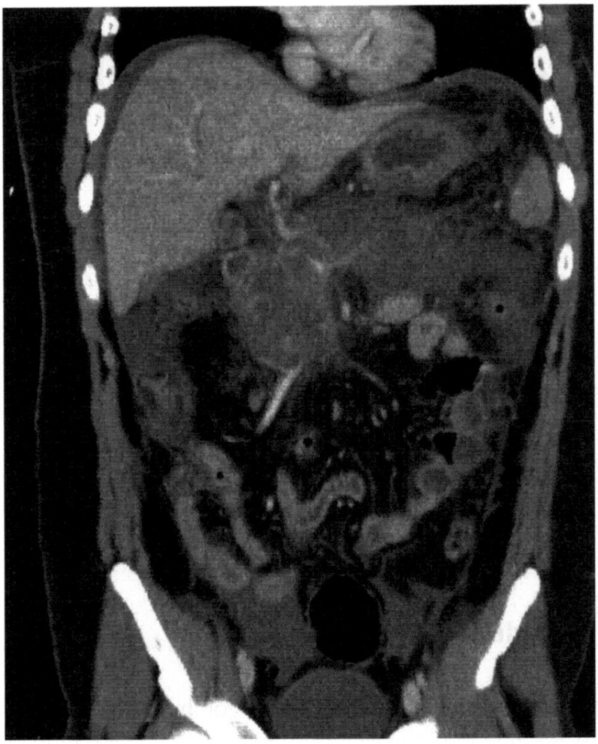

Fig. 15.1 Necrotizing acute pancreatitis

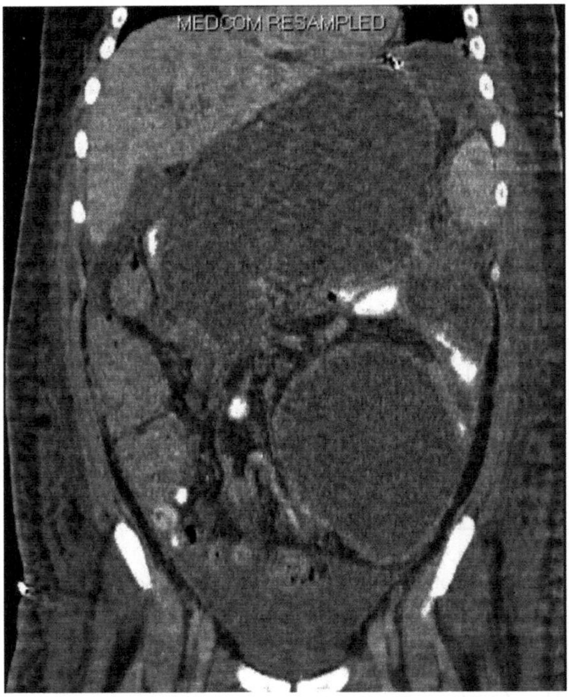

Fig. 15.2 After 3 weeks, liquefaction process

In around 30 % of patients, secondary infection of necrosis occurs, which, if left untreated, turns out to be fatal in nearly 100 % [3].

Interventional Treatment of Infected Necrosis

Since there is no causal treatment for acute pancreatitis, interventional treatment is restricted to complications of the disease. Organ failure – early or late – is a common and life-threatening complication and obviously needs adequate medical and supportive treatment. Treatment of organ failure is beyond the scope of this chapter and will not be dealt with in any detail.

If intra- and/or peripancreatic necrosis develops, this only needs treatment in case of infection or mechanical complications, like obstructive jaundice (when the necrotic collection leads to compression of the common bile duct) or mechanical ileus, due to compression of the duodenum or proximal jejunum.

Obstructive Jaundice or Mechanical Ileus

Since spontaneous resolution is well documented, an aggressive approach to necrotic collections causing mechanical complications is not justified. No controlled data, however, are available to guide the clinician through the period of expectative management in these patients. The risk of inducing infection by intervention in sterile necrosis should be weighed against the morbidity caused by protracted conservative management with stenting of the common bile duct or a long episode of enteral nutrition through a naso-jejunal tube, clinically or on an outpatient basis.

Infection of (Peri)pancreatic Necrosis

Acute pancreatitis runs a biphasic course. The first phase is characterized by a systemic inflammatory response syndrome (SIRS) and lasts about 2 weeks. The second phase is characterized by a counteractive anti-inflammatory response syndrome (CARS). Organ failure in the SIRS phase is usually not caused by infection but rather by severe inflammation. Organ failure in the CARS phase is related to infection of necrosis. Infections like bacteremia and (ventilator-associated) pneumonia, however, do occur in SIRS phase [4].

Necrosis can get infected in any stage of the disease, in a time interval ranging between the first week of disease and several months thereafter. Early infection is rare and over 50 % of the infections need treatment in the time period between 3 and 8 weeks after onset of disease. If after an episode of clinical stabilization or improvement, clinical signs of infection with sepsis, and organ failure develops, infection of necrosis is the cause of sepsis, once other sources have been ruled out. Infection of necrosis can induce a new episode of clinical signs of sepsis with or without organ failure. Organ failure developing early (first 2 weeks) in the course of disease is rarely caused by infection of necrosis [5].

Once infection of necrosis has been diagnosed and leads to signs of sepsis, intervention is the next step.

Intervention for Infected Necrosis

Recently the paradigm for treatment of infected necrosis has shifted from surgery – laparotomy or some of the available minimally invasive procedures – with removal of necrosis as the first step to catheter drainage as the first line of treatment.

In a randomized controlled study it was shown that around 30 % of patients with infected necrosis and signs of sepsis were effectively treated by catheter drainage only. In these patients, apparently drainage of pus under tension suffices and the patient is capable to get rid of the necrosis (resorption, liquefaction, spontaneous evacuation into the digestive tract) without further intervention, surgically or endoscopically.

In the remaining 70 %, removal of the necrosis is necessary and several techniques are currently applied, like open necrosectomy by laparotomy, videoscopic-assisted retroperitoneal debridement (VARD) [6–8], several laparoscopic techniques [9], and endoscopic transgastric necrosectomy [10–12].

One-stage open necrosectomy followed by postoperative lavage is widely accepted and still considered a valid option by many experienced centers and surgeons [13, 14]. Morbidity is considerable and mortality in around 15 % in expert centers.

VARD was developed in Seattle and consists of a retroperitoneal, small-incision approach to the necrotic collection with video-assisted direct (intentionally, one stage, complete) removal of the necrosis. Mortality ranges from 0 to around 20 % in recent series. Morbidity seems to be lower than in open necrosectomy.

Laparoscopic and endoscopic techniques as developed in Glasgow, Liverpool, Germany, and Rochester, respectively, are less invasive than VARD but need several sessions to totally or subtotally remove the necrosis. Probably the learning curve is longer than in case of VARD or open necrosectomy, although there is no controlled data on this topic.

Perioperative Care

Step 1: Percutaneous or Endoscopic Drainage

A percutaneous drain is placed in the peripancreatic collection under guidance of CT or ultrasound (step 1a). In the previously mentioned controlled study, minimal drain size is 12 French and multiple drains were allowed but mostly not necessary. The preferred route is of course dependent on the next step in case of drainage failure. If VARD is considered, the preferred route is through the left retroperitoneum, thereby facilitating minimally invasive retroperitoneal necrosectomy at a later stage. Transabdominal drainage can be performed if a retroperitoneal access route for drainage is not possible or if open necrosectomy is the next step. If neither retroperitoneal nor transabdominal drainage is possible or if endoscopic transgastric necrosectomy is the procedure of choice of the responsible team, transgastric drainage is performed. For irrigation the drains are flushed with a bolus of 250 cc of normal saline four times a day

Step 2: Necrosectomy

VARD, and all other current minimally invasive techniques, use the retroperitoneal drain for guidance. Only loosely adherent necrosis is removed with videoscopic assistance and two large-bore drains are inserted.

Postoperative Management

Continuous postoperative lavage amounting up to at least 10 L per 24 h on the third postoperative day will be performed both after open necrosectomy and minimally invasive surgery. Patients undergo contrast-enhanced CT 1 week after intervention; other CT scans are performed on demand, either to detect insufficiently drained collections or to control collapse of the necrotic cavity.

Complications of Surgery for Infected Necrosis

Complications after surgery can be divided into three subgroups: first, complications after surgery in critically ill and septic patients; second, complications in relation to the operation or intervention as such; and third, complications reflecting to what extent surgery has affected pancreatic function.

Complications of Surgery in Critically Ill Patients

New-onset organ failure induced probably by the release of the contents of the infected collection into the systemic circulation results in fever and signs of sepsis. This event can be called "new-onset organ failure" and is defined as organ failure directly after intervention and not already present at any time in the 24 h before this intervention, with two or more organs (pulmonary, circulatory, or renal failure) failing at the same time. From the literature, it is difficult to extract the exact incidence because definitions are different. Figures are ranging between 12 % for minimally invasive techniques and 56 % for open necrosectomy.

Organ failure may or may not be associated with disseminated intravascular coagulation, severe metabolic derangement with critical decrease of serum calcium level, and gastrointestinal bleeding.

Complications in Relation to the Operation or Intervention as Such

Enterocutaneous fistula, perforation of a visceral organ requiring intervention, and intra-abdominal bleeding requiring intervention are the best-documented type of complications. Enterocutaneous fistula is present if fecal material is produced from a percutaneous drain or drainage canal after removal of drains or from a surgical wound, from either small or large bowel, to be confirmed with imaging or during surgery and requiring surgical or endoscopic treatment.

The incidence of this type of complications ranges between 10 and 20 % in open surgery and between 7 and 15 % for the minimally invasive techniques.

Appropriate treatment strategies are usually not described and range from partial colectomy with end-to-end anastomosis to the construction of a loop ileostomy to be taken down at a later stage, with or without partial colectomy with restoration of continuity.

Intra-abdominal bleeding requiring intervention is defined as any bleeding needing surgical, radiological, or endoscopic treatment. Strategies in the different studies are again different with incidences ranging between 15 and 25 %.

Pancreatic fistula is a well-recognized complication of surgery for acute necrotizing pancreatitis and difficult to treat if persisting. Incidences are different for minimally invasive procedures (3–30 %) and open surgery (7–38 %). Treatment varies and consists of a conservative approach sometimes ending up with a pancreatic pseudocyst to partial pancreatectomy or pancreaticogastrostomy or pancreaticojejunostomy. The approach is highly dependent on the local intra-abdominal, anatomical situation and the preference and experience of the surgeon in charge.

All components of major morbidity tended to occur more frequently after primary open necrosectomy, although in the previous PANTER trial the difference was significant only for new-onset multiple organ failure and multiple systemic complications [15]. In this study the difference was mainly driven by the occurrence of organ failure.

Mortality after open and minimally invasive necrosectomy seems to be higher after open necrosectomy, even twice as high in a recent comparative but uncontrolled series. This has not been confirmed in controlled studies, where no difference has been documented so far. Probably selection or referral bias explains for the difference reported.

As expected, the rate of incisional hernia is higher after open necrosectomy than after VARD or other minimally invasive procedures. The same holds for the rate new-onset diabetes and use of pancreatic enzymes. More "liberal" debridement in case of open surgery with a higher tendency to also remove vital pancreas, looking necrotic on the outside but representing functional gland tissue on the inside, may be the cause but histological data to support this assumption are lacking.

Health Care Utilization and Costs

It is inappropriate in this era to exclude health care utilization in the scope of surgical treatment of acute pancreatitis. There is a distinct relation between the severity of complications, the outcome of treatment, the experience of the local team, and the costs to be considered in patients with infected necrotizing pancreatitis. In a recent randomized controlled trial, health care consumption was lower in the so-called step-up approach than after primary open necrosectomy. After primary open necrosectomy, more than twice as many of patients needed new ICU admission after surgical intervention compared to the step-up approach.

The mean total direct medical and indirect costs per patient during admission and 6 months follow-up were €78,775 ($116,016) for the step-up approach and €89,614 ($131,979) for open necrosectomy, resulting in a mean absolute difference of €10,839 ($15,963) per patient. Therefore, the step-up approach reduced costs by 12 %. This obviously constitutes an additional reason to prefer the "step-up" approach when patients reach the stage of infected necrosis with signs of sepsis [15].

How to Reduce the Rate of Complications?

Any attempt to reduce the rate of complications of the disease itself has failed so far, and early intervention by medical means definitely needs novel approaches.

Complications of intervention at a later stage – the stage of infected (peri)pancreatic necrosis – like enteric fistula and bleeding are related to the experience of the team responsible for treatment of these patients. Looking at recent literature, it seems as if the complication rate and mortality are lowest in expert units. Many of these series are retrospective and comparison between studies and centers is flawed because bias cannot be ruled out. More detailed analysis of recent data, for instance, by performing individual patient data meta-analysis (IPDMA) potentially corrects for bias and needs to be done, but the conclusion that centralization for these highly complex cases will improve results will be inevitable.

Pancreatic fistula is probably not experience dependent, and centralization will not help reducing this difficult notorious complication. The same holds for secondary onset diabetes mellitus and exocrine insufficiency.

Summary

Much progress has been made in the understanding of the course of necrotizing pancreatitis. Nomenclature and classification of the disease is in discussion, and when successfully completed, description of patients for clinical studies will improve.

New techniques and new strategies for intervention have improved the outlook, with mortality stabilizing between 15 and 20 % for the subgroup where necrosis gets infected and needs intervention. Possibly endoscopic transluminal necrosectomy will further reduce the complication rate with a positive impact on mortality.

References

1. Fagenholz PJ, Fernandez-del Castillo C, Harris NS, Pelletier AJ, Camargo CA. Direct medical costs of acute pancreatitis hospitalizations in the United States. Pancreas. 2007;35:302–7.
2. Shaheen NJ, Hansen RA, Morgan DR, Gangarosa LM, Ringel Y, Thiny MT, et al. The burden of gastrointestinal and liver diseases, 2006. Am J Gastroenterol. 2006;101:2128–38.
3. Banks PA, Freeman ML. Practice guidelines in acute pancreatitis. Am J Gastroenterol. 2006;101:2379–400.
4. Besselink MG, Van Santvoort HC, Boermeester MA, Nieuwenhuijs VB, van GH, Dejong CH et al. Timing and impact of infections in acute pancreatitis. Br J Surg 2009;96:267-73

5. Petrov MS, Shanbhag S, Chakraborty M, Phillips AR, Windsor JA. Organ failure and infection of pancreatic necrosis as determinants of mortality in patients with acute pancreatitis. Gastroenterology. 2010;303:202–7.
6. Horvath K, Freeny P, Escallon J, Heagerty P, Comstock B, Glickerman DJ, et al. Safety and efficacy of video-assisted retroperitoneal debridement for infected pancreatic collections: a multicenter, prospective, single-arm phase 2 study. Arch Surg. 2010;145:817–25.
7. Horvath KD, Kao LS, Wherry KL, Pellegrini CA, Sinanan MN. A technique for laparoscopic-assisted percutaneous drainage of infected pancreatic necrosis and pancreatic abscess. Surg Endosc. 2001;15:1221–5.
8. Van Santvoort HC, Besselink MGH, Horvath KD, Sinanan M, Bollen TL, Ramshorst B, et al. Videoscopic assisted retroperitoneal debridement in infected necrotizing pancreatitis. H P B. 2007;9:156–9.
9. Raraty MG, Halloran CM, Dodd S, Ghaneh P, Connor S, Evans J, et al. Minimal access retroperitoneal pancreatic necrosectomy: improvement in morbidity and mortality with a less invasive approach. Ann Surg. 2010;251:787–93.
10. Papachristou GI, Takahashi N, Chahal P, Sarr MG, Baron TH. Peroral endoscopic drainage/debridement of walled-off pancreatic necrosis. Ann Surg. 2007;245:943–51.
11. Seifert H, Biermer M, Schmitt W, Jurgensen C, Will U, Gerlach R, et al. Transluminal endoscopic necrosectomy after acute pancreatitis: a multicentre study with long-term follow-up (the GEPARD Study). Gut. 2009;58:1260–6.
12. Voermans RP, Bruno MJ, van Berge Henegouwen MI, Fockens P. Review article: Translumenal endoscopic debridement of organized pancreatic necrosis–the first step towards natural orifice translumenal endoscopic surgery. Aliment Pharmacol Ther. 2007;26:233–9.
13. Rau B, Bothe A, Beger HG. Surgical treatment of necrotizing pancreatitis by necrosectomy and closed lavage: changing patient characteristics and outcome in a 19-year, single-center series. Surgery. 2005;138:28–39.
14. Rodriguez JR, Razo AO, Targarona J, Thayer SP, Rattner DW, Warshaw AL, et al. Debridement and closed packing for sterile or infected necrotizing pancreatitis: insights into indications and outcomes in 167 patients. Ann Surg. 2008;247:294–9.
15. Van Santvoort HC, Besselink MG, Bakker OJ, Hofker HS, Boermeester MA, Dejong CH, et al. A step-up approach or open necrosectomy for necrotizing pancreatitis. N Engl J Med. 2010;362:1491–502.

Chapter 16
Prevention and Treatment of Major Complications after Surgery of the Spleen, Adrenal Glands, and Distal Pancreatectomy

Renske Konings, H. Jaap Bonjer, and Geert Kazemier

Keywords Laparoscopic Surgery • Spleen • Adrenal glands • Distal pancreatectomy • Spalenectomy • Adrenalectomy • Laparoscopic pancreatectomy • Portal vein thrombosis • Pancreatic fistula

Introduction

Safe and successful surgery of these three organs starts with a good indication to operate. Based on the symptoms of the patient, laboratory tests and imaging studies will be performed. Prior to surgery, a multidisciplinary meeting should take place to accept the patient for surgery, identify risk factors, and discuss treatment stratification to prevent major complications. Furthermore this chapter will guide you in practicing proper management of major complications.

Spleen

The majority of elective splenectomies will currently be performed laparoscopically [1]. Concerning the size of the spleen, indication for surgery can be divided into three groups: the normal spleen, the enlarged spleen, and the giant spleen in cases of malignant hematological diseases.

R. Konings • H.J. Bonjer, PhD, FRCSC (✉) • G. Kazemier
Department of Surgery, VU University Medical Center, Amsterdam, The Netherlands
e-mail: j.bonjer@vumc.nl

M.A. Cuesta, H.J. Bonjer (eds.), *Treatment of Postoperative Complications after Digestive Surgery*, DOI 10.1007/978-1-4471-4354-3_16,

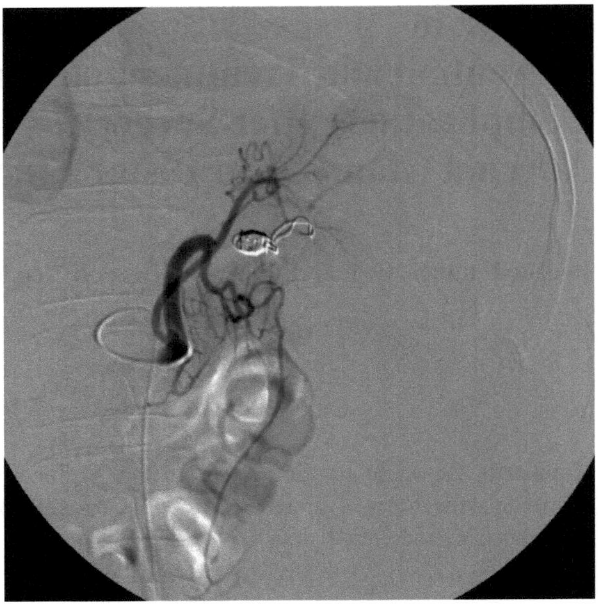

Fig. 16.1 Angiography and coiling splenic artery in spleen trauma

Examples for these are idiopathic thrombocytopenia (ITP), spherocytosis, and malignant hematological diseases such as myelodysplasia, myelofibrosis, and lymphomas. All these conditions require close collaboration with hematologists. Particular caution is necessary in patients with impaired formation of red and white blood cells, myelodysplasia, and myelofibrosis. In these patients, residual hemato- and leukopoiesis are located in the liver and the spleen. Removal of the spleen can be followed by fatal aplasia. In general, splenectomy should be avoided in patients with myelofibrosis.

In the first two groups, the spleen can be taken out by laparoscopy and fragmented (morcellated) in a bag, to be extracted in pieces without enlargement of any port. Morcellation of the spleen is best done by finger fracture inside the extraction bag. Employment of mechanical morcellators can cause inadvertent damage of intra-abdominal structures. During morcellation of the spleen, spill of fragments of the spleen should be avoided to prevent intraperitoneal seeding of splenic tissue. In the case of a giant spleen, this may be approached "hand assisted" and the organ as a whole is offered to the pathologist.

Currently, the clinical attitude and approach of the traumatic spleen is a point of discussion. Conservative treatment is first considered in hemodynamic stable patients. If interventional radiology expertise is available, an angiography should be done and the splenic artery or tributaries should be coiled if a blush is clear. If the patient is unstable, laparotomy and open splenectomy should be considered [2] (Fig. 16.1).

In the case of thrombocytopenia, preoperative intramuscular administration of immunoglobulin (IgG) can be used to increase the platelet count [3]. When platelet transfusions are considered, it is important to start transfusion only after the splenic artery has been ligated to maximize the effect [4].

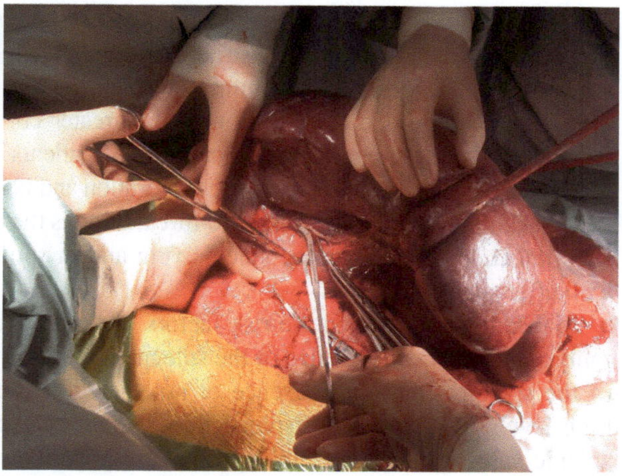

Fig. 16.2 Open splenectomy of giant spleen. Nowadays this operation will be performed laparoscopically

Patients undergoing laparoscopic splenectomy should be placed in a lateral decubitus position to expose the spleen and minimize the need for retracting surrounding organs. In lateral decubitus, the spleen hangs from its lateral attachments, while the stomach, splenic flexure, and pancreatic tail are displaced to the right of the patient due to gravity. Hence the splenic hilum is exposed rendering dissection simpler than in supine position. The key of safe splenectomy is atraumatic dissection, delicate traction on the tissues, and dissecting at least one centimeter away from the splenic parenchyma to leave some vessel length for ligation in case bleeding occurs. Large curved dissecting forceps facilitate isolating the large branches of the splenic hilum. Although suture ligation is possible, the use of mechanical staplers with vascular cartridges is preferable. It is of paramount importance to visualize the pancreatic tail and avoid central dissection of the splenic vessels to prevent pancreatic injury. During dissection and ligation of the short gastric vessels, utmost care should be taken to avoid diathermic injury of the gastric wall.

Assessment of the size of the spleen is important to determine whether laparoscopic removal will be possible (Fig. 16.2). While trocars can be placed closely to the left costal margin in normal or slightly enlarged spleens, trocar sites need to be placed further away from the costal margin when the spleen extends beyond the left costal margin. Giant spleens, those extending more than a hand's width from the costal margin, merit hand-assisted surgery. Most surgeons insert the left hand through a supraumbilical vertical incision. The hand facilitates atraumatic retraction of the spleen and digital compression of the splenic pedicle in case of bleeding.

Bleeding after splenectomy is rare when the splenic bed is inspected thoroughly after removal of the spleen. Lowering the insufflation pressure at the end of the procedure facilitates identification of venous bleeding. Thrombocytosis is normal after splenectomy, but if the number of platelets surpasses 1.2 million/mL, therapeutic anticoagulation should be considered [5].

Pancreatic fistula with formation of pancreatic fluid collection can occur when the pancreatic tail was severed during dissection of the splenic hilum. Vague upper abdominal pain, fever, and increased white blood cell count should alert the suspicion of such a complication. CT or ultrasound percutaneous drainage of such a collection suffices when there is no obstruction of the pancreatic duct. Administration of somatostatin is expensive and of unclear efficacy.

Gastric leakage due to laceration of the greater curvature during ligation of the short gastric vessels requires in the majority of patients repeat surgery, either laparoscopically or open, to close the gastric perforation and lavage the abdominal cavity [6].

Most complex and potentially life-threatening is the underreported, in most cases subclinical, thrombosis of the splenic vein and in some patients the portal vein as well after splenectomy.

Machado et al. studied the risk factors of portal vein thrombosis after splenectomy and identified large size of the spleen, myeloproliferative disorders, large size of the splenic vein, and presence of associated coagulopathy, including rebound high levels of platelets postsplenectomy. Giant spleens are associated with wide splenic veins. Occlusion of the splenic vein in patients with giant spleens leaves a venous stump ("cul-de-sac") laterally to the junction of the splenic vein and the inferior mesenteric vein which predisposes to turbulence and subsequent thrombosis [7]. Laparoscopic surgery seems associated with a higher rate of portal vein thrombosis, but the exact implication of the problem is not clear. It is important to define the risks of these complications and to find an adequate treatment. Administering anticoagulants in addition to routine thrombosis prophylaxis after removal of a large spleen should be considered. Once thrombosis has been confirmed by diagnostic imaging, therapeutic anticoagulation should be started in order to resolve the thrombus for 3–6 months [8]. Infarction of the gut, caused by venous thrombosis after splenectomy has been reported, is very rare and requires a laparotomy to resect the affected bowel segment [9].

Another major complication is "overwhelming postsplenectomy sepsis (OPSS)" or "postsplenectomy sepsis (PSS)." The most common cause is Streptococcus pneumoniae, Haemophilus influenzae type B, and Neisseria meningitides. Patients should be vaccinated 2 weeks preoperatively in elective surgery or 2 weeks after surgery in order to prevent this complication. Education of the patient includes recommendations concerning repeat vaccination and early use of antibiotics during respiratory infections [9]. We would like to emphasize its importance because the incidence of sepsis is 600× higher in postsplenectomy patients [9, 10].

Adrenal Glands

Managing patients with adrenal pathology requires close collaboration with endocrinology, nuclear medicine, and radiology. Good understanding of adrenal physiology, pathophysiology, and hormonal analysis is essential to select patients successfully for a conservative of surgical approach [11, 12].

Fine-needle aspiration biopsy of adrenal lesions is rarely helpful and can incur life-threatening hemodynamic instability in case of presence of a pheochromocytoma.

Adrenal incidentalomas are commonly referred to surgery. Hormonal analysis will determine whether these adrenal lesions are hormonally hyperactive which necessitates removal. Nonfunctional adrenal tumor greater than 4 cm in diameter requires surgery as well while smaller adrenal lesions can be followed by periodic imaging.

Distinguishing unilateral adrenal adenomas from bilateral hyperplasia in patients with hyperaldosteronism (morbus Conn) is done by imaging and progressively venous sampling. Hyperaldosteronism due to hyperplasia requires medical treatment. Removal of an aldosterone-producing adrenal adenoma (morbus Conn) is followed in all cases by normokalemia which eliminates the need to continue potassium-sparing medication postoperatively. Sixty percent of patients can discontinue all antihypertensive medications after removal of a Conn's adenoma. The remaining patients can either diminish medication or need to continue antihypertensive drugs in the same dosage.

In patients with hypercortisolism, differentiation between adrenal (Cushing's syndrome) or pituitary origin (Cushing's disease) is essential. Some neuroendocrine tumors such as carcinoids secrete ACTH and cause a non-pituitary ACTH-dependent adrenal hyperplasia. Primary therapy of morbus Cushing is pituitary surgery followed, if unsuccessful, by radiotherapy of the sella. Bilateral adrenalectomy is the ultimate intervention in refractory Cushing's disease.

Intravenous administration of corticosteroids needs to be started once the cortisol-producing adrenal tumor has been removed. Transition to oral corticosteroids can occur on the day after surgery.

Patients with pheochromocytomas require MIBG (mono-iodo-benzyl-guanidine) scintigraphy in addition to CT or MRI to identify multiple localizations. Adrenal pheochromocytomas can produce both adrenaline and noradrenaline, while extra-adrenal pheochromocytomas (paragangliomas) secrete noradrenaline or dopamine. Paragangliomas arise from the sympathetic chain and are mostly less amenable for minimally invasive surgery particularly when located between the caval vein and the aorta or in the renal hilum. These tumors tend to have multiple small venous branches which may require suture ligatures which are accomplished more easily through open surgery.

Patients with pheochromocytomas require thorough and timely control of hypertension prior to surgery. Alpha-blockers are administered clinically starting at least seven days before surgery striving for orthostatic hypotension. Beta-blockers are given when tachycardia arises.

Including anesthesiology in preoperative blood pressure management is advisable. Anesthesiologists experienced in medically controlling severe hypertension are invaluable in managing patients with pheochromocytomas intraoperatively. During surgery, the anesthesiologist needs to alert the surgeon when systolic blood pressures increase significantly. Cessation of dissection and retraction of the adrenal gland and desufflation are measures to reduce the release of catecholamines.

Postoperatively, these patients are monitored for at least 24 h in a critical care unit.

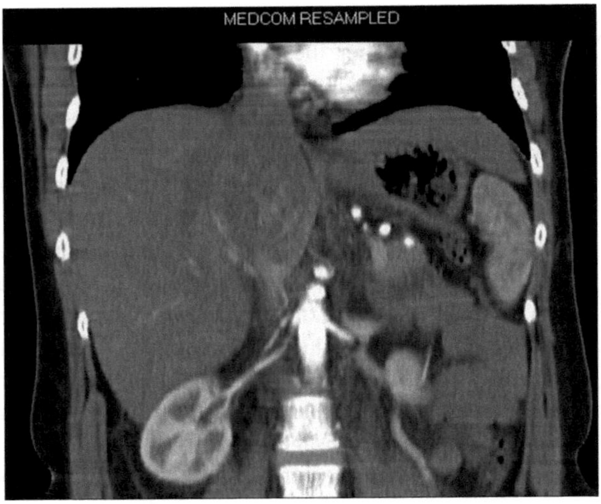

Fig. 16.3 Adrenal gland cancer with vena cava thrombus

Presence of an adrenocortical cancer needs to be considered in tumors larger than 6 cm in diameter, when different densities are present within the adrenal lesion, in case of irregular margins, and when pathological lymph nodes are identified [16]. Adrenocortical cancers may be associated with tumor thrombus in the adrenal vein. These thrombi can extend through the left renal vein and caval vein on the left side or directly through the caval vein on the right side into the right atrium (Fig. 16.3). Special attention is required to rule out the presence of tumor thrombus in patients with adrenal tumors suspect of adrenocortical cancer. Minimally invasive surgery is not advocated in these fragile tumors which render them susceptible to perforation and tumor spread during retraction and manipulation. Open surgery and, in case of tumor thrombus extending into the atrium, sternotomy are recommended.

Various minimally invasive approaches to the adrenal gland are employed [17]. General surgeons favor the transperitoneal approach with the patient in full lateral decubitus position. On the right side, the right lobe of the liver is liberally mobilized by incising the right triangular ligament. Cranial retraction of the right liver lobe and medial mobilization of the duodenum will expose the caval vein and right adrenal gland. Indirect retraction of the adrenal gland is utilized to avoid tearing the fragile adrenal gland. The right adrenal vein which drains into the caval vein is short and requires gentle retraction to prevent bleeding. Placement of clips on the side of the caval vein only suffices in case of limited length of the vein because venous back bleeding tends to be limited. An additional right adrenal vein may be present draining into a venous branch from the caudate lobe of the liver. Removal of the adrenal gland once it has been in a bag is necessary to avoid spill of adrenal tissue during extraction.

The transperitoneal approach to the left adrenal gland is performed with the patient in right lateral decubitus position. Mobilization of the lateral attachments of the spleen to the level of the left crus allows the spleen and the pancreatic tail to be displaced medially exposing the left adrenal gland. Mobilization of the splenic flexure exposed the upper pole of the kidney. The left adrenal vein is longer than the right adrenal vein which renders dissection and ligation less difficult. A branch of the left diaphragmatic vein joins the left adrenal vein and requires individual ligation.

Retroperitoneal adrenalectomy, favored by urologists, is done either with the patient in full lateral decubitus or prone position [13–15]. Anatomic landmarks are fewer than in transperitoneal surgery which render proper orientation more difficult. The retroperitoneal space is a virtual space which requires balloon dissection to establish a working space. The retroperitoneal approach obviates the need to mobilize and retract adjacent organs and avoids the peritoneal cavity which is advantageous in patients who had previous abdominal surgeries. Oppositely, prior renal or perirenal surgery is a contraindication for retroperitoneal adrenalectomy.

Retroperitoneal adrenalectomy in prone position allows bilateral adrenalectomy without the need for changing the position of the patient.

Postoperative complications are rare after adrenalectomy. Hematomas can occur in patients with hypercortisolism which is associated with coagulopathy.

Distal Pancreatectomy

Distal pancreatectomy is a complex procedure with a mortality rate ranging between 0 and 5 % in high-volume centers and a morbidity rate between 23 and 57 % [18, 19].

Pathology of the pancreatic tail includes adenocarcinoma, cystic neoplasm, mucinous cystic neoplasm, IPMN (intraductal papillary mucinous neoplasm), solid pseudopapillary neoplasm (SPPN), neuroendocrine tumors, pancreatic lymphomas, and metastases [20–22].

Careful assessment of CT and MRI images combined with ERCP or MRCP findings is crucial to determine the nature of the disorder. In patients with suspicion of malignancy, open surgery is recommended.

Preservation of the spleen is an important aspect of distal pancreatectomy. Isolation of the splenic artery which runs at the cranial margin of the pancreatic tail is feasible in most patients. However, dissecting the splenic vein can prove difficult particularly when the vein is entirely surrounded by pancreatic parenchyma. Several small fragile venous branches join the splenic vein. A combination of small clips, suture ligatures, and vessel sealing technology should be available to control these small branches.

Some surgeons transect both the splenic artery and vein and leave the spleen in situ relying on sufficient blood supply through the short gastric vessels [24].

Debate exists on whether to close the stump after distal pancreatectomy either with a stapler or with hand-sewn closure [25]. The DISPACT randomized study [26] randomized 450 patients in two groups (221 vs. 229) of whom finally 352 patients were analyzed. The pancreatic fistula rate or mortality did not differ between the two groups (32 % vs. 28 %), concluding that stapler closure did not reduce the rate of pancreatic fistula compared with hand-sewn closure for distal pancreatectomy.

Patients with BMI <27, without adenocarcinoma, and with pancreatic specimen length <8.5 cm had significant higher rates of fistulas after open than after laparoscopic surgery. In contrast no preoperatively evaluable variables were associated with a higher likelihood of significant fistula after laparoscopic versus open [23, 25].

Other alternative techniques are studied for prevention of postoperative pancreatic fistula. Examples given are stapling versus seromuscular patch or use of falciform ligament pedicle flap [27], ultrasonic dissection, and application of mesh or fibrin glue.

These studies show a variety of outcomes not providing a standard solution.

Cho et al. studied 693 patients after distal pancreatectomy, 439 open and 254 laparoscopic approached. On the multivariate analysis, variables associated with major complications and clinically significant fistulas (27 % open and 23 % laparoscopic) did not differ between open and laparoscopic surgery [23].

Pancreatic fistula and/or development of an abscess requires percutaneous or transgastric drainage and is associated with longer hospital stay and double costs in comparison with uncomplicated distal pancreatectomy [28]. In case of development of an abscess, this should be transgastrically or percutaneously drained [29, 30].

References

1. Targarona EM, Trias M. Laparoscopic surgery of the spleen. World J Surg. 2007;31:1363–4.
2. Van der Vlies CH, van Delden OM, Punt BJ, et al. Literature review of the role of ultrasound, computed tomography and transcatheter arterial embolization for the treatment of traumatic splenic injuries. Cardiovasc Intervent Radiol. 2010;33(6):1079–87.
3. Wu Z, Zhou J, Pankai P, Peng B. Laparoscopic splenectomy for immune thrombocytopenia (ITP) patients with platelet counts lower than 1x109/L. Int J Hematol. 2011;94:533–8.
4. Chen X, Peng B, Cai Y, et al. Laparoscopic splenectomy for patients with immune thrombocytopenia and very low platelet count: is platelet transfusion necessary? J Surg Res. 2011;170: e225–32.
5. Supe A, Parikh M, Prabhu R, et al. Post-splenectomy response in adult patients with immune thrombocytopenic purpura. Asian J Transf Sci. 2009;3:6–9. Postoperative treatment thrombocytosis.
6. Targarona EM, Espert JJ, Bombuy E, et al. Complications of laparoscopic splenectomy. Arch Surg. 2000;135:1137–40. Gastric perforation splenectomy.
7. Van 't Riet M, Burger JW, van Muiswinkel JM, et al. Diagnosis and treatment of portal vein thrombosis following splenectomy. Br J Surg. 2000;87:1229–33.
8. Pietrabissa A, Moretto C, Antonelli G, et al. Thrombosis in the portal venous system after elective laparoscopic splenectomy. Surg Endosc. 2004;18:1140–3.
9. Machado NO, Chopra PJ, Sankhla D. Portal vein thrombosis postlaparoscopic splenectomy presenting with infraction of the gut: review of risk factors, investigations, postoperative surveillance, and management. Surg Laparosc Endosc Percutan Tech. 2010;20:273–7.
10. Davies JM, Lewis MP, Wimperis J, et al. review of guidelines for the prevention and treatment of infection in patients with an absent or dysfunctional spleen: prepared on behalf of the British Committee for Standards in Haematology by a working party of the Haemato-Oncology task force. Br J Haematol. 2011;155:308–17.

11. Portfield JR, Thompson GB, Young WF, et al. Surgery for Cushing's syndrome: an historical review and recent ten-year experience. World J Surg. 2008;32:659–77.
12. Weingarten TN. cata JP, O'hara JF et al. Comparison of two preoperative medical management strategies for laparoscopic resection of pheochromocytoma. Urology. 2010;76:6–11.
13. Bonjer HJ, Sorm V, Berends FJ, et al. Endoscopic retroperitoneal adrenalectomy: lessons learned from 111 consecutive cases. Ann Surg. 2000;232:796–803.
14. Gagner M. Laparoscopic adrenalectomy. Surg Clin North Am. 1996;76:523–37.
15. Dickson PV, Alex GC, Grubbs EG, et al. Posterior retroperitoneoscopic adrenalectomy is a safe and effective alternative to transabdominal laparoscopic adrenalectomy for pheochromocytoma. Surgery. 2011;150:452–8.
16. Zini L, porpiglia F, Fassnacht M. Contemporary management of adrenocortical carcinoma. Eur Urol. 2011;60:1055–65.
17. Bergamini C, Martellucci J, Tozzi F, Valeri A. Complications in laparoscopic adrenalectomy: the value of experience. Surg Endosc. 2011;25:3845–51.
18. Soga K, Ochiai T. Sonoyama T et al Risk factors for postoperative pancreatic fistula in distal pancreatectomy. Hepatogastroenterology. 2011;58:1372–6.
19. Xie K, Zhu YP, Xu XW, et al. Laparoscopic distal pancreatectomy is a safe and feasible as open procedure: A meta-analysis. World J Gastroenterol. 2012;18:1959–67.
20. de Jong K, Bruno MJ, Fockens P. Epidemiology, diagnosis, and management of cystic lesions of the pancreas. Gastroenterol Res Pract. 2012;2012:147465. Epub 2011 Oct 11.
21. Morgan KA, Adams DB. Solid tumors of the body and tail of the pancreas. Surg Clin North Am. 2010;90:287–307.
22. Anaye A, Mathieu A, Closset J, et al. Successful preoperative localization of a small pancreatic insulinoma by diffusion-weighted MRI. JOP. 2009;10:528–31.
23. Cho CS, Kooby DA, Schmidt M, et al. Laparoscopic versus open left pancreatectomy. Can preoperative factors indicate the safer technique? Ann Surg. 2011;253:975–80.
24. Tien YW, Liu KL, Hu RH, et al. Risk of varices bleeding after spleen preserving distal pancreatectomy with excision of splenic artery and vein. Ann Surg Oncol. 2010;17:2193–8.
25. Goh BKP, Tan YM, Chung YFA, et al. Critical appraisal of 232 consecutive distal pancreatectomies with emphasis on risk factors, outcome and management of the postoperative pancreatic fistula. Arch Surg. 2008;143:956–65.
26. Diener MK, Seiler CM, Rossion I, et al. Efficacy of stapler versus hand-sewn closure after distal pancreatectomy (DISPACT): a randomised, controlled multicentre trial. Lancet. 2011;377:1514–22.
27. Walters DM, Stokes JB, Adams RB, Bauer TW. Use of falciform ligament pedicle flap to decrease pancreatic fistula after distal pancreatectomy. Pancreas. 2011;40:595–9.
28. Rodriguez JR, Germes SS, Pandharipande PV, et al. Implications and costs of pancreatic leak following distal pancreatic resection. Arch Surg. 2006;141:361–5.
29. Cronin CG, Gervais DA, Castillo C, et al. nterventional radiology in the management of abdominal collections after distal pancreatectomy: A retrospective review. ARJ. 2011;197:241–6.
30. Varadarajulu S, Trevino JM, Christein JD. EUS for the management of peripancreatic fluid collections after distal pancreatectomy. Gastrointest Endosc. 2009;70:1260–5.

Chapter 17
Prevention and Treatment of Complications after Small Bowel Surgery and Appendicectomy

Donald L. van der Peet and Miguel A. Cuesta

Keywords Small bowel surgery • Appendicectomy • Acute appendicitis • Small bowel • Crohn's disease • Appendectomy • Laparoscopic surgery

Small Bowel

Surgery involving small bowel is performed very frequently. The reasons are different such as involvement of small bowel loops growing in continuity with tumors of other organs, having to deal with perforations during the taking down of adhesions, or for resection of the ischemic loops found in an incarcerated hernia. These are distinct scenarios found in surgical practice each day. Moreover, resections have to be planned for treating specific diseases of the small bowel, such as Crohn's disease or the more rare small bowel cancers and lymphomas associated with celiac disease.

In elective surgery for Crohn's disease, it is important to plan the size of resection so to prevent short bowel syndrome, as in the case after recurrence of Crohn's disease. At least 1 m of small bowel with a whole colon is considered a minimum length for preventing the short bowel syndrome. During reoperation, extensive resection will have to be prevented, and eventually stricturoplasties of stenosis should be considered instead of resections.

The general principle during resection includes marking the mesentery to be resected in respect to the irrigation of mesentery to be left behind; doing so avoids unnecessary extensive resections. After resection, it is important to perform an adequate anastomosis. Meaning, an anastomosis will need to be performed with well-irrigated and with good color margins, not bluish, watertight, not under tension, and patent (Fig. 17.1). If in doubt, the anastomosis should be re-created. Queries about

D.L. van der Peet, MD (✉) • M.A. Cuesta, MD
Department of Surgery, VU University Medical Center, Amsterdam, The Netherlands
e-mail: dl.vanderpeet@vumc.nl

M.A. Cuesta, H.J. Bonjer (eds.), *Treatment of Postoperative Complications after Digestive Surgery*, DOI 10.1007/978-1-4471-4354-3_17,

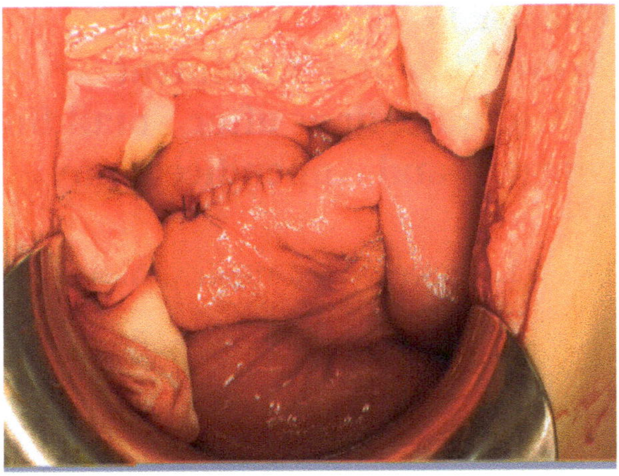

Fig. 17.1 Well-performed one-layer running small bowel anastomosis

types of anastomosis, end-to-end or side-to-side and mechanical or manual, are of lesser importance if certain principles are taken into account.

Concerning the types of anastomosis, single or double layer, in 1990, Irwin et al. published outcomes of a single-layer anastomosis in their institution during an 11-year period [1]. A total of 466 single-layer upper gastrointestinal anastomoses had been made in 349 patients, of which 1.3 % of the anastomoses had leaked. There were no leaks following 66 gastrojejunal anastomoses; one of 84 (1.2 %) gastroduodenal anastomoses leaked and that was converted to a gastrojejunal anastomosis. Two of 121 (1.7 %) biliary-enteric anastomoses leaked and both were successfully managed without reoperation. Two of 171 (1.2 %) enteroenteric anastomoses leaked, both holding for patients with established intraperitoneal sepsis, which proved fatal. Of the 349 patients, 13 (3.7 %) died in a hospital or within 30 days of their operation, but in only two cases could anastomotic leakage be implicated. Irwin et al. concluded that single-layer appositional upper gastrointestinal anastomoses are to be considered simple, safe, and economic.

In 2012, Sajid et al. performed a Cochrane systematic review of studies that compared single-layer (SGIA) versus double-layer suture anastomosis of the gastrointestinal tract [2]. SGIA can be performed quicker when compared to double-layer GIA. SGIA is comparable to DGIA in terms of anastomotic leak, perioperative complications, mortality, and hospital stay. SGIA may routinely be used for GIA following bowel resection. However, since this conclusion is derived from a study of a smaller number of patients recruited in relatively moderate quality trials, further trials should aim to reduce the limitations of this review.

An important intervention in daily practice is the reversal of a loop ileostomy and its complications. Luglio et al. reviewed a total of 944 patients undergoing reversal [3]. Ileostomy was created for several indications including ulcerative colitis (49.5 %) and rectal cancer (27.5 %) and compared different reversal techniques including sutured fold-over in 466 patients (49.4 %), stapled in 315 (33.4 %), and handsewn end-to-end in 163 (17.3 %). Handsewn cases had longer operative

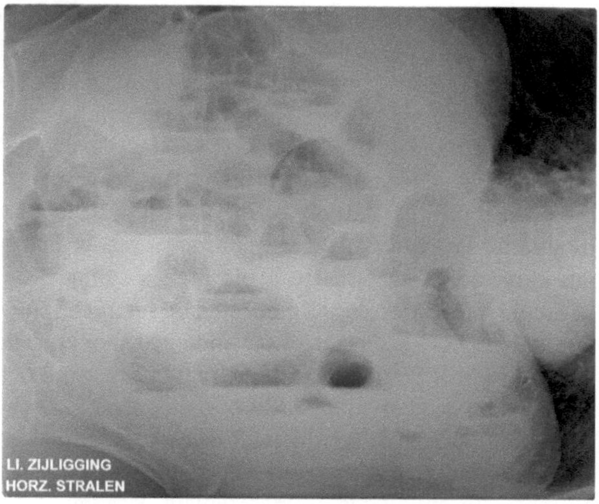

Fig. 17.2 Intestinal obstruction after reversal loop ileostomy

times, as well as longer times to bowel movement, to tolerance for soft diet, and to discharge. Overall, complications occurred in 203 patients (21.5 %), including 45 patients (4.8 %) who experienced a major complication; there were no deaths within 30 days (Fig. 17.2). Ileostomy closure should be reserved for patients who have a predicted postoperative major complication rate of 5 % or more without diversion. In a retrospective review by Giannakopoulos et al., the reversal of 119 loop ileostomies was analyzed [18]. The overall morbidity rate was 19 % with 12 % major complications. This study points out that the reversal of a loop ileostomy is associated with considerable risks. This should be kept in mind when thinking about applying it as a protective means in lower rectal surgery.

Acute Appendicitis

Indication for an appendectomy should be considered by way of (a) clinical assessment and physical examination, (b) laboratory tests especially leukocytes and differentiation and CRP, and (c) imaging techniques such as an ultrasonography and when in doubt by CT scan [4].

The current policy is to perform the appendectomy laparoscopically. Once it has been decided to operate the patient, prophylactic antibiotics (AB) should be administered. The combination of a cephalosporin with Metronidazol ® should be one dosage administered. In case of perforation or abscess, AB will need to be given for 5 days or according to the surgeon's opinion. Laparoscopy will start with inspection of the appendix, and if the appendix is normal, systematic inspection of the female genitalia and the rest of the abdomen will follow [5]. Special attention should be given to the presence of a Meckel's diverticulum. This is usually found within 1 m from the cecal at the antimesenterial side of the small bowel.

Prevention of complications start with the introduction of the trocars, especially those placed between the umbilicus and the left anterior spine, considering there always is a risk of damaging the inferior epigastric vessels with significant corresponding bleeding. Inspection of the artery during its introduction and control of trocar site at the end of intervention will help to avoid this complication.

During appendectomy, it is important to realize that the mobilization of the inflamed appendix takes place with an appropriate grasper, in order to avoid rupture by traction or perforations. Aspiration of pus or leakage material must be carried out immediately in order to avoid the spreading of infected materials. If general peritonitis or abscesses are present, then intervention will have to start with aspiration of the pus. The lavage of the abdomen should be done after the appendectomy. Dissection will be started with the mesentery using diathermia or clips. Dissection will then proceed up to the basis of the appendix. A known complication is leaving a long stump behind for this will cause a recurrent episode of acute appendicitis. An important issue at this point is how to handle the division of the appendix, either by means of endoloops or endostaplers. Kazemier et al. carried out a multi-analysis of four studies involving 427 patients [6]. Findings were that operative time was 9 min longer when using the endoloops. Also that superficial wound abscesses and postoperative ileus were significantly less frequent when the appendix stump was secured with staplers instead of with loops. Moreover, of the ten intraoperative ruptures of the appendix with contamination, seven cases occurred in loop-treated patients. Furthermore, hospital stay and postoperative intra-abdominal abscesses rate were also comparable in loop-treated and staple-treated patients. Beldi et al. studied a large cohort of prospectively acquired data of 6,486 patients, of which 60.5 % had been endoloop treated [7]. Intra-abdominal surgical-site infection rate and the rate of readmission to hospital were in this study found to be significantly less in the staple-treated cases. The only remaining problem turned out to be the cost of the endostapler.

In 2010, Sauerland et al. carried out the last Cochrane study comparing the morbidity of the procedure performed by laparoscopy or open appendectomy in 67 randomized studies [8]. Findings were that wound infections were less likely after laparoscopic appendectomy (LA) than after open appendectomy (OA), but the incidence of intra-abdominal abscesses was increased (Fig. 17.3). Comparatively, the duration of surgery for LA was 10 min longer than for OA. After LA, pain was on the first postsurgical day reduced by 8-mm on a 100-mm visual analogue scale. Hospital stay was shortened by 1.1 day, and return to normal activity, work, and sport occurred earlier after LA than following OA. While the operation costs for LA were significantly higher, the costs outside the hospital were reduced. Seven studies on children were included, but the results do not seem to be much different when compared to adults. Moreover, diagnostic laparoscopy reduced the risk of a negative appendectomy, but this effect was stronger in fertile women [5].

If the appendix is normal and the rest of the abdomen show no abnormalities, question arises what to do with the normal appendix? Since many years, this matter has remained controversial. Currently, this quandary has been addressed by Van den Broek et al., who studied the subject for a retrospective period of 4.4 years involving

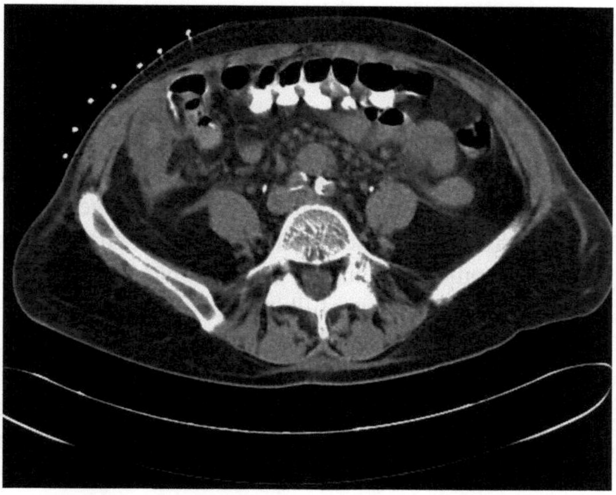

Fig. 17.3 Percutaneous drainage post-appendicectomy abscess

285 patients who had a normal appendix removed [9]. Findings show that different approaches were used and that complications occurred in 6 % of the cases, whereby 2 % of the patients requiring a reoperation. The extra hospital costs of a negative appendectomy were EUR 2712 per patient. The conclusion by Van den Broek et al. was that removal of a normal appendix entails considerable complications and costs. Therefore, when found, a normal appendix should be not removed. Moreover, it is important to perform adequate preoperative studies in order to establish a good diagnosis [4].

The policy concerning a carcinoid found in the appendectomy specimen has been addressed in one of the cases, but policy advised that "carcinoid tumours in the appendix smaller than 2-cm and radically operated do not need other complementary treatment whereas tumours >2-cm or not radical will need a right hemicolectomy to complete the completeness of the resection" [10].

Concerning diagnosis and treatment of postoperative complications, in the event that the patient should develop fever caused by wound abscess, this will need to be adequately drained. If the patient develops fever with a normal wound and has abdominal pain, then a CT scan of the abdomen should be done. An intra-abdominal abscess will need to be percutaneously drained.

Postoperative ileus after removal of a phlegmonous or perforated appendicitis may be related to inflammatory adhesions or the presence of an abscess at the ileocecal junction. Hence, it is important during an operation to ensure that the terminal ileum and Bauhin's valve are cleared of adhesions or of pus.

An interesting and sometimes difficult issue is how to deal with acute abdomen/acute appendicitis in pregnant women? For certain, a prompt diagnosis is crucial. Unal et al. studied a series of 20 pregnant patients [11]; they found that the use of ultrasound is limited for diagnosis, whereas the CT scan should not be used due to fetal radiation. Therefore, MRI is becoming more popular for the evaluation of such cases. Otto et al. have confirmed the valuable use of the MRI for pregnant patients involving a suspicion for acute appendicitis [12].

Is Laparoscopy Contraindicated in an Acute Abdomen During Pregnancy?

This subject remains controversial, especially if acute surgery has to be performed during the first trimester. Insufflation with CO_2 will induce during anesthesia a respiratory acidosis, yet not a decreased fetal oxygenation. Nonetheless, it will induce fetal acidosis and hypercapnia. Moreover, the Swedish register held on 720,000 pregnant women—including laparoscopically operated patients—led to the conclusion that no increase in stillbirths or birth defects and no difference in the type of delivery have been recorded in comparison with the control group [13]. The most important concerns remain twofold. Primarily, should in the event of an acute abdomen/acute appendicitis the operation be open or be laparoscopic? And secondarily, is the laparoscopic treatment risky for the fetus in terms of abortion and preterm labor? The SAGES guidelines address both points [14]. Regarding the first point, we read: "Risk and benefits of both procedures will be considered and discussed with the patient. Moreover, benefits of laparoscopy during pregnancy appear similar to the benefits in nonpregnant patients". Regarding the second point, their guideline is that "Recent literature has shown that pregnant patients may undergo laparoscopic surgery safely during any trimester without any increase of risks for mother or foetus" [14, 15]. Some general recommendations are pertaining to the following: the instruction that the pneumoperitoneum can be safely used between 10 and 14 mmHg; the advisable use of open-access laparoscopy in advanced pregnancy, in order to avoid mechanical lesions of the uterus and fetus; and finally the counsel to adequately monitor and correct gases during anesthesia. Moreover, the positions of trocars will be adapted to the size of the uterus.

Midterm complications

Concerning midterm complications after laparoscopic appendectomy, Swank et al. conducted a study on 755 patients operated in the open type (545 patients) and laparoscopic type (210 patients) [16]. In the long term, there were no differences between both groups concerning small bowel obstruction or incisional hernias.

Approach of an appendiceal phlegmon/mass

Traditional approach of an appendiceal phlegmon/mass has been conservative. A CT scan should be done in order to rule out the presence of an abscess, which should be percutaneously drained. Questions remaining after successful treatment are the following: (a) Should an interval elective appendectomy be performed? (b) How necessary is it to rule out a cecal cancer? Tekin et al. described 94 patients that had been diagnosed and treated because of appendicular mass [17]. In nine patients an abscess had to be drained and in five other patients a delayed operation was necessary because of intestinal obstruction or recurrence of abscess. The recurrence rate of mass or acute appendicitis after conservative treatment was 14.6 %. On view of these numbers, an interval elective appendectomy is not indicated if there has been no recurrence of complaints. Moreover, in patients older than 50 years, a routine colonoscopy should be done to rule out the presence of a cecal cancer.

References

1. Irvin ST, Krukowski ZH, Matheson NA. Single layer anastomosis in the upper gastrointestinal tract. Br J Surg. 1990;77:643–4.
2. Sajid MS, Siddiqui MR, Baig MK. Single layer versus double layer suture anastomosis of the gastrointestinal tract. Cochrane Database Syst Rev. 2012;1:CD005477.
3. Luglio G, Pendlimari R, Holubar SD, Cima RR, Nelson H. Loop ileostomy reversal after colon and rectal surgery: a single institutional 5-year experience in 944 patients. Arch Surg. 2011; 146(10):1191–6.
4. Poortman P, Oostvogel HJ, Bosma E, et al. Improving diagnosis of acute appendicitis: results of a diagnostic pathway with standard use of ultrasonography followed by selective use of CT. J Am Coll Surg. 2009;208:434–41.
5. Borgstein PJ, Gordijn RV, Eijsbouts QA, Cuesta MA. Acute appendicitis- a clear-cut case in men, a guessing game in young women. A prospective study on the role of laparoscopy. Surg Endosc. 1997;11:923–7.
6. Kazemier G, in t' Hof KH, Saad S, et al. Securing the appendiceal stump in laparoscopic appendectomy:evidence for routine stapling ? Surg Endosc. 2006;9:1473–6.
7. Beldi G, Vorburger SA, Bruegger LE, et al. Analysis of stapling versus endoloops in appendiceal stump closure. Br J Surg. 2006;93:1390–3.
8. Sauerland S, Jaschinski T, Neugebauer EA. Laparoscopic versus open surgery for suspected appendicitis. Cochrane Database Syst Rev. 2010;(10):CD001546. Review.
9. Bijnen CL, van den Broek WT, Bijnen AB, et al. Implications of removing a normal appendix. Dig Surg. 2003;20:215–9.
10. Butte JM, Garcia Huidobro MA, Torres J, et al. Long term survival in carcinoid tumor of the appendix. An analysis of 8903 appendectomies. Gastroenterol Hepatol. 2009;32:537–41.
11. Unal A, Sayharman SE, Ozel L, et al. Acute abdomen in pregnancy requiring surgical management: a 20 cases series. Eur J Obstet Gynecol Reprod Biol. 2011;159:87–90.
12. Otto A, Ernst RD, Ghulmiyyah LM, et al. MR imaging in the triage of pregnant patients with acute abdominal and pelvic pain. Abdom Imaging. 2009;34:243–50.
13. Reedy MB, Kallen B, Kuehl TJ. Laparoscopy during pregnancy: a study of five fetal outcome parameters with use of the Swedish Health Registry. Am J Obstet Gynecol. 1997;177:673–9.
14. Guidelines for diagnosis, treatment and use of laparoscopy for surgical problems during pregnancy. Practice/Clinical Guidelines published on 01/2011. By the Society of American Gastrointestinal and Endoscopic Surgeons (SAGES).
15. Oelsner G, Stockheim D, Soriano D, et al. Pregnancy outcome after laparoscopy or laparotomy in pregnancy. J Am Assoc Gynecol Laparosc. 2003;10:200–4.
16. Swank HA, Eshuis EJ, van Berge Henegouwen MI, Bemelman WA. Short- and long-term results of open versus laparoscopic appendectomy. World J Surg. 2011;35:1221–6.
17. Tekin A, Kurtoglu HC, Can I, Oztan S. Routine interval appendectomy is unnecessary after conservative treatment of appendiceal mass. Colorectal Dis. 2008;10:465–8.
18. Giannakopoulos GF, Veenhof AA, van der Peet DL, Sietses C, Meijerink WJ, Cuesta MA. Morbidity and complications of protective loop ileostomy. Colorectal Dis. 2009;11:609–12.

Chapter 18
Prevention and Treatment of Major Complications After Laparoscopic Ileocecal and Right Colectomy

W. Jeroen Meijerink

Keywords Perioperative complications • Laparoscopic ileocecal • Laparoscopic right colectomy • Ileotransversostomy • Anastomotic leakage • Duodenum lesion

Introduction

Laparoscopic colorectal surgery has been demonstrated to have superior outcome with earlier return of bowel function, decreased postoperative pain, shorter hospital admission, decreased morbidity, and favorable long-term outcome [1–4]. Laparoscopic ileocecal or right hemicolectomy is generally considered as one of the easiest to perform laparoscopic colectomies. Presumed easy access to vascular structures and presumed little danger of damage to adjacent organs and structures contribute to this conviction. But most experienced laparoscopic surgeons agree that a right hemicolectomy is not an easy procedure. A bulky colon, proximity of a right ureter, the duodenum, and a complex venous vascular structure when dissecting the transverse colon and omentum can make an ileocecal or right hemicolectomy to a real challenge, especially in the presence of a large malignancy, inflammation as seen in Crohn's colitis, or a complicated appendicitis.

W.J. Meijerink, MD
Department of Surgery, VU University Medical Center,
Amsterdam, The Netherlands
e-mail: j.meijerink@vumc.nl

M.A. Cuesta, H.J. Bonjer (eds.), *Treatment of Postoperative Complications after Digestive Surgery*, DOI 10.1007/978-1-4471-4354-3_18,

Safe Technique

Preoperative Preparations

Antibiotics, according to the hospital protocol, should be administered at least 30 min before starting the procedure. A catheter a demeure is inserted. Temporarily nasogastric tube is introduced in the stomach and removed at the end of the procedure. Other fast-track principles should be applied as much as possible and incorporated in the hospital protocols [5].

After general anesthesia and preferably a high epidural block, the patient is positioned in dorsal decubitus on a bean bag in French position with the left arm along the body. The right arm can be positioned according the anesthetists preference. Patient is slightly in anti-Trendelenburg position and tilted to the left. Typically there is a three-trocar access. The camera is positioned under the umbilicus, one trocar is placed in the left lower quadrant, and the third trocar can be positioned either suprapubical in the midline or in the midline in the upper abdomen, according to the surgeon's preference. The suprapubical position guarantees easy access to the terminal ileum and the right paracolic space; the upper midline trocar position facilitates the mobilization of the hepatic flexure and part of the transverse colon. The choice of the trocar position is dependent from the intended resection. For an ileocecal resection in Crohn's disease, the lower triangle configuration is the best choice. For a formal extended right hemicolectomy, the upper triangle configuration could be the preferred trocar position. An additional trocar should be placed without hesitation to the surgeon's preference and need.

The right hemicolectomy can be performed with basic laparoscopic instruments: one or two fenestrated graspers, dissector, scissor, and a diathermic hook. A sealing device as the harmonic scalpel or Ligasure device can be used if preferred. If no sealing devices are used, clips to ligate the vascular structures should be available.

A rinsing tube for irrigation and suction, straight endoscopic staplers (blue 60 or 80 mm), and reloads and wound protector should be readily available.

Proper Plane

As in all laparoscopic colectomies, identification of the proper planes is crucial to a successful procedure (Fig. 18.1). Opposite to the open procedures, the laparoscopic approach is from medial to lateral or mediocaudal to lateral. At the lateral side fascia of Toldt is the landmark. A thin white line typically identifies this fascia. Opening of this plane should be on the visceral side. One should stay close to the ascending colon and its mesocolon. As the medial-to-lateral or mediocaudal-to-lateral approach is advocated by most surgeons, dissection of the lateral peritoneum is one of the last steps of the resection. As the complete cecum and ascending colon are mobilized from the medial (caudal) side, this peritoneal reflection is a thin layer and easily identified.

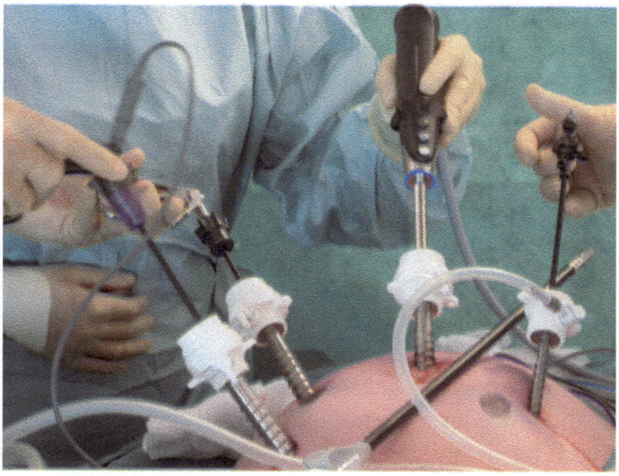

Fig. 18.1 Laparoscopic colectomy

Starting from lateral to medial, identification of the proper plane can be difficult, and it is easy to be lost in Gerota's fascia and eventually behind the kidney.

The medial landmark is the lateral border of the pars descendens of the duodenum. As the duodenum is a retroperitoneal organ, this structure is not always easily identified. A cautious approach from distally after opening the mesocolon the base of the ileocolic artery will show the duodenum just cranially from the ileocolic artery.

The upper limit of the resection is the caudal part of the liver. The hepatic flexure and ligaments are easily identified in the final phase when dissecting the peritoneum from lateral.

It is easy to be confused with the adhesions from the omentum to the transverse colon. Partial en bloc resection of the omentum is dependent from the diagnosis. In oncological resections in case of malignancy, as colon cancer, the omentum is taken with the specimen. In benign diseases the omentum can be dissected from the transverse colon in order to have a clear view on the transverse colon and hepatic flexure. The distal margin of the right hemicolectomy is formed by the ileocolic artery and the terminal ileum. The appendix is removed en bloc with the ileocecal resection or right hemicolectomy.

After dissection and anastomosis, the mesentery defect could either closed or left open. In open surgery the defect is historically always closed. Since the introduction of laparoscopic surgery, defects of the mesentery are left open. A recent study even showed that closure of the mesenteric defect was associated with a higher rate of complications [6].

Ileocecal Resection in Crohn's Disease

Despite novel medical treatment regimens in Crohn's disease, the rate and type of surgical resections have barely changed in the last decade [7]. Surgical therapy in Crohn's disease is indicated in case of complications of disease. Most frequently an ileocecal resection is performed, as this part of the bowel is most afflicted. Active disease can cause obstruction of the lumen with signs of a (sub-) ileus. One-third of patients have enteroenteric, enterocutaneous, enterosigmoid, or enterovesical fistulae at time of surgery.

If medical treatment fails, surgical resection of the inflamed part of the bowel is indicated. The timing of resection is in close collaboration with the gastroenterologist in a narrow equilibrium between optimal conservative treatment and surgery. The surgical procedure is characterized by a limited procedure to avoid the risk of short bowel at time of procedure or future procedures. Disease-free resection margins are not necessary, as there is no relationship between a (microscopic) disease-free margin and recurrence of disease. The surgeon's assessment of the diseased part of the bowel is generally longer than the histologist's judgement [8]. At the start of the procedure, the complete small bowels are inspected for additional lesions. Strictures in any part of the small bowel are treated with stricturoplasty. Resection is only needed in case of active disease with signs of obstruction.

Ileocecal resection in Crohn's disease is preferably performed by laparoscopy. Apart from faster functional recovery and less pain, there is a superior cosmetic result, which is important in often young patients. Less cicatrical hernia's and postoperative adhesions facilitate future surgical resections. Postoperative complications are common as most patients also use immunosuppressive medication. Anastomoses in inflamed tissue have a higher probability of leakage.

A laparoscopic ileocecal resection can be very demanding, especially in case of severe inflammation or presence of fistula formation between bowel loops or other organs.

Reoperation for recurrence of Crohn's disease is more complex than primary surgery. Often additional surgical interventions, e.g., extensive adhesions or associated with severity of disease, are required, and patients are prone to a higher morbidity rate and longer hospital stay. The need for temporary defunctioning stoma is higher [9, 10].

Technique

In uncomplicated cases of Crohn's disease, resection can be easily accomplished. The proximal margin has to be judged. The fatty overgrowth is one of the indications. Thickening of the mesentery and an inflammatory aspect of the bowel is another. The resection should be as close to the distal end of normal appearance of the small bowel. Here the small bowel should be supple, although prestenotic dilatation can be present. The small bowel is cut with a linear stapler. Dissection of the small bowel in the initial stage has the advantage that the afflicted bowel and mesentery can be inspected easily from both sides during dissection for the presence of fistulae or adhesions in the small pelvis. Another advantage is the fact that the inflamed bowel and mesentery have not to be exteriorized at the same time as the large cecum and ascending colon, limiting the extraction site. A sealing device can be used to dissect the mesentery close to the bowel. The cecum and ascending colon are mobilized from the lateral attachments. The ileocolic artery should be spared. An intra- or extracorporeal anastomosis can be made according to the preference and experience of the surgeon (see below). Laparoscopic intracorporeal anastomosis in ileocolic resection for Crohn's disease has to be demonstrated safe and feasible [11]. No influence on recurrence was found whether a side-side or end-end anastomosis is made [12].

The surgery of complicated Crohn's disease can be very demanding. Subtle and tedious dissection of adhesions can be necessary to free the inflammatory mass from other organs and bowel. The presence of (large) abscesses or fistulae can make a laparoscopic approach very difficult. Fistulae to the bladder can be very firm and fibrotic. In most case they can be cut, even with a sealing device. The orifice in the bladder can be sewn. If the fistula is not clear and not leaking when filling the bladder, a catheter a demeure is left for 7–10 days before removal.

Right Colectomy

Medial to Lateral

The patient is placed in mild Trendelenburg position and tilted to the left side. The omentum and transverse colon are retracted cephalad. The omentum is placed over the liver and stomach. The small bowels are moved to the left side of the abdomen.

The ileocecal fold is grasped with a fenestrated grasper close to the bowel. Traction is applied to ventrolateral direction. In most cases the fold of the ileocolic artery in the mesocolon is easily identified. At the base of the artery, the peritoneum is opened along the axis of the mesenteric vessels. The ileocolic artery, ileocolic veins, and superior mesenteric vein are identified. The ileocolic artery and ileocolic veins are transected with a sealing device or hemoclips. The mesocolon with the vascular trunk is lifted upwards. Below the mesocolon, the dissection is continued in an avascular plane by traction and countertraction technique. When in the proper plane, the white line of Toldt can be seen. Below this layer, the retroperitoneal structures as gonadal vessels and ureter can be seen. Dissection in this avascular plane is continued cephalad and lateral to the abdominal wall. Superior of this dissection plane, the posterior side of the ascending colon can be seen. In cranial direction, dissection is continued below the transverse colon up to the liver. Identification in an early stage of the duodenum is important to avoid damage to this structure. The duodenum is smoothly taken down from the mesocolon. Then the peritoneum is opened from the base of the trunk of the ileocolic vessels in an avascular thin layer just over the duodenum. The dissection along the superior mesenteric vein, medial of the duodenum, is continued to the base of the transverse colon. The head of the pancreas can be visualized. The right colic artery can be found in 30 % of cases. Then the base of the transverse mesocolon is dissected lateral to the branching of the middle colic artery. The right branch of the middle colic artery and vein are divided, preserving the left branch. The dissection of the mesocolon continued till the transverse colon. The transverse colon is divided with a straight linear stapler. The adjacent omentum is dissected as well preserving the gastroepiploic vein and Henlé's trunk. After completing the medial dissection, the mesenterium of the terminal ileum is dissected along the ileocolic vessels. The terminal ileum is divided with a straight linear stapler.

The last phase of the procedure is dissection of the lateral peritoneum from the appendix upwards to the hepatic flexure. If posterior dissection is carried out properly, the ascending colon is only attached with a thin layer of peritoneum to the lateral abdominal wall. Dissection of the hepatic flexure completes the dissection of the right colectomy.

Mediocaudal to Lateral

Some surgeons prefer the mediocaudal access to the vascular trunk of the ileocolic vessels. Patient position and exposure are the same as in the medial approach. The terminal ileum is lifted ventral. The peritoneum at the base of the cecum and appendix is dissected and the retroperitoneal space is identified. This avascular plane below the right mesocolon is dissected cephalad by traction and countertraction technique. The terminal ileum can be dissected at this point with a straight linear stapler. Dissection along the ileocolic vessels is carried out to the base at the mesenteric vessels. The ileocolic artery and vein are dissected and duodenum is identified. The dissection is then carried out in the same way as the medial approach.

In the laparoscopic-assisted technique, division of mesentery, ileocolic, and medial colic vessels as well as the division of bowel itself can be either intra- or extracorporeally. As the base of the mesocolon and vessels are located in the midline, surgeons argue that these structures can be easily exteriorized through a 4–6 cm midline incision. The base of these vessels is easily accessible for proximal ligation [13]. But in increasingly obese patients, exposure of the pedicles can be very limited, compromising optimal oncologic results. Many series, therefore, advocate intracorporeal ligation and transection of the mesentery with an extracorporeal anastomosis [2, 14, 15].

Intracorporeal vs Extracorporeal Anastomosis

Laparoscopic-assisted hemicolectomy involves externalization for bowel resection and anastomosis. A midline periumbilical or transverse incision can be used. The incision should allow a smooth externalization of small and large bowel and the adjacent mesocolon. If dissection is completed intracorporeally, a small Pfannenstiel or umbilical incision for removal of the specimen is needed. The incision length should be appropriate to the size of the tumor. A stapled side-to-side intracorporeal anastomosis is created with a linear stapler. The common opening is sutured with a running suture. Some authors advocate a second running seromuscular suture around the entire anastomosis to reinforce the staple line [16].

In comparison to the extracorporeal resection, superior results in intracorporeally completed resection and anastomosis with earlier return of bowel function, decreased postoperative pain, morbidity, and hospital stay have been claimed [16–18], although debated by others [19]. In experienced hands intracorporeal anastomosis is associated with equal or even shorter operative time [20, 21], as compared to open or extracorporeal anastomosis. Less mobilization and less tension applied to the colon, mesentery and incision with better preserved blood supply to the bowel and wound could be contributing factors for this superior result. There is also a reduced risk of twist of the small bowel at time of the anastomosis. The advantages of a laparoscopic-assisted hemi-right compared to open resection have been doubted. Since intracorporeal anastomosis was introduced in laparoscopy colon programs, authors claim augmented benefits compared to both open and laparoscopic-assisted procedures [16, 19–21].

In case of an extracorporeal anastomosis, a good orientation at the base of the mesentery, after transection of bowels, is extremely difficult. A twisted small bowel loop can occur, resulting in prolonged postoperative ileus or even small bowel obstruction. An extracorporeal anastomosis harbors also potential danger of traction on vascular pedicles with bleeding. Recognition and awareness of this bleeding is often late as the extraction site is blocked by exteriorized bowel loops. A laparoscopic check at the end of the procedure can both control for possible twists of bowel loops and bleeding of vascular pedicles. A safe intracorporeal anastomosis requires good dexterity and superior laparoscopic suturing skills.

Perioperative Complications

The complications of an ileocecal or right colectomy are essentially the same as for open colectomy, except for specific laparoscopic complications as trocar site hernia and pneumoperitoneum-related complications. Opposite to open surgery, overview during surgery is limited to an often bulky cecum and ascending colon. Identification of the proper planes is easy, but once one fails to identify the proper planes, it can be very difficult to identify the crucial structures. Gonadal vessels have been cut assuming them as ileocolic or right colic vessels. Dissection behind the duodenum or (thermal) injuries to the duodenum has occurred, failing to recognize the duodenum at an early stage.

Structures at Risk

Ureter at the right side is usually less at risk as the left ureter in left sided colectomies. Resection planes are above the level of the iliac crossing of the ureter. The ureter and gonadal vessels are in the retroperitoneal space. When dissection is in the proper plane, both ureter and gonadal vessels are below Gerota's fascia. In inflammatory bowel resections, identification of the proper planes can be extremely difficult. Explicit identification of the ureter in these cases is mandatory. Also in advanced cancer with involvement of the posterior planes, the ureter can be incorporated in the process. Careful dissection of the ureter in these situations, preferably after inserting a pre- or perioperative splint in the ureter, can avoid damage to the ureter. Special devices as double J ureteral stents or a ureter infrared illuminated stent can be helpful in identifying the ureter, especially in surgical therapy in inflammatory bowel disease or advances cancer cases.

Small lesions to the ureter detected during surgery can be sutured over a laparoscopic-inserted double J ureteral stent. Complete transection and dissection of part of the ureter require complex reconstruction in cooperation with the urologist. Not recognized lesions are typically detected second or third postoperative day. Fluid leakage from trocar incisions or intra-abdominal drains may be observed. A (large) intra-abdominal or retroperitoneal fluid collection on sonography or CT scan indicates a urinoma. Puncture of the fluid collection and determination of the creatinine content can proof urinary leakage. Small lesions detected with an intravenous pyelography can be treated with a transurethral double J catheter for some weeks. Larger defects need surgical repair.

Ileocolic Artery and Mesenteric Artery

The ileocolic pedicle and the right branch of the middle colic artery are divided close to their origin. Failure to identify the proper vascular structures potentially endangers the blood supply of the small bowel or remaining transverse and left colon. When isolating and dissecting the ileocolic artery at the origin, proper identification of the superior mesenteric artery and vein is mandatory. Failure to recognize the superior mesenteric artery potentially leads to ischemic alterations and subsequent necrosis of (parts of) the small bowel. Dissection of the pedicle of the middle colic artery leaves the entire colon depending on a patient's Drummond arcade. An incomplete arcade at Griffith's point or an absent arcade of Riolan is present in up to 30 % of patients. Dissection of the middle colic artery could lead to severe ischemia and subsequent necrosis of the transverse and left colon.

Duodenum and Small Bowel Injuries

The duodenum is one of the structures most at risk in a right colectomy. After dissection of the vessels and going upwards below the right mesocolon, the duodenum has to be identified clearly. By careful traction, counter-traction technique, the duodenum should be cleared from the mesocolon.

Unrecognized small bowel or duodenal lesions leads to significant and severe postoperative morbidity and even mortality. Damage to the electrical isolation of the shaft of laparoscopic instruments causes cauterization injuries to small bowel and other intra-abdominal organs without being notified during surgery. Leakage test of all laparoscopic instruments is mandatory in some countries. Adhesiolysis at the start of the procedure has to be performed with great care to avoid serosal lesions and full-wall perforations. Leakage of thermal and serosal injuries is typically on second or third postoperative day. Clinical signs depend on severity of spillage and resemble anastomotic leakage or intra-abdominal abscess formation. Gross spillage of bowel content usually requires reintervention. As the lesion is not recognized during surgery, exact localization of the perforation is unclear, even in case of clear extraluminal contrast at a CT scan. A diagnostic laparoscopy can be performed, but often fails to localize the focus, due to postoperative adhesions, protein deposits, and fecal content. A formal midline laparotomy is necessary in most cases. As the bowel often has a limited injury, the perforation can be oversewn. In case of severe damage to the bowel, resection and anastomosis might be indicated.

Duodenal perforations are not limited to the retroperitoneal space due to the dissection at surgery. Duodenal perforation presents similar to small bowel injuries and is treated similarly. In severe duodenal injuries, a jejuno-duodenostomy can be performed.

Postoperative Complications

Anastomotic Leakage

Anastomotic leakage has a profound and severe influence on postoperative outcome. It is one of the most serious complications in colorectal surgery with a reported incidence of between 1 and 17 %. The incidence of leakage is higher in inflammatory disease and Crohn's disease. Dedicated centers claim 3–6 % as an acceptable overall leakage range. Mortality rates after anastomotic leakage up to 40 % have been reported. Reoperation and redo of the anastomosis or dismantling the anastomosis and a temporary ileostomy are nearly always necessary.

A tension-free and well-vascularized anastomosis is the base of any bowel anastomosis. A proper blood supply of both remaining ends of the bowel is the result of a proper knowledge of the vascular anatomy (and its variations) and positive perioperative identification of the remaining pedicles.

Emergency surgery, prolonged surgical procedures, perioperative radiotherapy or chemotherapy, and immunosuppressive medication (e.g., steroids) have a negative influence on the healing of the anastomosis. Patient-related factors as diabetes, malnutrition, cardiovascular and hepatic comorbidity, high ASA score, or male gender have all been associated with a higher rate of anastomotic leakage. Resection in case of inflammation generally has higher leakage ratios than in cancer surgery. In a nationwide German survey, anastomotic leakage in 28,271 colorectal cancer patients was 3 %. Multivariate analysis identified long duration of surgery, a high ASA score, male gender, obstruction, left sides tumor, cardiovascular hepatic comorbidity, single-layer hand suture, biofragmentable ring anastomosis, intraoperative complications, and BMI >30 kg/m^2 as risk factors for postoperative leakage [22].

Anastomotic leakage not only increases postoperative morbidity and hospital stay but also has been associated with nearly threefold higher recurrence rates and reduced survival after curative resection of colon cancer [23–25].

Management of anastomotic leakage should be individualized to the patient's need. Early detection of anastomotic leakage is crucial and improves outcome. Early signs of leakage are often nonspecific and should be interpreted within the context of the postoperative course. Rise in heart rate, subfebrile temperature, decreasing urinary output and rising infection parameters (white blood cell count, sedimentation rate and C-reactive protein) in the blood, and increasing (local) tenderness are all indicative of an intra-abdominal problem or infection. They are nonspecific indicators as other sources of infection have similar signs. If leakage is suspected, a CT scan with oral and i.v. contrast is made. Observation and bowel rest, percutaneous drainage of abscess or fluid collection, surgical revision of the anastomosis, and diversion are available strategies. Re-anastomosis in cases with limited contamination should be considered. In selected cases early anastomotic leakage can be solved laparoscopically, even in the presence of a limited postoperative ileus. Additional sutures in small leaks or complete revision of anastomosis is challenging, and conversion to open revision should be without hesitation.

If there are signs of a generalized peritonitis with or without septic shock, prompt resuscitation, antibiotics, and surgical intervention are mandatory. Revision of anastomosis is dependent from the degree of peritonitis and condition of the bowel.

In case of anastomotic leakage, fistula formation, or intra-abdominal abscess related to anastomotic leakage after resection for Crohn's disease, revision of the anastomosis is debated. It has been claimed that surgical outcome is better with a lower rate of recurrence of postoperative Crohn's disease after dismantling the anastomosis with an end stoma [26].

Abscess

Intra-abdominal postoperative abscess is a frequent observation in colon cancer. Incidence is reported up to nearly 40 % in colon cancer patients. Clinical manifestation is depending from size and localization. Subfebrile or spiking temperature, local tenderness, prolonged postoperative ileus, and rising infection parameters are indicative, but are similar to those observed in anastomotic leakage or other postoperative infections. A CT scan is preferred over sonography to prove the presence of an abscess, as percutaneous drainage of larger abscesses can be performed in the same session. Small abscess (<3–4 cm) can be treated with prolonged antibiotic regimen only.

Prolonged Postoperative Ileus

Bowel function normally is restored within 24–48 h after right colectomy. A prolonged ileus can indicate surgical-related complications as a twisted anastomosis or stenosis of the anastomosis.

In case of an extracorporeal anastomosis, the choice of the extraction site is limited. Proper intestinal alignment after extraction can be difficult. An intestinal twist can be the result of lack of proper orientation of the bowel alignment. Intracorporeal anastomosis may reduce this risk.

References

1. Schwenk W, Haase O, Nudecker JJ, Muller JM. Short term benefits for laparoscopic colorectal resection. Cochrane Database Syst Rev. 2005;20(3):CD003145. Review.
2. Clinical Outcomes of Surgical Therapy Study Group. A comparison of laparoscopically assisted and open colectomy for colon cancer. N Engl J Med. 2004;350:2050–9.
3. Colon Cancer Laparoscopic or Open Resection Study Group. Laparoscopic surgery versus open surgery for colon cancer: short-term outcomes of a randomized trial. Lancet Oncol. 2005;6:477–84.
4. Duepree H-J, Senagore AJ, Delaney CP, Fazio VW. Does means of access affect the incidence of small bowel obstruction and ventral hernia after bowel resection? Laparoscopy versus laparotomy. J Am Coll Surg. 2003;197:177–81.
5. Kehlet H. Fast track colorectal surgery. Lancet. 2008;371:791–3.
6. Causey MW, Oguntoye M, Steele SR. Incidence of complications following colectomy with mesenteric closure versus no mesenteric closure. does it really matter? J Surg Res. 2011;171:571–5.
7. Jones DW, Finlayson SR. Trends in surgery for Crohn's disease in the era of infliximab. Ann Surg. 2010;252:307–12.
8. Pelletier A, Stefanescu C, Vincent C, Etienney I, Mentre F, Soule JC. Is the length of postoperative recurrence on the neo terminal ileum predictable in Crohn's disease? J Crohns Colitis. 2011;5:24–7.
9. Brouquet A, Blanc B, Bretagnol F, Valleur P, Bouhnik Y, Panis Y. Surgery for intestinal Crohn's disease recurrence. Surgery. 2010;148:936–46.
10. Holubar SD, Dozois EJ, Privitera A, Cima RR, Pemberton JH, Young-Fadok T, Larson DW. Laparoscopic surgery for recurrent ileocolic Crohn's disease. Inflamm Bowel Dis. 2010;16:1382–6.
11. Bergamaschi R, Haughn C, Reed III JF, Arnaud J-P. Laparoscopic intracorporeal ileocolic resection for Crohn's disease: is it safe? Dis Colon Rectum. 2009;52:651–6.
12. McLoad RS, Wolff BG, Ross S, Parkes R, McKenzie M, Investigators of the CAST Trial. Recurrence of Crohn's disease after ileocolic resection is not affected by anastomotic type: results of a multicenter, randomized, controlled trial. Dis Colon Rectum. 2009;52:919–27.
13. Young-Fadok TM, Nelson H. Laparoscopic right colectomy: five-step procedure. Dis Colon Rectum. 2000;43:267–71.
14. Senagore AJ, Delaney CP, Brady KM, Fazio VW. Standardized approach to laparoscopic right colectomy: outcomes in 70 consecutive cases. J Am Coll Surg. 2004;199:675–9.
15. Lezoche E, Feliciotti F, Paganini AM, Guerrieri M, De Sanctis A, Minervini S, Campagnacci R. Laparoscopic cs open hemicolectomy for colon cancer. Surg Endosc. 2002;16:596–602.
16. Grams J, Tong W, Greenstein AJ, Salky B. Comparison of intracorporeal anastomosis in laparoscopic-assisted hemicolectomy. Surg Endosc. 2010;24:1886–91.
17. Bergamaschi R, Teutch JJ, Pessaux P, Arnaud J-P. Intracorporeal vs laparoscopic assisted resection for uncomplicated diverticulitis of the sigmoid. Surg Endosc. 2000;14:520–3.
18. Bergamaschi R, Schochet E, Haughn C, Burke M, Reed III JF, Arnaud J-P. Standardized laparoscopic intracorporeal right colectomy for cancer: short term outcome in 111 unselected patients. Dis Colon Rect. 2008;51:1350–5.
19. Bernstein MA, Dawson JW, Reissman P, Weiss EG, Nogueras JJ, Wexner SD. Is complete laparoscopic colectomy superior to laparoscopic assisted colectomy. Am Surg. 1996;62:507–11.

20. Franklin ME, Gonzalez JJ, Miter DB, Mansur JH, Trevino JM, Glass JL, Mancilla G, Abrego-Medina D. Laparoscopic right hemicolectomy for cancer: 11-year experience. Rev Gastroenterol Mex. 2004;69:65–72.
21. Hellan M, Anderson C, Pigazzi A. Extracorporeal versus intracorporeal anastomosis for laparoscopic right hemicolectomy. JSLS. 2009;13:312–7.
22. Kube R, Mroczkowski P, Steinert R, Sahm M, Schmidt U, Gastinger I, Lippert H. Anastomotic leakage following bowel resections for colon cancer: multivariate analysis of risk factors. Chirurg. 2009;80:1153–9.
23. Mirnezami A, Mirnezami R, Chandrakumaran K, Sasapu K, Sagar P, Finan P. Increased local recurrence and reduced survival from colorectal cancer following anastomotic leak: a systematic review and meta-analysis. Ann Surg. 2011;253:890–9.
24. Marra F, Steffen T, Kalak R, Warschkow I, Tarantino I, Lange J, Zund M. Anastomotic leakage as a risk factor for the long-term outcome after curative resection for colon cancer. Eur J Surg Oncol. 2009;35:1060–4.
25. McArdle CS, McMillan DC, Hole DJ. Impact of anastomotic leakage on long-term survival of patients undergoing curative resection for colorectal cancer. Br J Surg. 2005;92:1150–4.
26. Iesalnieks I, Kilger A, Kalisch B, Obermeier F, Schlitt HJ, Agha A. Treatment of the anastomotic complications in patients with Crohn's disease. Int J Colorectal Dis. 2011;26:239–44.

Chapter 19
Prevention and Treatment of Major Complications After Left Colon, Sigmoid, and Rectal Surgery

Cesar Reategui, Badma Bashankaev, and Steven D. Wexner

Keywords Complications • Left colon • Sigmoid • Rectal surgery • Fecal peritonitis • Intra-abdominal abscess • Presacral abscess • Stenosis • Low anterior resection (LAR) • Anastomotic leakage

Leakage of Anastomosis with Fecal Peritonitis

Anastomotic complications after colorectal surgery are unfortunate. The determinants of anastomotic healing include both general patients and disease-related conditions. Malnutrition (especially albumin <2.0 g/dl or recent weight loss >15 %), DM, radiation, shock, blood loss, and immune deficiency are among the many factors for anastomosis leak. These conditions should be taken into account when deciding whether or not to perform a primary anastomosis or an end colostomy and Hartmann's stump or mucous fistula.

Most leaks become apparent between the 5th and 10th postoperative day. Early leaks present with fever, leukocytosis, localized or generalized tenderness, ileus, and sepsis. If a leak is suspected but not apparent, a water-soluble contrast enema is the initial test of choice to identify it. Abdominal CT can help in the identification of collections which are suggestive of leaks. If there are signs of peritonitis with or

C. Reategui • B. Bashankaev
Department of Colorectal Surgery, Digestive Disease Center, Cleveland Clinic Florida, Weston, FL, USA

S.D. Wexner, MD, PhD (Hon), FACS, FRCS, FRCS(Ed) (✉)
Department of Colorectal Surgery, Digestive Disease Center, Cleveland Clinic Florida, Academic Affairs Florida Atlantic University College of Medicine, Clinical Education Florida International University College of Medicine, Weston, FL, USA
e-mail: wexners@ccf.org

M.A. Cuesta, H.J. Bonjer (eds.), *Treatment of Postoperative Complications after Digestive Surgery*, DOI 10.1007/978-1-4471-4354-3_19,

without septic shock, resuscitation, broad-spectrum antibiotics and urgent laparotomy are indicated. If findings show a small leak (<1 cm) and the bowel is healthy, local repair with proximal fecal diversion might be feasible. If ischemia and necrosis ≥1/3 of the circumference are noted, the anastomosis should be resected and either re-done or exteriorized as an end stoma.

Technical considerations are fundamental to a successful anastomosis. Blood supply should be ensured by transecting the mesentery close to the anastomosis and by preserving the vascular arcade supplying the respective area. Anything less than pulsatile bleeding at the cut edge after bowel transaction is unacceptable, and resection should be proximally extended until bleeding is encountered. Fatty tissue should not be cleared more than 5–6 mm from the edge. Tension is another key factor, as it may compromise blood flow.

Tension-free anastomosis in the left colon can be facilitated by:

1. Complete mobilization of the splenic flexure
2. Separation of the omentum from the distal transverse colon and mesocolon
3. High ligation of the inferior mesenteric artery (IMA)
4. Division of the inferior mesenteric vein (IMV) at the lower edge of the pancreas

The bowel ends must be viable. Inflamed or thickened bowel must be resected until it is soft and thin colon is encountered. Single or double layer, interrupted or continuous sutured, or manual or stapled anastomotic techniques are all acceptable variants. Most anastomotic leaks occur after rectosigmoid surgeries with low anastomosis. The anastomosis can be tested by occluding and submerging the anastomosis under saline while insufflating air through the rectum. The absence of bubbles confirms anastomotic integrity.

A Cochrane data base review [1] of 1,233 patients enrolled in randomized clinical trials (RCTs) compared stapled and handsewn colorectal anastomosis. There was insufficient evidence to demonstrate any superiority of one technique over the other, regardless of the level of the colorectal anastomosis.

Intraoperative flexible sigmoidoscopy is a valuable tool during left colon surgeries to assess the anastomosis for air leaks or anastomotic bleeding. This intraoperative procedure has been studied to assess its usefulness in preventing anastomotic leaks and bleeding after colorectal surgery. In a study of patients undergoing colorectal resection with distal anastomosis [2], 107 patients who underwent routine intraoperative endoscopy (RIOE) were compared to 137 who underwent selective intraoperative endoscopy (SIOE). The results showed more postoperative anastomotic complications including staple line bleeding and anastomotic leakage in the SIOE as compared to the RIOE group.

The long-term oncological impact after anastomotic leaks was recently reviewed by Mirnezami et al. [3]. He performed a meta-analysis of 21,902 patients with anastomotic leakage (AL) after restorative surgery for colorectal cancer. They found an OR (OR) of 2.9 for developing a local recurrence for articles describing rectal anastomoses. Those describing both colon and rectal anastomoses showed an OR of 2.9. Distant recurrence and long-term cancer-specific mortality after AL showed an OR 1.38 and 1.75, respectively.

Intra-abdominal Abscess

Intra-abdominal abscess can result from anastomotic leaks, enterotomies, or spillage from bowel contents at the time of the surgery. Its incidence varies. Eberhardt et al. [4] analyzed the impact of leaks and intra-abdominal abscesses on cancer recurrence and survival in patients undergoing resections for colorectal cancer. Besides concluding that neither leaks nor abscesses are associated with worsened survival or recurrence at 5 years, they showed an incidence of intra-abdominal abscess of 38.9 % for colon cancer patients vs. 14.4 % for the rectal cancer group. Symptoms are highly variable. They may present 5–7 days after surgery with persistent abdominal or pelvic pain, focal tenderness, spiking fever, prolonged ileus, and/or leukocytosis. Intermittent polymicrobial bacteremia suggests an intra-abdominal abscess in patients who have had abdominal surgery. If an abscess is located deep in the pelvis, classic signs and symptoms might be absent. Abdominal CT scan with IV, oral, and possible rectal contrast is the modality of choice as it provides more than a 95 % diagnostic accuracy rate. A fluid collection with a thickened enhancing rim and surrounding inflammatory stranding is diagnostic.

Most intra-abdominal abscesses can be percutaneously drained under CT guidance with an efficacy of 65–90 % depending on size, complexity, etiology, and microbial flora.

Leakage of Distal Rectal Anastomosis

The incidence of leaks in left side colorectal anastomosis varies according to the distance of anastomosis from anal verge. Vignali et al. [5] reported an overall leak rate of 2.9 % in a series of 1,014 colorectal anastomosis. Eight percent of low anastomosis <7 cm from anal verge leaked compared to 1 % of anastomosis >7 cm from anal verge. Ileal pouch-anal anastomosis has the greatest risk for leak with a reported incidence of 5–10 %. Other identified risk factors are male gender, increased BMI, previous surgery, distal rectal cancer [6], albumin <3.5 g/dl, operative time >200 min, blood loss >200 cc, transfusion requirement [7], and "after hours" construction of anastomosis [8] . As previously mentioned technical factors included an ample blood supply and tension-free anastomosis. A leak may present in 3 ways:

Dramatic Early Leak

Presents with acute abdominal pain, distension, fever, tachycardia, diffuse peritonitis, oliguria, and shock within several days of surgery. These symptoms usually predict a large uncontained leak.

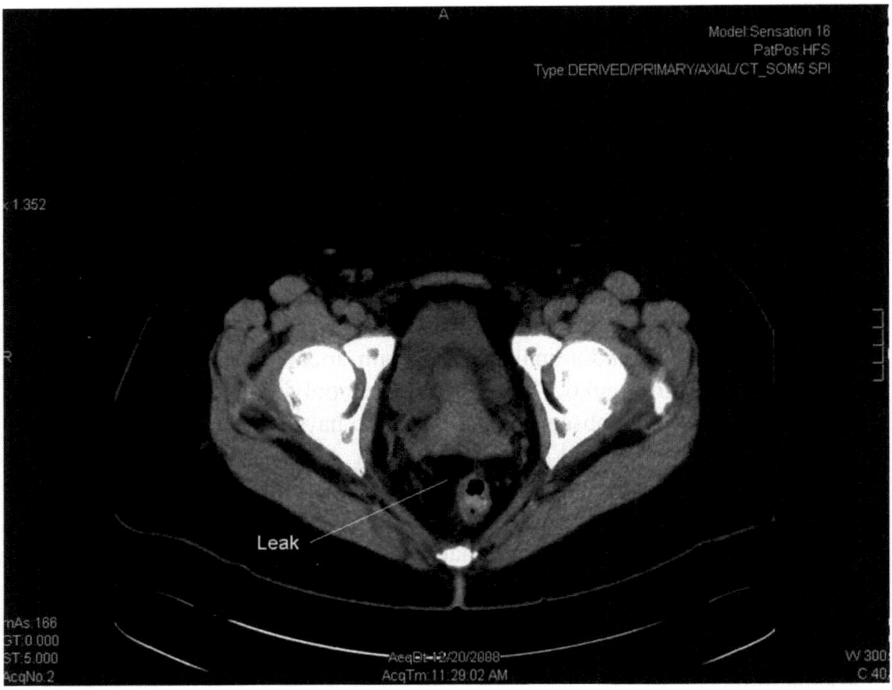

Fig. 19.1 Anastomotic leak following distal colorectal anastomosis

Subtle Insidious Leak

Can present with mild leukocytosis, protracted ileus, and failure to thrive. Such leaks typically present 5–14 days following surgery; by this time adhesions have formed and contain the process. Because of nonspecific signs, detection may be difficult.

Asymptomatic Leak

Is usually harmless, is incidentally discovered by radiologic studies weeks to months after surgery, and consists of a walled-off sinus. Treatment is rarely necessary.

Initial management in patients without signs of peritonitis is aimed to identify and localize the process. Water-soluble enema is usually the first test ordered, although CT scan with triple contrast (oral, intravenous, and rectal) has become the imaging modality of choice (Fig. 19.1). During this period, an infectious process may be difficult to differentiate from acute postoperative inflammation and fluid collection. Collections >4 cm can often be drained via a transabdominal, transgluteal, or transanal image-guided catheter. If the abscess cavity is small

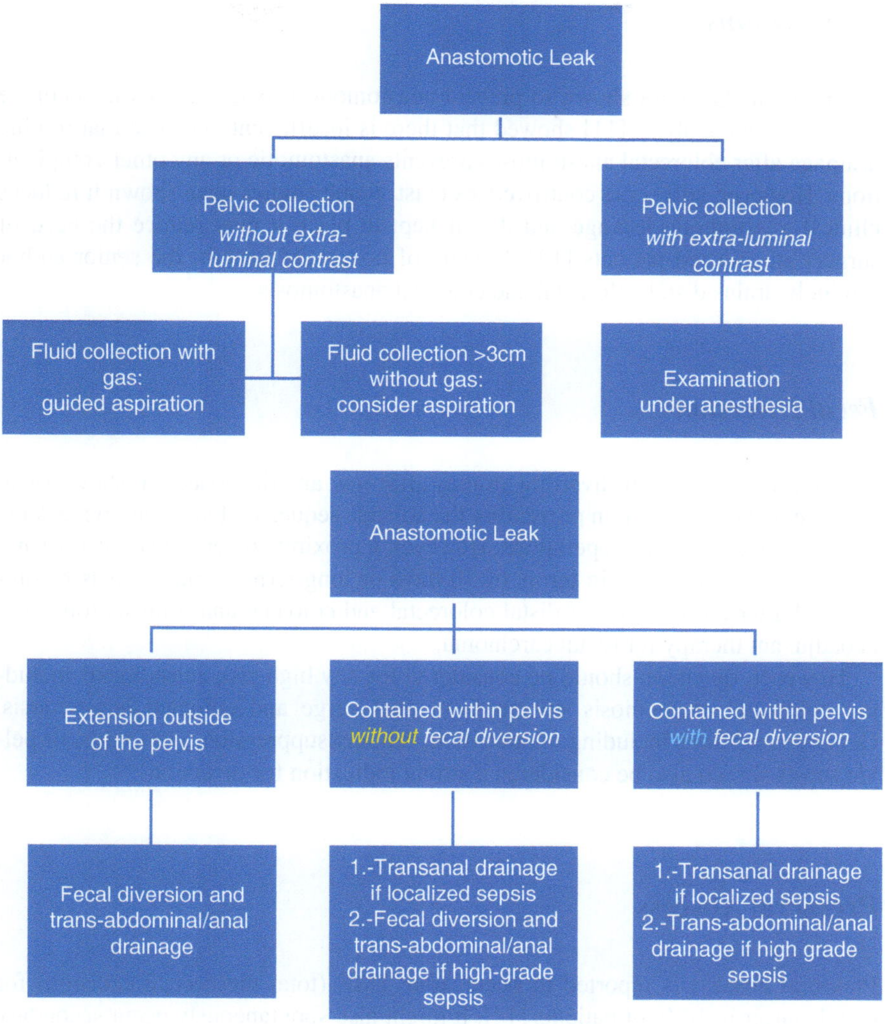

Fig. 19.2 Standardized algorithms for management of anastomotic leaks (Adapted from Phitayakorn et al. [9])

and contrast flows freely back into the lumen, conservative management with intravenous antibiotics and bowel rest may suffice. An algorithm to manage leaks has been proposed [9] Fig. 19.2.

A vacuum-assisted endosponge is a new approach to treat patients with anastomotic dehiscence following anterior resection for rectal cancer. It has been shown useful in treating pelvic sepsis following anastomotic dehiscence or rectal stump insufficiency [10]. Management of persistent sinuses involves observation, sinus unroofing, debridement, and instillation of fibrin glue.

Pelvic Drains

Pelvic drains have not shown to prevent anastomotic leakage. In fact a Cochrane database meta-analysis [11] showed that there is insufficient evidence that routine drainage after colorectal anastomoses prevents anastomotic or any other complications. However, still some controversies exist. Some studies have shown it reduces clinical anastomotic leakage and that if kept in place it may reduce the need of surgery in selected patients [12]. In spite of no agreed benefit, the senior author routinely drains distal colorectal and coloanal anastomosis.

Fecal Diversion

A recent review [13] of diverting stomas after low anterior resection showed that they seemed to be useful in preventing the adverse sequelae of anastomotic leakage and consequent urgent reoperations. However, a proximal diverting stoma does not seem to offer advantage in terms of 30 days or long-term mortality. It is recommended after construction of distal colorectal and coloanal anastomosis following neoadjuvant therapy for rectal carcinoma.

However, diversion should be considered for any high-risk anastomosis including colorectal anastomosis <6 cm from anal verge and coloanal anastomosis. General conditions including malnutrition, immunosuppression, peritonitis, or pelvic sepsis should also be considered a strong indication for diversion.

Presacral Abscess

Presacral abscess is reported to occur after TME (total mesorectal excision) for rectal cancer in 10 % of patients [14]. It might also spontaneously occur secondary to Crohn's disease. The large defect created by the total mesorectal excision (TME) is filled by the neorectum or the colonic J pouch. In case of a leak, this cavity may turn into an abscess. Patients in poor general health, who have received neoadjuvant radiation therapy ($p<0.003$), or who have large tumors (median 38 mm [$p<0.04$]) are at risk for developing a presacral abscess [14]. The clinical picture is sometimes insidious; thus, vigilance and clinical suspicion are important as a delay in diagnosis may increase morbidity. Collections can be drained via transgluteal approach by CT guidance, transrectal approach under ultrasonography (US) guidance, or a dorsal transsacral approach. Probably the most promising indication for vacuum-assisted closure is the treatment of para-anastomotic presacral abscesses following anastomotic leakage after total mesorectal excision. In a multicenter [15] study which aimed to evaluate the use and success of the endosponge for treating the presacral cavity due to leakage, the authors concluded that the success of this treatment is not dependent on the time interval between surgery and treatment. Nine of their 16 patients (56 %) achieved definite resolution. Six of the 8 patients achieved resolution when the sponge was placed within 6 weeks of surgery compared to only 3 out of 8 patients (38 %) in whom it was placed at a later time point.

Stenosis of the Anastomosis After Low Anterior Resection

Benign strictures after low anterior resection (LAR) are a common complication with an incidence ranging from 5.8 to 22 %. They can be defined as a narrowing of the anastomosis of less than 12 mm, thus preventing the passage of a 12 mm sigmoidoscope. Symptoms vary according to the degree of stenosis, from asymptomatic to constipation, tenesmus, abdominal pain, and even large bowel obstruction. Risk factors promoting this problem include ischemia, dehiscence, and radiation therapy. In a study of 24 patients [16], symptoms developed at a mean of 6.8 (range3 to 19) months. Diagnosis is clinically suspected and then subsequently confirmed by a water-soluble contrast enema and endoscopy. A variety of modalities of treatment have been reported, although therapy is based on 3 main procedures: (1) dilation with finger, anal dilators, or endoscopy, (2) electroincision, and (3) resection and reanastomosis. A method utilizing a transanal circular stapler has also been reported [17, 18]. The most commonly used method is digital dilation although the most common method reported in the literature is endoscopic dilation. A recent study [19] showed no difference with regarding the number of dilations needed, stenosis-free time intervals, and complications between endoscopic balloon dilation when compared to Eder-Puestow metal olive dilators. An indisputable advantage regarding the cost favors the Eder-Puestow technique (22.30 Euros vs. 680 Euros; $p<0.001$). Surgical resection with reanastomosis is associated with a more demanding procedure with higher morbidity and mortality than endoscopic procedures and is usually performed after failure of the later.

Denoya et al. [20] reviewed the records of 16 patients who developed an anastomotic stricture after colorectal resection and anastomosis. Results showed that 94 % of patients had incomplete left colonic mobilization. The authors concluded that lack of complete mobilization of the left colon is associated with anastomotic stricture formation.

Stenosis of Anastomosis After Sigmoid Resection

Anastomotic strictures after sigmoid resection are an interesting topic although reported series are heterogeneous due to patient selection. The incidence of symptomatic anastomosis stricture with double-stapling technique has been reported as 18 % [21]. Stenosis can present several months after surgery and may occur after primary resection and anastomosis or after Hartmann's reversal. Fistula, leak, or

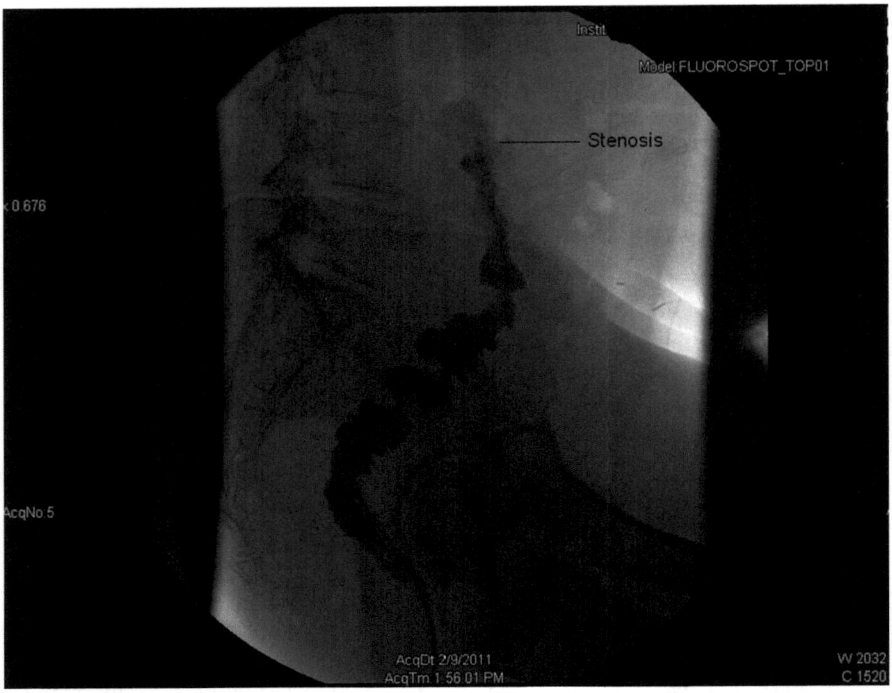

Fig. 19.3 Stenosis after sigmoid resection

inclusion of remnants of sigmoid in the anastomosis might be related to its development. Arterial preservation, double- or single-stapled techniques, and stapler diameter do not seem to influence the risk of anastomotic stenosis. Symptoms include lower abdominal pain when passing gas or stool, abdominal distension, fractional evacuation, constipation, and/or ribbonlike stools. Diagnostic evaluation includes contrast enema (Fig. 19.3) and flexible sigmoidoscopy. Ambrosetti reported a mean diameter of 7 mm (4–10) in 22 patients with stenosis after sigmoid resection for diverticular disease [21]. Management involves endoscopic balloon dilatation as the initial option when the stenosis is short, which is the most common presentation. Success rate ranges between 59 and 88 % after an average of 2.5 sessions (1–13) [22]. If anastomosis is short and needs to be re-done, surgery can be simplified by the use of a circular stapler introducing the anvil through a proximal enterotomy. Anastomosis resection and reanastomosis is reserved for those patients who fail balloon dilation or who have a long stricture. Re-resection is associated with increased morbidity and mortality. Ureteral stents should be placed to help in the identification of the ureters. Although this practice does not decrease the ureteral injury rate, it helps with its identification and management.

Boutros et al. [23] reported 9 ureteral injuries (23 %) out of 3,950 patients who underwent colorectal surgery. In 1,038 patients (26 %) ureteral stent placement (USP) was performed. Laparoscopy and pelvic dissection were more commonly

Table 19.1 Leakage of ileoanal pouch anastomosis

Year	Author	*N* patients enrolled	% Leakage IAA
1995	Fazio	1,005	Early 2 % Late 0.9 %
1997	Bauer	392	10.7 %
1999	Billeveau	239	Early 3.3 %
2003	Fabrizio	391	Early 3.3 %
2003	Michalessi	391	6.4 %
2005	Krausz	174	4.8 %
2007	Manoj	141	[b]With abscess 2 % [b]Without abscess 3.1 %
2007	Von Roon	189	12.6 %
[a]2009	Rink	131	0.76 %

[a]Preserving mesorectal tissue. Follow-up at a median of 85 (14–169) months
[b]All early leaks. Early = within 30 days after surgery

performed in this group of patients ($p<0.002$ and $p<0.001$, respectively). They were also significantly older ($p<0.01$), had an increased BMI ($p<0.02$), a diagnosis of diverticular disease, Crohn's disease, fistula, and a history of radiation therapy ($p<0.001$ each). All ureteral injuries (UI) were recognized intraoperatively. Eight of them occurred in the USP group. The authors concluded that the use of prophylactic USP may aid in the intraoperatively UI identification as well as promptly and successful repair.

The last meta-analysis comparing open sigmoid resection (OPR) vs. laparoscopic sigmoid resection (LSR) [24] showed no differences in incidence of strictures. This type of stricture is avoidable by performing a complete distal sigmoid resection and anastomosis of the proximal colon to the rectum rather than any residual sigmoid colon [25].

Leakage of an Ileoanal Pouch Anastomosis

The ileal pouch-anal anastomosis (IPAA) has become the standard of care for patients with mucosal ulcerative colitis (MUC) and familial adenomatous polyposis (FAP) who require total proctocolectomy (TPC) and do not wish a permanent ileostomy. Leakages at the ileoanal anastomosis (IAA) are associated with the development of pelvic or abdominal sepsis and subsequently with pouch-cutaneous or pouch-vaginal fistulas. Handsewn anastomosis has been reported to be a risk factor for its development; this fact may be due to increased tissue trauma, leading to poor healing or increased tension at the anastomosis resulting in ischemia [26]. Tension in the anastomosis and current steroid use has also been identified as risk factors [27]. The incidence of this complication is shown in Table 19.1.

Ileoanal pouch leaks usually present within 30 days after surgery. Raval at al. [29] showed a median time from pouch construction to the diagnosis of pouch leak of 19 (1–336) days. In 68 % of patients, the leak was recognized within 30 days of surgery. Symptoms included fever (67 %), abdominoperineal pain (38 %), and abdominal abscess (6 %). The diagnosis is made usually by radiologic studies including pouchogram and pelvic CT, although occasionally, endoscopy is the method of identification. Proximal diversion is a matter of debate since recent data show that it can be safely omitted in selected patients. A recent survey among ASCRS members [28] concluded that the majority of surgeons create a temporary loop ileostomy at the time of ileal pouch-anal anastomosis for ulcerative colitis. Different approaches for treatment have been proposed depending upon whether or not the patient is diverted. Non-diverted patients with peritonitis need immediate diversion. Non-diverted patients who develop a leak might be initially treated without diversion. In a recent study [29] 80 % (33/42) of patients were successfully treated without diversion. A trial of conservative therapy with pouch drainage, antibiotics, and abscess drainage can be attempted before surgery. If leak persists after a week, diversion is undoubtedly needed. Leaks identified in diverted patients can be managed depending on the severity of the leak. Local attempts may include debridement with installation of fibrin glue and pouch advancement. The latter method consists of mobilizing the pouch transperineally or utilizing a combined abdominoperineal approach. Regardless of the technical approach selected at the time of pouch advancement, infected tissue must be excised and granulation tissue curetted. Omentopexy to separate tissues can be performed. Pouch reconstruction or excision may be necessary. An algorithm has been proposed for the management of leak after IPAA Fig. 19.4.

Late Ileoanal Pouch Fistulas

Timewise ileoanal pouch fistulas can be classified according to its appearance after surgery as either early (<12 months) or late (>12 months). The etiology in late developing fistulas although still poorly understood might be related to undiagnosed Crohn's disease. However, leaks, pelvic sepsis, experience, and techniques have been linked to the development of early fistulas. In general the incidence of pouch fistulas varies from 4 to 16 %. Nisar J et al. [30] classified them according to their severity in major and minor fistulas. Major fistulas including complex fistulas which extend to or originate from 2 or more sites: abdominal wall, vagina, peritoneal cavity, or urological structures. Minor fistulas involve the buttocks, perineal or perianal skin, or presacral space. They concluded that the presence of major fistulas is associated with pouch failure. Fistulas can present as external fistulas (most common presentation), with pelvic or abdominal sepsis and/or pelvic or abdominal pain. The diagnosis can be made clinically or with imaging studies. Time and frequency distribution vary and are shown in Fig. 19.5.

Treatment should be individualized. The decision to perform a specific procedure is based on the etiology and anatomy of the problem, the surgeon's preference, and patient-related factors. Fistulas, leaks, and strictures are the most common

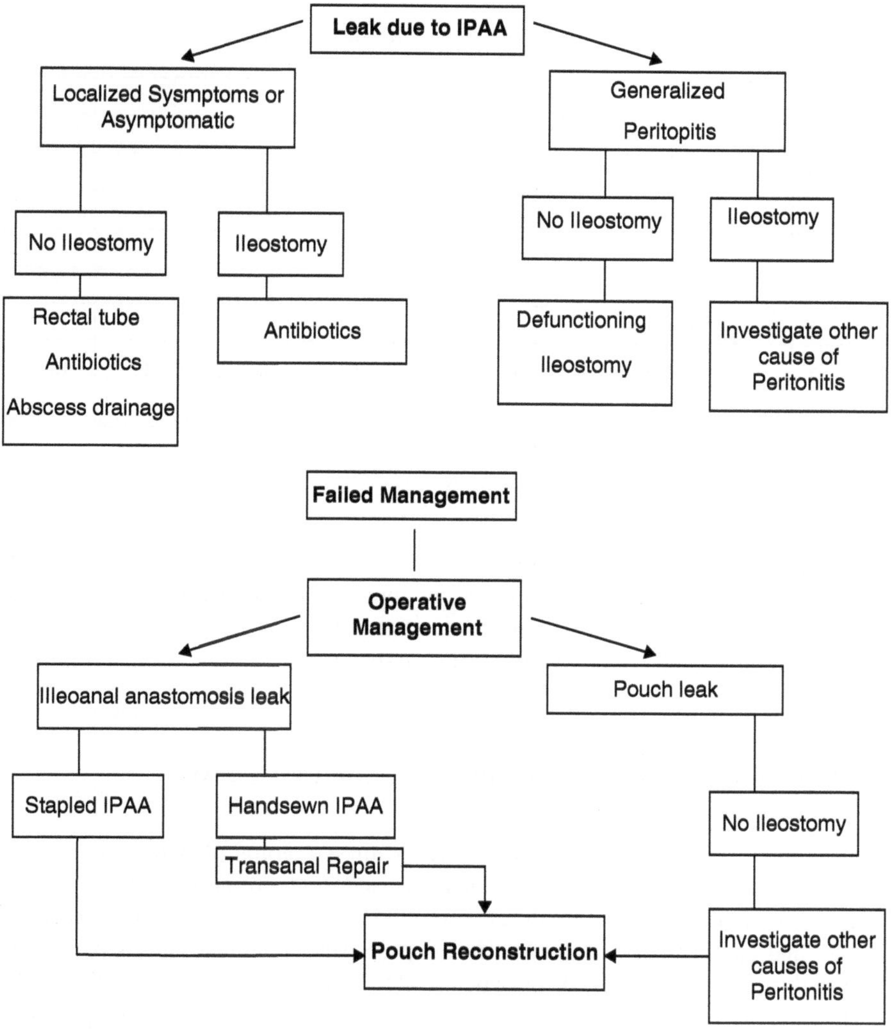

Fig. 19.4 Suggested algorithm for the management of IPAA by Raval et al. [29]

causes for redo abdominal pouch surgery. Drainage, correction of strictures, and loop ileostomy are usually the first steps. Local repair if feasible includes endoanal ileal advancement flap, pouch advancement, and muscle interposition techniques. Salvage pouch surgery can be safe and successful in avoiding pouch excision and permanent ileostomy. Pouch salvage procedures are mostly performed on early appearing fistulas, whereas anoperineal procedures are most common performed on their late counterparts.

In an effort to assess outcomes and predictors of success after re-operative ileo-anal pouch surgery and pouch excision, Shawki et al. [31] reviewed the records of 51 and 17 patients, respectively. The re-operative group consisted of patients with

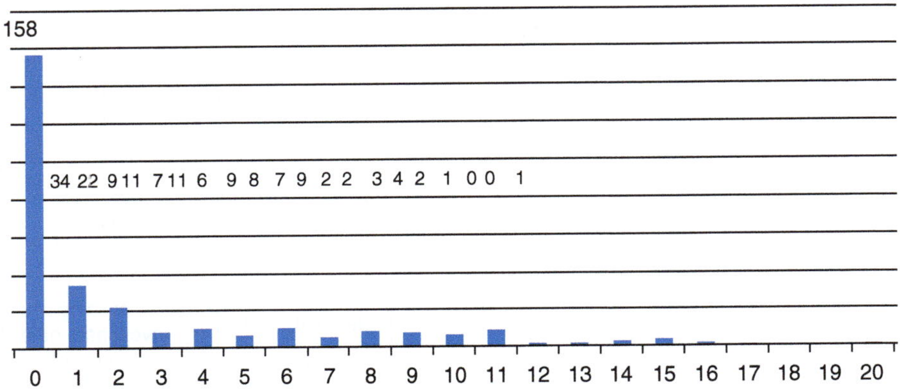

Fig. 19.5 Time of onset of pouch-related fistulas after ileal pouch-anal anastomosis creation. Number of patients and years provided

diagnosis of ulcerative colitis, (44) familial adenomatous polyposis (6), and indeterminate colitis (1). While in this group 38 (74.4 %) of patients had a successful outcome, Crohn's disease was diagnosed in more than half of the patients who underwent primary pouch excision. In general prevention of this complication is aimed to reduce contamination and tension in the pouch.

Rectovaginal Fistula After Low Anterior Resection

Rectovaginal fistulas (RVFs) are suspected with symptoms of flatus and/or malodorous discharge per vagina, incontinence episodes, recurrent, urinary tract infections, and vaginitis. They are not a common complication after rectal surgery for cancer and can present early or late in the postoperative course. RVFs have been reported to occur in 0.9–2.9 % of patients after LAR (low anterior resection). The early variant has been classically associated with the involvement of the posterior vaginal wall in the staple line at the moment of firing the circular stapler and therefore depends on the individual surgeon's experience and skills using the stapler. Recurrent tumor, radiation history, and devascularized vagina in close proximity to the anastomosis have also been proposed as risk factors [32]. The delayed variant as reported by Shin et al. usually presents after 30 days [33]; they studied 1,838 patients who underwent sphincter-preserving surgery for rectal cancer to investigate the characteristics of those who developed delayed anastomotic leaking (DAL). They found 10 delayed anastomotic-vaginal fistulas (0.54 %) which were detected at a median of 37 postoperative days. Female gender, low colorectal anastomosis (<4 cm from anal verge), and a history of preoperative chemoradiation therapy were independent risk factors for the development of DAL. The authors proposed that leakage at the colorectal anastomosis with subsequent tracking to the vaginal wall is a more plausible explanation than incorporating the posterior vaginal wall in the

Table 19.2 Surgical management of RVF after LAR

	Success rate
A. Management with diversion ($n=28$)	
1. Diversion only ($n=17$)	35 %
2. Diversion with staged endoanal repair ($n=8$)	62 %
3. Diversion with reanastomosis (3)	100 %
B. Management without diversion	
1. Endoanal repairs	66 %
2. Reanastomosis	100 %
C. Pull-through operation ($n=2$)	
D. Abdominal perineal resection ($n=3$)	

Adapted from Rex Jr. et al. [32]

anastomosis since no vaginal tissue was found in the doughnut rings from the EEA stapler. Diagnosis is made clinically and by physical examination. In an earlier study by Rex et al. [32], a questionnaire was sent to 990 members of the American Society of Colon and Rectal Surgery of which 300 (30 %) surgeons answered. Of 57 RVFs/year identified, only 4 occurred after handsewn anastomosis. In this study fistulas presented at an average of 20 days after surgery (1–90). The management by the respondents is outlined in Table 19.2.

Overall conservative therapy should be considered first before diversion or surgical repair especially if the fistula is small. Transvaginal approach with simple closure or advancement flap has also been reported by some authors. Prevention of this complication aims to the need of dissecting free the rectum from the posterior wall of the vagina and to angle the stapler so that the vagina is kept out of the staple line. Good visualization of the operative field in the deep pelvis is mandatory, and a simple digital vaginal examination before firing the stapler has been found to prevent this complication.

Infection Perineal Wound After APR

Unhealed wounds typically occur more frequently in the perineal region after APR with an incidence of 11–50 %. Neoadjuvant radiation therapy especially including the perineum, prolonged operative time, intraoperative hypothermia, fecal contamination during perineal dissection [34], DM, and increased BMI [35] have been identified as risk factors. Besides good surgical technique, good blood supply, nutritional status, and smoking may be the only modifiable factors at the time of proctectomy. Avoiding the external sphincter during intersphincteric dissection has been proposed for benign diseases. This maneuver allows better hemostasis and multiple layer closure. The use of drains has been associated with an improved rate of perineal healing, especially transabdominal drains compared to perineal drains; they should be kept 2–5 days. Perineal muscle flaps have provided little improvement in perineal wound healing. If infection occurs, the skin should be opened to allow drainage, and a program of wet to dry packing should be started followed by a vacuum-assisted closure device. If perineal sinus develops, wound debridement and myocutaneous flap reconstruction with gracilis, inferior gluteus, or rectus abdominis muscle might ultimately be necessary.

Perineal Hernia

A perineal hernia is a protrusion of intra-abdominal contents through a pelvic floor defect as a result of surgery. They reportedly occur in 0.1–7 % of patients after APR, although most of them are asymptomatic and <1 % needs repair. Symptomatic herniation is estimated to be <1 %. Coccygectomy, previous hysterectomy, pelvic irradiation, excessive length of small bowel mesentery, large pelvis, failure to close perineal defect, and excision of the levators seem to be risk factors. Bulging feeling, pain when sitting, and discomfort in the perineum are sometimes referred by patients. These symptoms can be controlled with a T bandage or a firm pair of underpants. The diagnosis is usually made clinically and subsequently confirmed with imaging modalities. Surgical management is based on the same principle of other hernias repair. The aim is to reconstruct the pelvic floor using synthetic mesh or autogenous tissue such as grafts or muscle flaps. The operative approach can be perineal, abdominal, or a combination of both. The perineal approach seems to be preferable since the abdominal cavity is not entered although all approaches seem to have similar results. The transabdominal approach is reserved for patients with recurrent hernias or those who need abdominal entry for any reason. This technique allows suturing a mesh to the bony pelvis under direct vision. Recently the laparoscopic transabdominal approach has been described. However, it can be difficult to approach the levators after cancer surgery since the defect may be quite large. Using the perineal approach, a mesh can be secured to the musculofascial tissue or the periosteum of sacrum (Fig. 19.6a, b). Care should be taken to avoid large vessels. Ureteral stents and an obturator in the vagina can be preoperatively inserted to aid in these structures identification. Its main disadvantage is the limited exposure and higher rate of hernia recurrence. So et al. [36] reported an incidence of 0.62 % following APR and a recurrence of 16 % after 12-month follow-up (all had undergone perineal repair). It may be also advisable to work combined with plastic surgery for the transposition of healthy tissue to fill large anatomical defects.

Abscesses After Hartmann Procedure

Hartmann's procedure may be performed when making a colorectal anastomosis is considered unsafe. Thus, not surprisingly Hartmann's operation is associated with high morbidity and mortality if severe peritonitis of sigmoid diverticular origin occurs. Unfortunately the rectal stump may postoperatively leak.

This complication is not frequently reported in the literature. Symptoms are usually related to intra-abdominal infection. Cherukuri et al. [37] reported 4 leaks

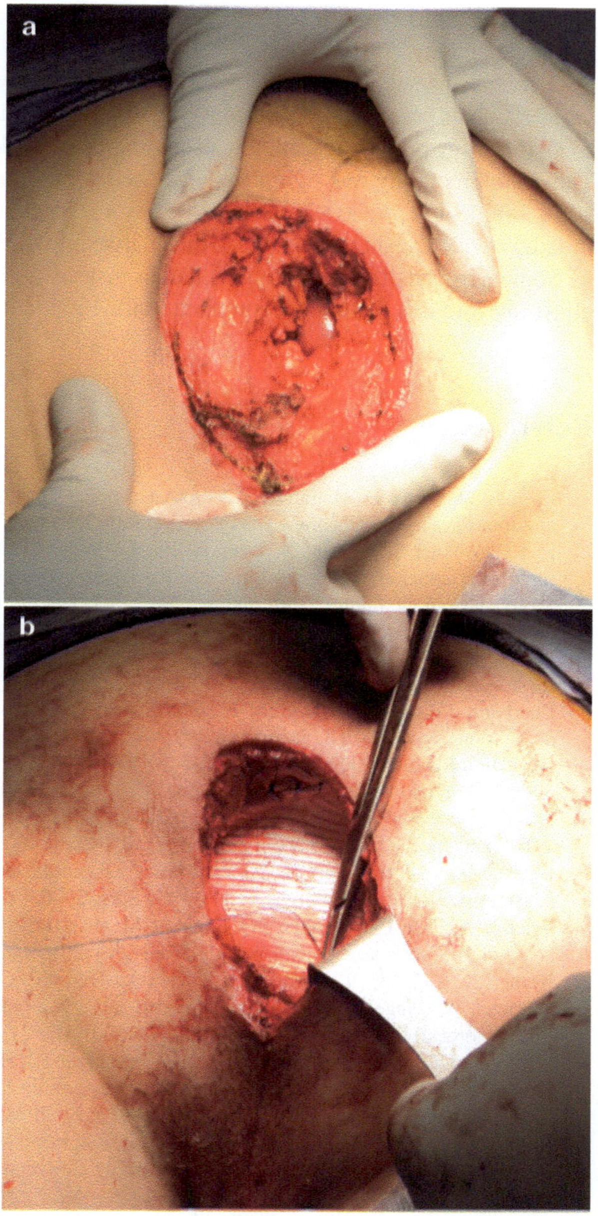

Fig. 19.6 (**a**) Perineal hernia. (**b**) Perineal hernia with mesh in place (Courtesy of Cleveland Clinic Florida)

(2 symptomatic) in 84 patients who underwent contrast-enhanced radiography of the pouch after Hartmann's procedure to evaluate for postoperative abnormalities. Schein et al. [38] have reported so far the biggest series of patients with clinical leak of the rectal stump.

Management basically consists of a washout with or without refashioning of the rectal stump. The washout system is based on 2 observations: leaving the rectal stump open and irrigate it before the repair, avoiding further contamination of the abdominal cavity.

A recent review [39] of 15 studies to compare primary resection with anastomosis vs. Hartmann's procedure in nonelective surgery for diverticulitis included 963 patients, 57 % following primary resection with anastomoses and 43 % Hartmann's procedures. The overall mortality was significantly reduced with primary resection and anastomosis (4.9 vs. 15.1 %; odds ratio = 0.41). Leaks from the rectal stump were not included in the study, which again may be due to the relative infrequency of this problem.

Some surgeons fashion a mucus fistula instead of Hartmann's procedure in an effort to avoid this theoretical complication.

References

1. Lustosa SA, Matos D, Atallah AN, Castro AA. Stapled versus handsewn methods for colorectal anastomosis surgery. Cochrane Database Syst Rev. 2001;(3):CD003144.
2. Li VK, Wexner SD, Pulido N, Wang H, Jin HY, Weiss EG, Nogueras JJ, Sands DR. Use of routine intraoperative endoscopy in elective laparoscopic colorectal surgery: can it further avoid anastomotic failure? Surg Endosc. 2009;23(11):2459–65. Epub 2009 Mar 20.
3. Mirnezami A, Mirnezami R, Chandrakumaran K, Sasapu K, Sagar P, Finan P. Increased local recurrence and reduced survival from colorectal cancer following anastomotic leak: systematic review and meta-analysis. Ann Surg. 2011;253(5):890–9.
4. Eberhardt JM, Kiran RP, Lavery IC. The impact of anastomotic leak and intra-abdominal abscess on cancer-related outcomes after resection for colorectal cancer: a case control study. Dis Colon Rectum. 2009;52(3):380–6.
5. Vignali A, Fazio VW, Lavery IC, Milsom JW, Church JM, Hull TL, Strong SA, Oakley JR. Factors associated with the occurrence of leaks in stapled rectal anastomoses: a review of 1,014 patients. J Am Coll Surg. 1997;185(2):105–13.
6. Lipska MA, Bissett IP, Parry BR, Merrie AE. Anastomotic leakage after lower gastrointestinal anastomosis: men are at a higher risk. ANZ J Surg. 2006;76:579–85.
7. Telem DA, Chin EH, Nguyen SQ, Divino CM. Risk factors for anastomotic leak following colorectal surgery: a case-control study. Arch Surg. 2010;145(4):371–6; discussion 376.
8. Komen N, Dijk JW, Lalmahomed Z, Klop K, Hop W, Kleinrensink GJ, Jeekel H, Ruud Schouten W, Lange JF. After-hours colorectal surgery: a risk factor for anastomotic leakage. Int J Colorectal Dis. 2009;24(7):789–95. Epub 2009 Mar 21.
9. Phitayakorn R, Delaney CP, Reynolds HL, Champagne BJ, Heriot AG, Neary P, Senagore AJ. Standardized algorithms for management of anastomotic leaks and related abdominal and pelvic abscesses after colorectal surgery. World J Surg. 2008;32(6):1147–56.
10. Riss S, Stift A, Meier M, Haiden E, Grünberger T, Bergmann M. Endo-sponge assisted treatment of anastomotic leakage following colorectal surgery. Colorectal Dis. 2010;12(7 Online):e104–8. Epub 2009 Apr 13.
11. Jesus EC, Karliczek A, Matos D, Castro AA, Atallah AN. Prophylactic anastomotic drainage for colorectal surgery. Cochrane Database Syst Rev. 2004;4, CD002100.
12. Tsujinaka S, Kawamura YJ, Konishi F, Maeda T, Mizokami K. Pelvic drainage for anterior resection revisited: use of drains in anastomotic leaks. ANZ J Surg. 2008;78(6):461–5.
13. Montedori A, Cirocchi R, Farinella E, Sciannameo F, Abraha I. Covering ileo-or colostomy in anterior resection for rectal carcinoma. Cochrane Database Syst Rev. 2010;12(5), CD006878.
14. Veenhof AA, Brosens R, Engel AF, van der Peet DL, Cuesta MA. Risk factors and management of presacral abscess following total mesorectal excision for rectal cancer. Dig Surg. 2009;26(4):317–21. Epub 2009 Aug.

15. Van Koperen PJ, van Berge Henegouwen MI, Rosman C, et al. The Dutch multicenter experience of the endo-sponge treatment for anastomotic leakage after colorectal surgery. Surg Endosc. 2009;23:1379–83.
16. Alonso A, Sergio E, Costa A. Efficacy and safety of endoscopic balloon dilation of benign anastomotic strictures after oncologic anterior rectal resection: report on 24 cases. Surg Laparosc Endosc Percutan Tech. 2008;18(6):565–8.
17. Nissotakis C, Sakorafas GH, Vugiouklakis D, Kostopoulos P, Peros G. Transanal circular stapler technique: a simple and highly effective method for the management of high-grade stenosis of low colorectal anastomoses. Surg Laparosc Endosc Percutan Tech. 2008;18(4):375–8.
18. Gentilli S, Balbo M, Sabatini F, Fronticelli CM, Villata E. Cicatricial stenosis of colorectal anastomosis. Transanal treatment with circular stapler. Minerva Chir. 1999;54(12):905–7.
19. Xinopoulos D, Kypreos D, Bassioukas SP, Korkolis D, Mavridis K, Scorilas A, Dimitroulopoulos D, Loukou A, Paraskevas E. Comparative study of balloon and metal olive dilators for endoscopic management of benign anastomotic rectal strictures: clinical and cost-effectiveness outcomes. Surg Endosc. 2011;25(3):756–63. Epub 2010 Oct.
20. Denoya P, Shawki S, Sands D, Nogueras J, Weiss E, Wexner S. Colorectal anastomotic stricture: is it associated with inadequate colonic mobilization? Colorectal Dis. 2008;10 Suppl 1: 28, abstract 85.
21. Ambrosetti P, Francis K, De Peyer R, Frossard JL. Colorectal anastomotic stenosis after elective laparoscopic sigmoidectomy for diverticular disease: a prospective evaluation of 68 patients. Dis Colon Rectum. 2008;51(9):1345–9. Epub 2008 May 3.
22. Suchan KL, Muldner A, Manegold BC. Endoscopic treatment of postoperative colorectal anastomotic strictures. Surg Endosc. 2003;17(7):1110–3. Epub 2003 May 6.
23. Boutros M, Kalaskar S, da Silva G, Weiss E, Wexner S. Ureteral injury in colorectal surgery: incidence, risk factors and role of prophylactic ureteral stents. Poster presented at: the American Society of Colon and Rectal Surgeons meeting, 2011 May 14–18, Vancouver.
24. Siddiqui MR, Sajid MS, Qureshi S, Cheek E, Baig MK. Elective laparoscopic sigmoid resection for diverticular disease has fewer complications than conventional surgery: a meta-analysis. Am J Surg. 2010;200(1):144–61.
25. Thaler K, Baig MK, Berho M, Weiss EG, Nogueras JJ, Arnaud JP, Wexner SD, Bergamaschi R. Determinants of recurrence after sigmoid resection for uncomplicated diverticulitis. Dis Colon Rectum. 2003;46(3):385–8.
26. Macrae HM, McLeod RS, Cohen Z, et al. Risk factors for pelvic pouch failure. Dis Colon Rectum. 1997;40:257–62.
27. Heuschen UA, Hinz U, Allemeyer EH, Autschbach F, Stern J, Lucas M, Herfarth C, Heuschen G. Risk factors for ileoanal J pouch-related septic complications in ulcerative colitis and familial adenomatous polyposis. Ann Surg. 2002;235(2):207–16.
28. de Montbrun SL, Johnson PM. Proximal diversion at the time of ileal pouch-anal anastomosis for ulcerative colitis: current practices of North American colorectal surgeons. Dis Colon Rectum. 2009;52(6):1178–83.
29. Raval MJ, Schnitzler M, O'Connor BI, Cohen Z, McLeod RS. Improved outcome due to increased experience and individualized management of leaks after ileal pouch-anal anastomosis. Ann Surg. 2007;246(5):763–70.
30. Nisar PJ, Kiran RP, Shen B, Remzi FH, Fazio VW. Factors associated with ileoanal pouch failure in patients developing early or late pouch-related fistula. Dis Colon Rectum. 2011;54(4):446–53.
31. Shawki S, Belizon A, Person B, Weiss EG, Sands DR, Wexner SD. What are the outcomes of reoperative restorative proctocolectomy and ileal pouch-anal anastomosis surgery? Dis Colon Rectum. 2009;52(5):884–90.
32. Rex Jr JC, Khubchandani IT. Rectovaginal fistula: complication of low anterior resection. Dis Colon Rectum. 1992;35(4):354–6.
33. Shin US, Kim CW, Yu CS, Kim JC. Delayed anastomotic leakage following sphincter preserving surgery for rectal cancer. Int J Colorectal Dis. 2010;25(7):843–9.

34. Nissan A, Guillem JG, Paty PB, Douglas Wong W, Minsky B, Saltz L, Cohen AM. Abdominoperineal resection for rectal cancer at a specialty center. Dis Colon Rectum. 2001;44(1):27–35; discussion 35–6.
35. Christian CK, Kwaan MR, Betensky RA, Breen EM, Zinner MJ, Bleday R. Risk factors for perineal wound complications following abdominoperineal resection. Dis Colon Rectum. 2005; 48(1):43–8.
36. So JB, Palmer MT, Shellito PC. Postoperative perineal hernia. Dis Colon Rectum. 1997;40(8): 954–7.
37. Cherukuri R, Levine MS, Maki DD, Rubesin SE, Laufer I, Rosato EF. Hartmann's pouch: radiographic evaluation of postoperative findings. AJR Am J Roentgenol. 1998;171(6):1577–82.
38. Schein M, Kopelman D, Nitecki S, Hashmonai M. Management of the leaking rectal stump after Hartmann's procedure. Am J Surg. 1993;165(2):285–7.
39. Constantinides VA, Tekkis PP, Athanasiou T, Aziz O, Purkayastha S, Remzi FH, Fazio VW, Aydin N, Darzi A, Senapati A. A Primary resection with anastomosis vs. Hartmann's procedure in nonelective surgery for acute colonic diverticulitis: a systematic review. Dis Colon Rectum. 2006;49(7):966–81.

Chapter 20
Prevention and Treatment of Major Postoperative Complications After Laparoscopic Colorectal Resections

Willem A. Bemelman

Keywords Postoperative complications • Laparoscopic colorectal resections • Ureter damage • Trocar hernia • Bowel ischemia • Internal herniation • Anastomotic leakage

Introduction

Colorectal surgery for benign and malignant disease comprise of the majority of the abdominal operations. It is generally done either by colorectal surgeons or gastrointestinal surgeons. The implementation of the laparoscopic approach, since its introduction in 1991, has rapidly expanded particularly over the last 5 years. Patient demands, surgeon's preference, broad acceptance, and above all training programs have been responsible for this explosive growth. In most surgical units the laparoscopic approach is the preferred one in primary surgery for colorectal disease. With the introduction of the laparoscopic approach specific complications have emerged, e.g., trocar herniation, nonexisting in open surgery. In this chapter we will focus on the prevention, diagnosis, and treatment of major complications associated with laparoscopic colorectal surgery, e.g., "late" conversion, peroperative major bleeding, bowel ischemia, and anastomotic leakage.

W.A. Bemelman, MD
Department of Surgery, Academic Medical Center,
Amsterdam, The Netherlands
e-mail: w.a.bemelman@amc.uva.nl

M.A. Cuesta, H.J. Bonjer (eds.), *Treatment of Postoperative Complications after Digestive Surgery*, DOI 10.1007/978-1-4471-4354-3_20,

General Remarks

Key in the prevention of complications is surgical proficiency and case selection irrespective of the approach or type of procedure. With the introduction of laparoscopic surgery, the "learning curve" was introduced as if it did not exist in open surgery. Different outcome parameters have been used to assess the learning curve of a specific procedure; operating time, conversion rate, hospital stay, and morbidity were the most common parameters. Probably hospital stay and morbidity are the outcome parameters that really matters. The learning curve for colorectal resections depend on the complexity of the resection increasing from ileocecal resection, right colectomy, low anterior resection to restorative proctocolectomy. The difficulty of the operation also depends on the type of laparoscopic approach, e.g., facilitated (laparoscopic mobilization only), laparoscopic assisted (intracorporeal mobilization and devascularization, and extracorporeal anastomosis), and total laparoscopic. A surgeon should tailor the type of procedure, the type of laparoscopic approach, the extent of the pathology, and the patient characteristics to his or her laparoscopic skills. Literature data indicate that the numbers for the learning curve vary from 15 to more than 100 laparoscopic cases before proficiency is reached [1]. Experienced laparoscopic surgeons know that learning goes on long after having done 100 cases. In the prevention of complications, case selection is therefore of paramount importance. In the beginning of the learning curve, the surgeon should select a patient with a low BMI, preferably women (little abdominal fat), no prior major open surgery, requiring a relatively simple resection, and done either facilitated (e.g., ileocecal resection) or laparoscopic assisted [2–4]. The procedure is done with the assistance of a more experienced colleague.

Each procedure must be succinctly planned and prepared. In left-sided resection one or two enemas are required to empty the bowel to prevent stapling problems in a stool-loaded bowel. If bowel preparation is indicated because off, for instance, when a defunctioning ileostomy is planned, bowel preparation should be started timely. Late initiation of bowel preparation will result in a fluid-loaded small and large bowel jeopardizing exposure of the surgical field. Proper position on the table with the legs in French position or the Lloyd Davis boots is of great importance enabling transanal access. Optimal equipment preferably chip on the tip or high-definition technology is a prerequisite for advanced laparoscopic procedures. The ability to use vessel sealing equipment (ligasure, ultracision), endoscopic staples, and wound protectors is basic in advanced laparoscopic surgery.

A huge amount of evidence exists nowadays that "late" conversion is associated with increased morbidity and mortality. "Late" conversion meaning conversion because of a peroperative complication or due to lack of progression of the procedure should be prevented and is a reflection of a mismatch of surgical skill required for this particular patient to complete the procedure [3].

Some have shown that implementation of recovery after surgery programs ("fast-track programs") have reduced the morbidity rate. It is therefore advised to train the medical and nursing staff in the fast-track principles [5, 6].

Key in diagnosis is early suspicion. Patients having laparoscopic colorectal surgery without complications are mobilized and have a regular oral intake within 2–3 days after surgery. If this is not the case, there must be a high level of suspicion that something is wrong. Increasing instead of a decreasing C-reactive protein (CRP) might precede the clinical manifestation of the complication [7, 8]. CT scanning with enteral and intravenous contrast is the first line diagnostic tool.

Key in treatment is even more surgical experience. Depending on the type of complication, the treatment options are external drainage by intervention radiology, relaparoscopy, or open surgery. In contrast to open surgery, laparoscopic reintervention after prior laparoscopic operation is rarely hampered by early adhesions to the abdominal wall. If a surgical reintervention is required, this is preferably done laparoscopically provided small bowel distension is limited and provided a sufficiently experienced surgeon is available.

Conversion

Late conversion must be considered as a complication and must therefore be prevented. Within 15 min after the start of the laparoscopic procedure, the surgeon has to decide whether there is a fair chance that he or she can complete the procedure laparoscopically within a reasonable operating time. When in doubt, a more experienced laparoscopic surgeon must be asked to help out, or it is decided to "convert early."

Bowel Ischemia and Bleeding

The introduction of vessel sealing equipment made life easier for the laparoscopic surgeons. Superior homeostasis even of large vessels is obtained and obviates the need of meticulous dissection. However, careless dissection taking unidentified structures can lead to major damage to important blood vessels and ureters.

During right-sided dissection the superior mesenteric artery can be mistaken for the ileocolic artery particularly when an anterior medial approach of the mesentery is applied. When in doubt, a submesenteric tunnel beneath the mesentery of the right colon must be created to clarify the vascular anatomy. Pulling at the cecum will show the ileocolic trunk discriminating it from the superior mesenteric trunk (Fig. 20.1a, b). If the superior mesenteric trunk is damaged, the small bowel is devascularized, and immediate conversion and reconstruction by the vascular surgeon must be attempted.

During left-sided resections care must be taken to preserve the left branch of the middle colic artery, particularly when it is decided to perform a high tie ligation to obtain maximum bowel length as in coloanal anastomosis. Applying transmesenteric transbursal dissection and mobilization of the left flexure, it is possible that the window towards the lesser sac is opened anteriorly from the left branch of the middle colic. Freeing the mesentery of the pancreas, another structure either not

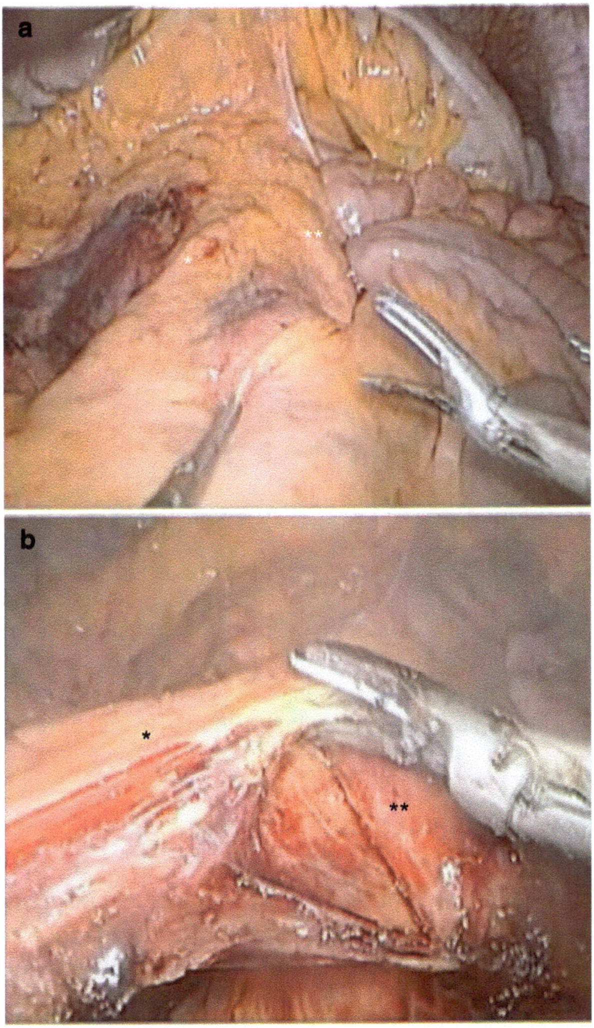

Fig. 20.1 (**a**) (*) Ileocolic pedicle. (**) Superior mesenteric pedicle. (**b**) (*) Ileocolic pedicle. (**) superior mesenteric vein

recognized or identified as "an aberrant" vessel might be cut devascularizing the entire left colon. To prevent this, one should stick on the anterior surface of the pancreas opening the transmesenteric window to the lesser sac (Fig. 20.2).

Another pitfall of the medial to lateral mobilization of the left colon is that while expanding the submesenteric tunnel cranially, the plane behind the pancreas is opened. The splenic vein on the posterior part of the pancreas can be damaged (Fig. 20.3).

Creating the submesenteric tunnel, the gonadal vessels are encountered. If the submesenteric plane is opened correctly, the gonadal vessels will remain in their retroperitoneal position. If the vessels are crossing the submesenteric tunnel or are stuck to the posterior surface of the mesentery, they will detach and left retroperitoneal.

Dealing with a major bleeding, one should start with control of the bleeding using an adequate irrigation and suction system and effort must be done to grasp the bleeder

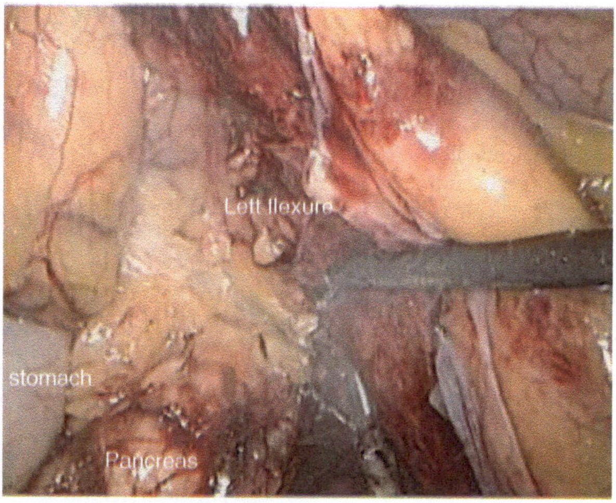

Fig. 20.2 Transmesenteric transbursal medial to lateral left flexure mobilization. Stick to the pancreas

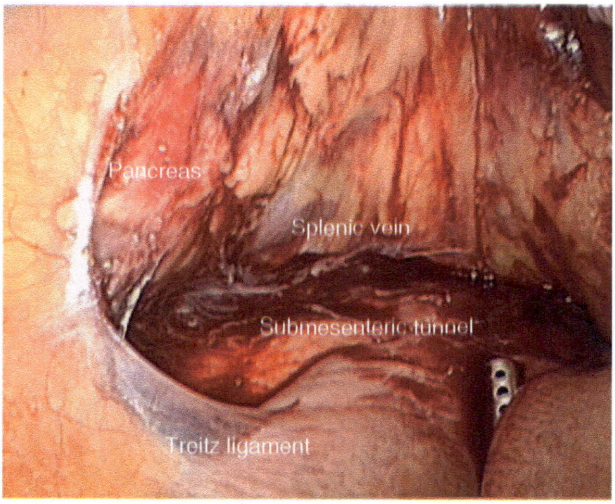

Fig. 20.3 Exposed splenic vein on the posterior part of the pancreas

with a fenestrated grasper. Sometimes, it is helpful to insert additional trocars and to ask for assistance. The bleeder can only be controlled with suture of vessel sealing device if it is clear what the origin of the vessel is, otherwise conversion is warranted.

Ureter Damage

It is estimated that ureter damage occurs in 1 % of the laparoscopic colorectal resections [9]. The best way to prevent ureteral damage is to clear the ureter at the beginning of the procedure by creating the submesenteric tunnel in the proper plane and freeing the mesentery from the retroperitoneum. In this way the ureter remains behind a connective tissue layer, and the ureter cannot be damaged in case of more anteriorly located

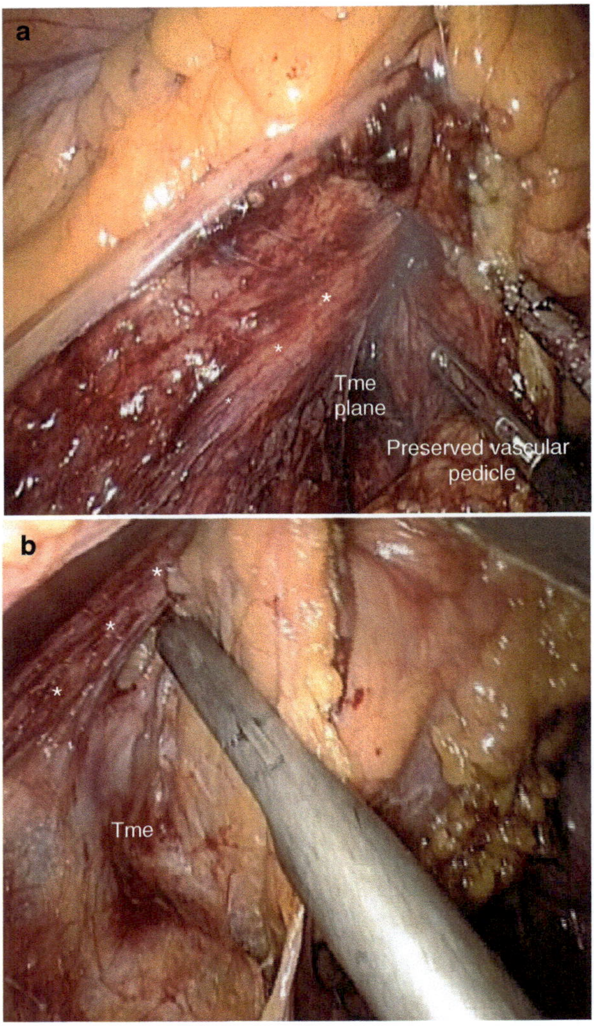

Fig. 20.4 Two window technique (**a**) in superior rectal artery saving sigmoidectomy for diverticulitis (*Tme* total mesorectal excision). The left ureter (*) is freed from medial to lateral as far as possible into the pelvis (**b**)

inflammatory mass like in diverticulitis (Fig. 20.4). Before taking the superior rectal artery or the inferior mesenteric artery at its root, it is important to free the vessel circumferentially. The ureter might be pulled up behind the vessel. Otherwise the left ureter can be damaged if the artery is stapled or taken care of with a vessel dealing device.

Postoperatively, ureteral damage can be diagnosed by creatinine level in the drain fluid, ultrasound of the kidneys, or intravenous pyelogram.

Internal Herniation

There are clear literature data with respect to the incidence of internal herniation [10, 11]. Occasional case reports indicate that it occurs incidentally. Particularly in the medial to lateral approach with central vascular ligation, a large mesenteric defect is created. In

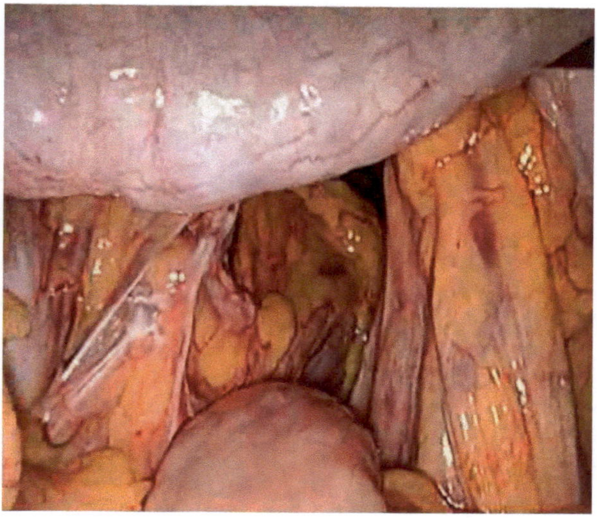

Fig. 20.5 Mesenteric defect after laparoscopic left-sided colectomy responsible for intermittent small bowel obstruction. The small bowel is repositioned

anterior resections, the remaining mesentery of the colon anastomosed to the rectum will run parallel to the retroperitoneum and will close the opening. After the anastomosis is stapled, the small bowel must be checked for its position in relation to the mesentery and if necessary repositioned. In left colectomy with transverse-sigmoidal anastomosis, the first loop of small bowel will very likely herniate unless the large bowel mesentery is closed meticulously reconstructing Treitz ligament (Fig. 20.5). The likelihood of internal herniation is probably lower after right-sided resection. The mesenteric defect is large and herniation remains a small but significant a risk provided it is closed. Unexplained small bowel obstructing shortly after surgery must raise the suspicion. CT scan can be used to establish the diagnosis. Sometimes the diagnosis can only be established by relaparoscopy. The bowel needs to be repositioned and the mesentery closed meticulously. Another subset of patients might prevent late complaining of intermittent small bowel obstruction. Since adhesions are rare after laparoscopic bowel resection, an internal herniation requiring relaparoscopy must be suspected.

Trocar Hernia

The adoption of laparoscopy in surgical practice has resulted in the emergence of incisional hernia at the trocar site (Fig. 20.6). Trocar site hernia (TSH) can be asymptomatic, but occasionally presents with ileus or intestinal strangulation, requiring emergency surgery.

Trocar site hernia can be classified into early- and late-onset dehiscence. In the case of early dehiscence, intestine or omentum herniates through the peritoneum, within several days after surgery. The herniation can be at the level of the preperitoneal fat, at the level of abdominal musculature, underneath the external fascia, or full thickness. In the case of late dehiscence, the peritoneum is intact, yet there is dehiscence of the abdominal musculature or fascia. In these cases the intestine or

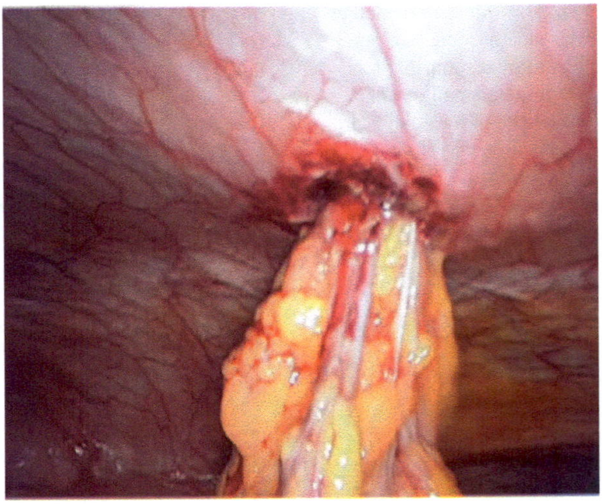

Fig. 20.6 Trocar site hernia

omentum herniates through the musculature and fascia along with the peritoneum, typically several months after surgery.

In a systematic review [12], 22 articles were included, of which one randomized controlled trial, five prospective cohort studies, and sixteen retrospective cohort studies. The prevalence of TSH is low, with a pooled estimate of 0.5 % (range 0–5.2 %). No meta-analysis could be performed on the risk factors. Pyramidal-shaped sharp trocars, 12 mm trocars, and a long duration of surgery were identified as the most important technical risk factors for TSH. Higher age and a higher BMI were found to be patient-related risk factors.

It is advised to close trocar sites larger than 10 mm. Full-thickness closure with devices like the Endoclose (Covidien®) is probably superior to closure of the anterior fascia only. In the latter, partial abdominal wall or subfascial herniation can still occur.

Symptoms of trocar site hernia consist of a painful lump at the trocar site. Sometimes it is accompanied by ileus due to small bowel occlusion or torsion (Fig. 20.7). Subfascial hernia is difficult to diagnose because it does not present with a lump. CT scan or ultrasound imaging should make the diagnosis.

Trocar hernia's can be best treated laparoscopically, freeing the fixed viscus or omentum. Full-thickness closure is advised to prevent the recurrence of subfascial hernias.

Anastomotic Leakage

Anastomotic leakage is the most important surgical complication following colorectal resection with intestinal anastomosis. The reported clinical leakage rate after colorectal resection depends on the site of anastomosis and ranges from 2 to 21 %. Anastomotic leakage after colorectal surgery is associated with a high morbidity rate and is the most important causative factor for postoperative death. Leakage may

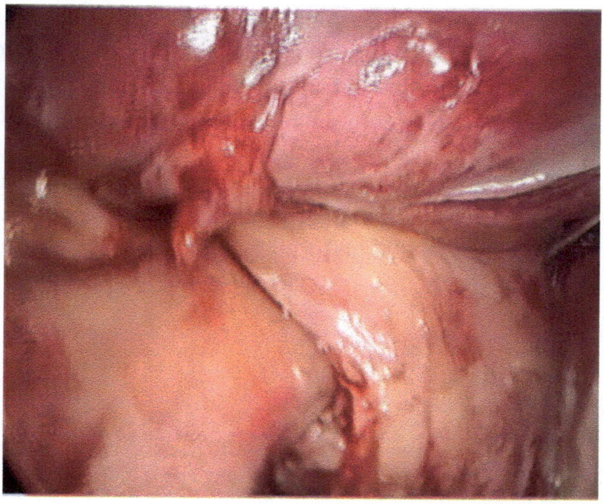

Fig. 20.7 Internal herniation after anterior resection causing anastomotic leakage in colorectal anastomosis

result in a long stay in intensive care, sepsis, and abdominal wall complications due to reinterventions and wound infections. Furthermore, the risk of permanent stoma ranges from 10 to 100 %. The rate of anastomotic leak after laparoscopic colorectal surgery is similar to that after open surgery [13]. Prevention of leakage consists of preservation of the vascular supply of the two bowel parts and tension free anastomosis. Low anastomosis is generally checked by applying the air bubble test. Coloanal anastomoses, preoperative chemoradiation, high doses of steroid, and prior irradiation are risk factors for leakage warranting a defunctioning ileostomy. If a defunctioning ileostomy is scheduled, Rullier et al. [14]. indicated that bowel preparation is superior to the non-prepared bowel with respect to the occurrence of pelvic sepsis.

Anastomotic leakage must be suspected if a patient cannot tolerate a normal diet within a couple of days and has signs of infection. For this reason, earlier diagnosis and reintervention might be expected after a laparoscopic operation. This earlier reintervention might prevent severe generalized peritonitis and systemic sepsis.

Confirmation of an anastomotic leak is best done by CT scan with intravenous and enteral contrast.

During laparoscopic reintervention, the previous trocar wounds are used for insertion of a blunt trocar, e.g., TrocDoc trocar (Storz, Tubingen, Germany), establishing the pneumoperitoneum [15]. The whole reintervention is performed laparoscopically, and the minilaparotomy used for specimen retrieval at the first operation can be opened only when necessary.

The operative procedure consists of inspection and exploration, then culturing and rinsing of the abdominal cavity. Ileoanal, coloanal, and low colorectal anastomoses are diverted by creating a loop ileostomy and irrigation of the rest of the colon. In patients with intra-abdominal located anastomoses with major breakdown, the afferent loop needs to be exteriorized as an end stoma. An end colostomy is created in those with anastomotic leakage after left-sided resections, and an end ileostomy is created after right-sided resections.

If long-standing peritonitis with pus pockets and inflammatory adhesions precludes adequate irrigation, an option is to insert a hand port via the (earlier used) Pfannenstiel incision to facilitate irrigation and blunt separation of the bowel loops.

Wind et al. [16] showed that laparoscopic reintervention for anastomotic leakage after primarily laparoscopic surgery is feasible and safe, with no conversions or intraoperative complications observed. They demonstrated that a laparoscopic reintervention tends to be associated with less postoperative morbidity, a faster recovery, and fewer abdominal wall complications.

References

1. Tekkis PP, Senagore AJ, Delaney CP, Fazio VW. Evaluation of the learning curve in laparoscopic colorectal surgery: comparison of right-sided and left-sided resections. Ann Surg. 2005; 242(1):83–91.
2. Chew MH, Ng KH, Fook-Chong MC, Eu KW. Redefining conversion in laparoscopic colectomy and its influence on outcomes: analysis of 418 cases from a single institution. World J Surg. 2011;35(1):178–85.
3. Tan PY, Stephens JH, Rieger NA, Hewett PJ. Laparoscopically assisted colectomy: a study of risk factors and predictors of open conversion. Surg Endosc. 2008;22(7):1708–14.
4. Thorpe H, Jayne DG, Guillou PJ, Quirke P, Copeland J, Brown JM, Medical Research Council Conventional versus Laparoscopic-Assisted Surgery In Colorectal Cancer Trial Group. Patient factors influencing conversion from laparoscopically assisted to open surgery for colorectal cancer. Br J Surg. 2008;95(2):199–205.
5. Laparoscopy and/or Fast Track Multimodal Management Versus Standard Care (LAFA) Study Group, Wind J, Polle SW, Fung Kon Jin PH, Dejong CH, von Meyenfeldt MF, Ubbink DT, Gouma DJ, Bemelman WA, Laparoscopy and/or Fast Track Multimodal Management Versus Standard Care (LAFA) Study Group, Enhanced Recovery after Surgery (ERAS) Group. Systematic review of enhanced recovery programmes in colonic surgery. Br J Surg. 2006; 93(7):800–9.
6. Vlug MS, Wind J, Hollmann MW, Ubbink DT, Cense HA, Engel AF, Gerhards MF, van Wagensveld BA, van der Zaag ES, van Geloven AA, Sprangers MA, Cuesta MA, Bemelman WA, Collaborative LAFA study group. Laparoscopy in combination with fast track multimodal management is the best perioperative strategy in patients undergoing colonic surgery: a randomized clinical trial (LAFA-study). Ann Surg. 2011;254:868–75.
7. MacKay GJ, Molloy RG, O'Dwyer PJ. C-reactive protein as a predictor of postoperative infective complications following elective colorectal resection. Colorectal Dis. 2011;13(5):583–7. doi:10.1111/j.1463-1318.2010.02236.x.
8. Matthiessen P, Henriksson M, Hallböök O, Grunditz E, Norén B, Arbman G. Increase of serum C-reactive protein is an early indicator of subsequent symptomatic anastomotic leakage after anterior resection. Colorectal Dis. 2008;10(1):75–80.
9. Nam YS, Wexner SD. Clinical value of prophylactic ureteral stent indwelling during laparoscopic colorectal surgery. J Korean Med Sci. 2002;17(5):633–5.
10. Cabot JC, Lee SA, Yoo J, Nasar A, Whelan RL, Feingold DL. Long-term consequences of not closing the mesenteric defect after laparoscopic right colectomy. Dis Colon Rectum. 2010; 53(3):289–92.
11. Sereno Trabaldo S, Anvari M, Leroy J, Marescaux J. Prevalence of internal hernias after laparoscopic colonic surgery. J Gastrointest Surg. 2009;13(6):1107–10.
12. Swank HA, Mulder IM, la Chapelle CF, Reitsma JB, Lange JF, Bemelman WA. Trocar site hernia: a systematic review. Br J Surg. 2011;99:315–23.

13. Reza MM, Blasco JA, Andradas E, Cantero R, Mayol J. Systematic review of laparoscopic versus open surgery for colorectal cancer. Br J Surg. 2006;93:921–8.
14. Bretagnol F, Panis Y, Rullier E, Rouanet P, Berdah S, Dousset B, Portier G, Benoist S, Chipponi J, Vicaut E, French Research Group of Rectal Cancer Surgery (GRECCAR). Rectal cancer surgery with or without bowel preparation: the French GRECCAR III multicenter single-blinded randomized trial. Ann Surg. 2010;252(5):863–8.
15. Bemelman WA, Dunker MS, Busch OR, Den Boer KT, de Wit LT, Gouma DJ. Efficacy of establishment of pneumoperitoneum with the Veress needle, Hasson trocar, and modified blunt trocar (TrocDoc): a randomized study. J Laparoendosc Adv Surg Tech A. 2000;10(6):325–30.
16. Wind J, Koopman AG, van Berge Henegouwen MI, Slors JF, Gouma DJ, Bemelman WA. Laparoscopic reintervention for anastomotic leakage after primary laparoscopic colorectal surgery. Br J Surg. 2007;94(12):1562–6.

Chapter 21
Prevention and Treatment of Postoperative Complications After Stoma Surgery

Han C. Kuijpers and Sigrun Klok

Keywords Postoperative complications • Stoma surgery • Enterostomies • Colorectal • Loop enterostomy • End ileostomy • Bowel • Postoperative • Peristomal sepsis • Necrosis • Retraction • Prolapse

Intestinal stomas or enterostomies are an important and essential part of a colorectal surgeon's repertoire. Their function is to divert the fecal stream when necessary. Indications are the prevention of complications in anorectal sepsis or low rectal anastomosis, the treatment of fecal incontinence and severe proctocolitis, and the avoidance of an anastomosis in intra-abdominal sepsis.

Creation of an enterostomy should be considered as a major component of the surgeon's armamentarium. Complications of enterostomies lead to stomal dysfunction resulting in leakage and skin excoriations and an unfavorably adjustment to the new situation. Complications have been reported in up to 50 %, and surgical revision is required in approximately 30–40 %, which is often due to poorly siting and construction by an inexperienced surgeon. Since poorly sited stomas may seriously hinder adequate stoma care and are associated with a high complication rate, selection of the optimal stoma site by enterostomal nurses is of utmost importance. It is imperative for any abdominal surgeon to have this skill too since a stoma therapist may not always be available and counseling is not possible for patients who need emergency surgery. Occupation, clothing style, abdominal wall contour, and physical limitations and disabilities such as bad sight or rheumatoid arthritis should be considered. In complex cases, test placement should be performed with the

H.C. Kuijpers, MD, PhD (✉)
Department of Gastrointestinal Surgery, Gelderse Vallei Hospital,
Ede, Gelderland, The Netherlands
e-mail: jhckuijpers@hotmail.com

S. Klok
Stoma Care, Gelderse Vallei Hospital, Ede, Gelderland, The Netherlands

M.A. Cuesta, H.J. Bonjer (eds.), *Treatment of Postoperative Complications after Digestive Surgery*, DOI 10.1007/978-1-4471-4354-3_21,

appliance full of water and the patient fully clothed. In obese patients stoma management may only become possible by the use of a mirror. The selected site should be marked with indelible ink. Preoperative counseling is also mandatory in properly preparing the patient for life with a stoma. With proper preoperative education and training, earlier hospital discharge is possible [1].

The ideal stoma site is a flat surface on the abdomen supported by the rectus abdominis without folds or scars. Construction of the trephine is essential. The preferred site is in the center of a 100 cm^2 flat skin surface over the rectus muscle, between the umbilicus and the anterior superior iliac spine, just below the midline and well away from the pubis and costal margins, free of scars and skin folds since an irregular skin surface leads to a poor seal and subsequent leakage. The apex of the infraumbilical fat mound should be used. The trephine for a permanent stoma should be constructed before opening the abdomen so as to ensure a straight course from the peritoneal cavity to the abdominal wall. A midline incision should always be used since it leaves both iliac fossae undisturbed for possible future stoma resiting.

The trephine should run through the rectus muscle. Placement outside the rectus muscle more often leads to parastomal herniation of the small bowel causing loosening of the appliance and subsequent leakage. A 3–4 cm skin disk is excised leaving all of the subcutaneous fat to minimize the chance on dead space and accumulation of a parastomal seroma or abscess. A vertical fascial incision is preferred to a cruciate incision since more fascia will remain intact. The rectus muscle is split in the direction of its fibers and the posterior fascia and peritoneum incised.

The trephine should allow admission of one finger for an end ileostomy and two fingers for a double-loop ileostomy or an end colostomy. A too narrow trephine may interfere with adequate blood supply, leading to necrosis and stenosis, or cause obstruction. When too wide it will allow the passage of small bowel loops creating a parastomal hernia. In a floppy abdominal wall, implantation of a mesh is an effective procedure to narrow the trephine opening and decrease the risk of prolapse although it bears the risk of infection.

The vascular supply of the bowel should be adequate. In a loop enterostomy this will not be a problem since vessels are not ligated, but in an end enterostomy, too much dissection may impair mesenteric circulation leading to stoma necrosis, stricture formation, and stoma retraction. It is fairly easy to bring out enough small bowel, but for a colostomy, mobilization of the proximal colon, especially the splenic flexure, is often necessary. The mesentery should not be stretched for fear of rendering the stoma ischemic.

The end of the bowel, normally closed by a stapling procedure, is grasped with an Ellis or Babcock clamp and gently pulled through the trephine to avoid tearing of the mesentery. Maturation of an enterostomy is performed after closing the abdominal wound to avoid spilling intestinal content in the abdominal wound in order to prevent wound infection. After opening the bowel, the vascularization of its edge and the mucosal color should be checked both before and after stoma construction. Any blackening is suspect and a clear invitation for reconstruction.

The ileum should protrude 3–4 cm to create a spigot effect. The eversion will drain the liquid output directly into the stoma bag minimizing leakage and skin

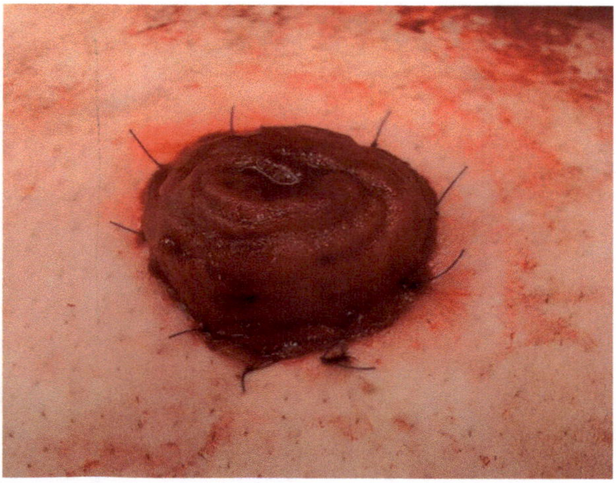

Fig. 21.1 Well-created eversion colostomy

irritation. This is also preferred in colostomy formation despite the presently prevailing opinion that the more solid nature of the stool does not damage the skin. A 1–2 cm protrusion performed similarly to ileostomy maturation is beneficial for appliance placement. The preferred height should be 15 mm since it causes 35 % less care problems [2]. When the intestinal contents are liquid such as after a previous small bowel resection or when little proximal colon is left, an eversion colostomy is preferable (Fig. 21.1).

An end-ileostomy maturation is performed by grasping the internal bowel wall at 3–4 cm from the edge and folding back the distal bowel wall. In a loop ileostomy an ileal segment at 15–20 cm from the ileocecal valve is pulled up 3–4 cm. This provides enough distal ileum to create an ileoileal anastomosis when, in restoring continuity, a small resection has to be performed due to bowel wall damage. The segment is gently pulled through the abdominal wall with the afferent loop distally, which will provide the best spigot. Twisting of the bowel should be avoided to ensure that the afferent loop remains distally. The efferent loop is incised about 5 mm above skin level transecting 80 % of the circumference. If the incision is flushed with the skin, mucus may escape from the recessive limb and cause a faulty seal with the appliance. Eversion is done as in an end ileostomy.

Fixation in this position is performed by placing four sutures through the skin edge, the seromuscular layer of the ileum at skin level, and the seromuscular and mucosal edge of the bowel, the so-called tripartite sutures. Supporting the limb in a loop ileostomy by a plastic rod is not necessary since the eversion is kept in place by the tripartite sutures. A rod may be responsible for bowel damage and skin excoriation. Suturing the bowel serosa to the posterior abdominal fascia is not necessary for fixation either and may lead to bowel perforation and stomal fistulae. One or two sutures are placed in between to further approximate the mucocutaneous junction.

Visual inspection of the stoma in the early postoperative period is of utmost importance. When stoma viability is doubtful, the extent can be judged by mucosal

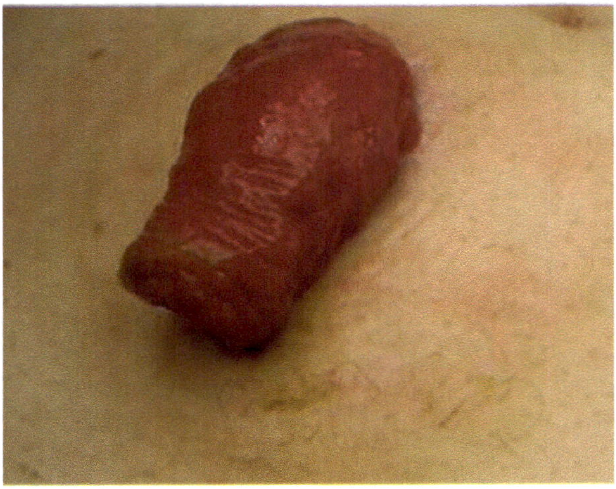

Fig. 21.2 Well-created loop ileostomy

inspection through a glass tube inserted into the stoma. Nurses charged with post-operative care must be well trained to detect early stoma complication. Early post-operative inspection may prevent late complications.

Closure of the lateral gutter between the bowel and the abdominal wall is not necessary since internal herniation rarely occurs. Routine prophylactic placement of a mesh patch around the stoma to decrease the incidence of parastomal herniation is controversial because of the risk of infection.

In extreme obesity the fashioning of an enterostomy may be extraordinary difficult. When the mesentery is fatty, a generous (8–10 cm) incision may be made in the peritoneum and posterior rectus sheath so that the bowel can be brought out through the abdominal wall easily. Sutures are previously placed on each side of the extended incisions and tied after the bowel has been brought out. The surgeon should watch for any ischemic effects on the bowel produced by tying these sutures. It may also be difficult to bring the end of the ileum beyond skin level due to the thick abdominal wall and the shortened mesentery. A loop-end ileostomy may then be fashioned. The terminal ileum is delivered through the trephine approximately 5 cm from the closed bowel end, incised and everted at the proximal side. Adequate blood supply is thus guaranteed.

For temporary diversion, a loop ileostomy is usually preferred (Fig. 21.2). A right-sided loop colostomy (at the right side of the arteria colica media) is an alternative but has a higher overall stoma-related morbidity and reoperation rate. Loop ileostomy causes less skin excoriations, is less bulky, is associated with a lower incidence of peristomal sepsis and parastomal herniation or prolapse, and is easier to close, whereas a loop transversostomy has a much larger lumen, rarely stays everted, is usually inconveniently placed in the epigastrium, is quite malodorous, and frequently needs a rod. The rod is necessary to hold the loop colostomy in position, to prevent retraction, and to achieve complete defunctioning. It should be in place for at least 5–6 days. A left-sided loop colostomy should never be constructed since it bears the risk of damage to the marginal artery during construction or

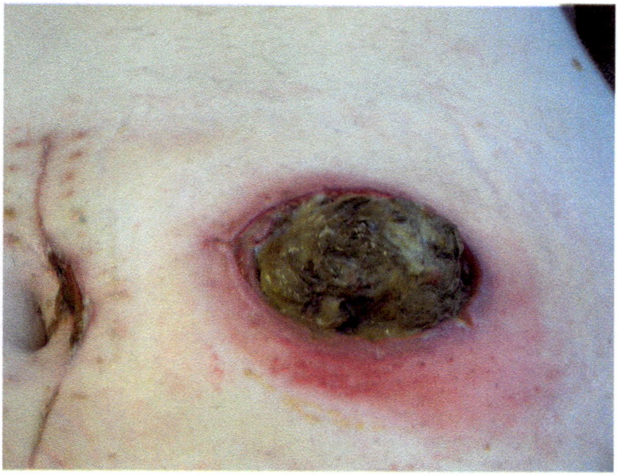

Fig. 21.3 Necrosis of colostomy

closure and, hence, to the distal colonic blood supply after previous ligation of the inferior mesenteric artery. Construction of an end or split enterostomy for temporary use should be avoided when possible since restoration of continuity requires a regular laparotomy instead of a local procedure. An alternative is a side-to-side end ileostomy which does not require a regular laparotomy for closure. The bowel is completely divided, the proximal part everted as in an end ileostomy, and the distal end closed sutured to the side of the emerging bowel and at fascial or subcutaneous level. A cecostomy has become obsolete. It never completely diverts and often does not close spontaneously. A loop ileostomy usually remains adequately everted, but some spillover may occur. Complete defunctioning is obtained only by a split or side-to-side end ileostomy, but this is hardly ever necessary. When diversion is performed for anastomotic dehiscence, the colon has to be washed out to prevent persisting contamination from the leaking site. A Foley catheter is inserted through the efferent loop with both legs of the patient in stirrups and 3–6 l of warm saline is irrigated. If a stoma gives rise to leakage and skin irritation, correction may be necessary. A well-trained stomatherapist can resolve many stoma complications. Most ileostomy complications can be managed by experienced stoma care, but 30–40 % requires surgical revision. Evaluation of the appropriate refashioning procedure involves careful clinical assessment between the surgeon and the stomatherapist.

Early complications are peristomal sepsis, necrosis, and retraction (Figs. 21.3, 21.4, 21.5, and 21.6). They are usually the result of abdominal sepsis, too extensive mesenteric dissection and stretching of the bowel in order to reach the abdominal wall, or entrapment of the mesentery in the abdominal wall opening. In peristomal sepsis a protective barrier may be built to separate the stoma from the drainage site until granulation tissue has been formed. Skin barrier dressings such as hydrofiber and alginate can be used. Stomal intubation is an alternative. Adequate drainage of the subcutaneous layer can be achieved by placing a small flat drain around the stoma perforating the skin beyond the edge of the appliance. This could also be done as a prophylactic measure in abdominal sepsis. Resiting and proximal

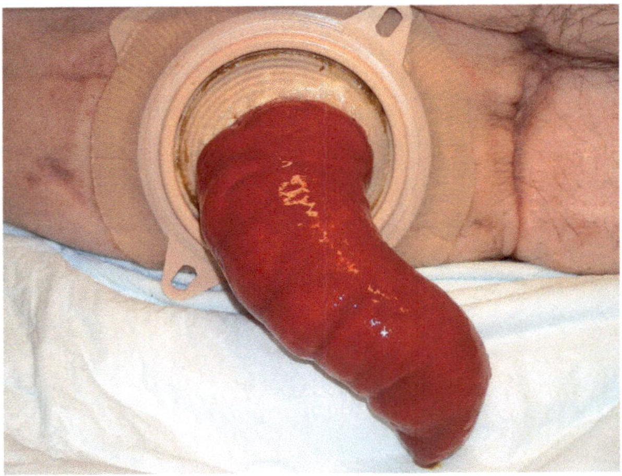

Fig. 21.4 Prolapse end ileostomy

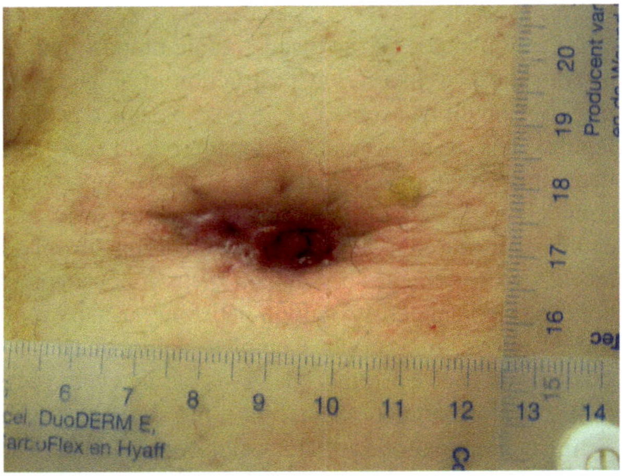

Fig. 21.5 Stenosis of colostomy

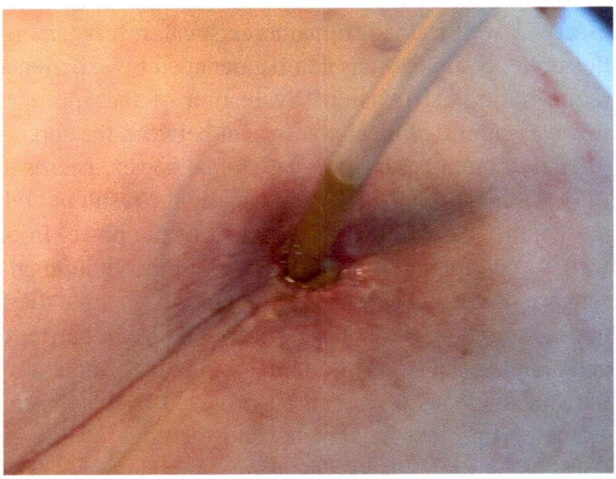

Fig. 21.6 Dilatation of stenosis

deviation are other alternatives. Another cause of stomal sepsis is subcutaneous bowel perforation caused by fixation sutures. After healing a fistula will remain. The fistula opening is normally adjacent to the mucocutaneous junction and can be incorporated into the pouching system. Necrosis and retraction may lead to contamination of the abdominal wall and cavity with peristomal sepsis, occasionally life-threatening fasciitis necroticans, and secondary peritonitis. The extent of the necrosis should be assessed by mucosal inspection through a glass tube inserted into the stoma. Any sign of necrosis or retraction is suspect, should be assessed, and be an invitation for reconstruction. An early, aggressive approach, even in mild cases, will be rewarded. When, in mild cases, surgery is delayed too long, the patient will suffer from frequent leakage and painful skin irritation for months since stomal refashioning should not be attempted within the first 10–12 weeks of the last laparotomy since the risk of damage to the small bowel with subsequent resection is considerable.

Intestinal obstruction occurs in about 10 % after an abdominal intervention. When combined with an ileostomy, a too narrow trephine could be the cause of the intestinal obstruction. Insertion of a Foley catheter could be both a diagnostic and therapeutic intervention. It should be considered as an alternative when relaparotomy is considered. When the obstruction is at fascia level, the catheter will start to produce immediately after intubation and symptoms of obstruction will disappear within a few hours. The balloon should not be inflated and the catheter removed after 24 h to avoid small bowel perforation due to pressure.

References

1. Chaudhri S, Brown L, Hassan I, Horgan AF. Preoperative intensive, community-based vs. Traditional stoma education: a randomized, controlled trial. Dis Colon Rectum. 2005;48:504–9.
2. Cottam J, Richards K, Hasted A, Blackman A. Results of a nationwide prospective audit of stoma complications within 3 weeks of surgery. Colorectal Dis. 2007;9:834–8.

General Literature

van Lanschot JJB, Gouma DJ, et al (editors). Integrated medical and surgical gastroenterology. Bohn StafleuVan Loghum Houten, Stuttgart: Germany Thieme; 2004. p. 449–57.

Keighley MRB, Williams NS, editors. Surgery of the anus, rectum and colon. 3rd ed. London: WB Saunders Compant Ltd; 2008.

Beck DE, Wolff BG, Fleshman JW, et al., editors. The ASCRS textbook of colon and rectal surgery. New York: Springer; 2007.

Chapter 22
Prevention and Treatment Complications in Proctology

Christopher Thorn and Janindra Warusavitarne

Keywords Proctology • Complications • Hemorrhoids • Fissure in ano • Fistula in ano • Fecal incontinence • Anal pain • Disruption anorectal function

This chapter will cover three of the most common proctological disorders encountered in practice, hemorrhoids, fissure in ano, and fistula in ano. Numerous procedures are advocated for their effective treatment, which relates in part to the difficulty of minimizing disruption to anorectal function. Due to the many symptoms which may be attributed by patients to anal conditions, a clear history and a discussion of realistic outcomes are paramount.

This is particularly important in the treatment of hemorrhoids which are highly prevalent and may be asymptomatic. After controlling for preoperative symptoms and postoperative complications in a series of 350 patients, patient dissatisfaction was independently related to recurrent or residual anal pain. It was noted that the dissatisfied group (16 %) were more likely to have a preexisting history of irritable bowel syndrome [1]. It is important therefore to distinguish between true complications and those relating to unrealistic expectations or inadequate diagnosis.

Hemorrhoids

Introduction

Established operative interventions for the treatment of hemorrhoids include open (Milligan-Morgan) and closed (Ferguson) hemorrhoidectomy which may be

C. Thorn (✉) • J. Warusavitarne
Department of Colorectal Surgery, St Marks Hospital Harrow, London, UK
e-mail: christhorn77@yahoo.com

M.A. Cuesta, H.J. Bonjer (eds.), *Treatment of Postoperative Complications after Digestive Surgery*, DOI 10.1007/978-1-4471-4354-3_22,

performed using bipolar energy devices (e.g., LigaSure). More recent techniques include stapled hemorrhoidopexy (PPH) and Doppler hemorrhoidal artery ligation (HAL) with or without rectoanal mucopexy. This array of techniques testifies to the inadequacy of a single technique for the treatment of all cases. The range of clinical manifestations of hemorrhoidal disease requires the surgeon to select an appropriate technique. Rubber band ligation, injection sclerotherapy, and photocoagulation will not be covered in this section.

Conventional hemorrhoidectomy, including open, closed, submucosal, and LigaSure variants, is less likely to result in residual hemorrhoidal symptoms compared with a stapled approach which has been shown to result in a threefold increase in overall recurrence and a higher long-term reoperation rate [2, 3]. However, PPH (procedure for prolapse and hemorrhoids) and HAL result in reduced postoperative pain and a more rapid return to activity. A recent Cochrane review also reported no significant difference between conventional and stapled techniques for other reported outcomes including recurrent bleeding, pruritus, passive fecal incontinence or urgency, residual/recurrent skin tags, anal stenosis, quality of life, or recurrent pain [3]. LigaSure hemorrhoidectomy reduces early postoperative pain and time off work compared with diathermy excision [4]. Postoperative pain scores with LigaSure are equivalent to stapled hemorrhoidectomy with a reduction in recurrent hemorrhoidal prolapse when compared with PPH [5, 6]. The decrease in pain is thought to be related to improved control of thermal energy transmission to the tissues (Figs. 22.1 and 22.2a, b).

It is generally accepted that in elderly patients, the contribution of hemorrhoidal tissue to continence may be significant, and consideration should be given to nonoperative management in this group, particularly when only minor symptoms are present. Although hemorrhoidectomy has not been described as a risk factor for fecal incontinence in a recent US federal report, the fine balance of continence vs. incontinence in the elderly, especially women, should alert the clinician to avoid surgery in this group where possible [7].

Major complication following hemorrhoidectomy is rare. Pelvic sepsis may complicate rubber band ligation, injection sclerotherapy, and conventional hemorrhoidectomy although the frequency appears to be lower than with stapled techniques [8]. Pruritus ani may result from iatrogenic internal anal sphincter (IAS) injury, from the loss of hemorrhoidal tissue in the elderly, or rarely due to mucosal ectropion resulting from the suturing of anorectal mucosa below the level of the IAS, as can occur after an incorrectly performed Whitehead's procedure. Reactive bleeding is an avoidable complication and wounds must be carefully inspected for bleeding at the end of the procedure and under run if required. Secondary hemorrhage is managed conservatively if at all possible.

In the case of the acutely thrombosed but not gangrenous hemorrhoid, every attempt should be made to avoid surgery. Ice packs, adequate analgesia, and a hygroscopic agent (such as honey) facilitate a conservative approach. Following resolution of the acute episode, the appropriate operative or nonoperative management option can be administered based on the clinical scenario after the acute inflammation has settled.

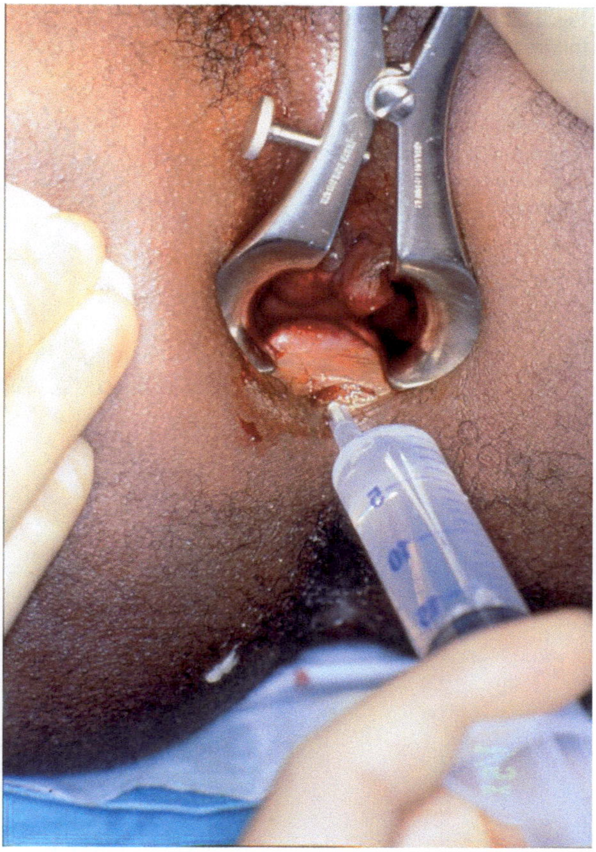

Fig. 22.1 Injection into the submucosa space of a dilution of 1:200,000 adrenaline in saline to facilitate a clear views of the dissection plane.

Prevention and Treatment of Complications

Conventional Hemorrhoidectomy

During the procedure, it is recommended that the right posterior (7 o'clock) and left lateral (3 o'clock) hemorrhoids are excised prior to the right anterior (11 o'clock) hemorrhoid in order to minimize disruption of the field with bleeding.

Minor continence disturbance is common after hemorrhoidectomy (50 %) but usually settles within 6 weeks [9]. It results from the replacement of sensate anorectal epithelium with fibrosis and generally occurs in the elderly who may have a history of incontinence.

Postoperative pain is a major concern of patients if not strictly a complication of hemorrhoidectomy. Ambulatory hemorrhoidectomy has significant advantages and has been widely adopted but is not compatible with the use of epidural morphine. The use of GTN ointment 0.2 % and ketorolac have been demonstrated to reduce pain in randomized trials, whereas the use of long-acting local anesthetic

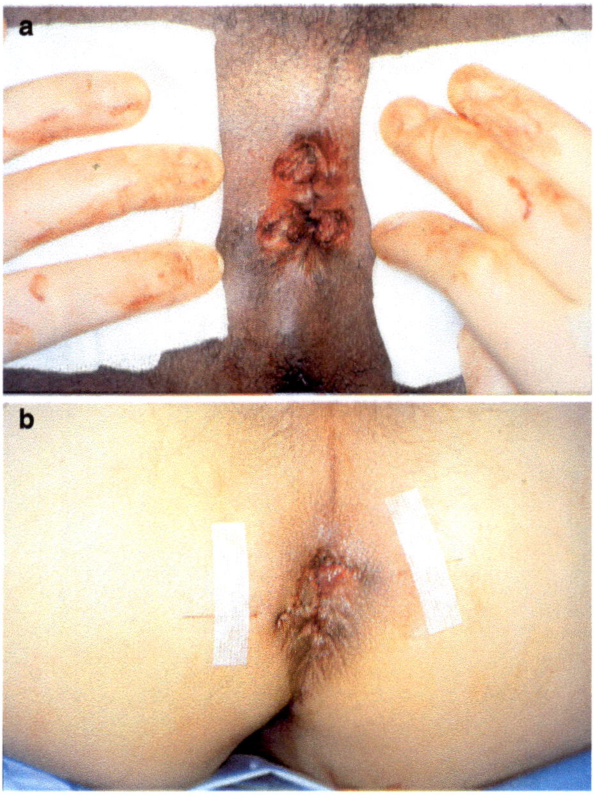

Fig. 22.2 (**a**, **b**) Wounds following open (Milligan-Morgan) and closed (Ferguson) haemorrhoidectomy, undertaken using diathermy and scissor dissection respectively.

is not supported. The evidence for botulinum toxin and metronidazole is conflicting.

Massive reactive hemorrhage reflects a technical error and relates to inadequate ligation of the arterial pedicle. This complication is reduced with the use of suture ligation. Delayed hemorrhage occurs between 3 and 14 (most frequently 4 and 6) days postoperatively at a frequency of 2 % and relates to sepsis around or erosion of the pedicle suture. It is not considered to be a preventable complication and should be managed with conservative measures including balloon tamponade with a Foley catheter in severe cases.

The prevalence of postoperative urinary retention has been described to be as high as 20 % in historical series. These rates have reduced dramatically after the introduction of ambulatory hemorrhoidectomy. Perianal pain results in a failure of urinary sphincteric relaxation which is partially mitigated using day surgery anesthetic techniques. Intravenous fluid overload has also been described to be an important predictor of retention. Urinary voiding should not be considered a prerequisite for discharge, except in those with known bladder outflow disease. Postprocedural constipation relates to pain and narcotic analgesia which should be treated actively with stimulant and bulk laxatives in titrated doses.

The incidence of severe sepsis following conventional hemorrhoidectomy is extremely rare and restricted to case reports alone. It may manifest as Fournier's gangrene or systemically due to translocation. It is prudent to give prophylactic antibiotics to immunocompromised patients in whom these complications are more common.

Anal stricture will not occur provided adequate skin bridges are preserved. Submucosal veins spared beneath skin bridges may become engorged and manifest as a "recurrence" which can be avoided by ligating vessels beneath skin bridges to avoid the need for a Whitehead's procedure in extensive disease. The vast majority of anal strictures, which may follow any hemorrhoidectomy procedure, respond to simple dilatation. For mild to moderate stenoses, unilateral or bilateral VY or house advancement flaps are appropriate. However, in severe cases where more than 50 % of the anal canal requires reconstruction, rotational flap reconstruction, which covers a greater surface area without tension, may be required. Acute hemorrhoidal thrombosis with supervening gangrene requires the surgeon to denude the anal canal circumferentially and is not a recommended technique. Conservative treatment as detailed earlier is the best option. In situations where it is absolutely necessary to perform surgery in the acute setting and where the anal canal is completely denuded, delayed anoplasty will be required. The stricture is completely excised, and thereafter, the rectal mucosa is sutured to a sphincterotomized internal anal sphincter in order to widen the anal canal. Prophylactic antibiotics and preoperative phosphate enema are indicated, particularly when extensive skin flaps are to be raised. Ectropion may complicate open hemorrhoidectomy or anoplasty since the anorectal mucosa can migrate to cover the denuded area, below the anal canal. This may be prevented by suturing excess mucosa to a level above the caudal extent of the IAS.

Stapled Hemorrhoidectomy

Acute postoperative pain is less frequent after PPH than conventional hemorrhoidectomy [3]. Complications, including severe postoperative pain at 1 week, are significantly more frequent in those patients who had squamous (but not merely transitional) epithelium identified within the resection "doughnut" [10, 11]. There was no significant association between the inclusion of rectal muscle wall and these complications. Chronic pain of unknown origin has been termed the PPH syndrome and although uncommon can be extremely disabling and difficult to treat. It has some features in common with the low anterior resection syndrome [12]. Its etiology is unknown but has been postulated to relate to the formation of a rectal pocket or rectal inclusion cysts caused by the purse string partially cutting through the rectal mucosa prior to the deployment of the staples. An intramural or submucosal diverticulum thus formed may be complicated by local infection and require a further surgery to lay open the pocket. It has been suggested that staple line irritation of branches of the pudendal or sacral nerve spindles in the pelvic floor may mediate the symptoms. The chronic pain associated with PPH syndrome may respond to oral nifedipine in some circumstances and may be effective after topical GTN has failed, suggesting an etiology outside the anal canal. Agrapphectomy or staple line revision by excision and hand suture is also advocated as an effective treatment. More conservative measures such as transanal electrostimulation, topical steroids, and local anesthetics are useful in some but not all cases [13].

Complete rectal obliteration has been reported at least six times and on one occasion has led to a patient's death. It is thought to result from anvil placement to the side of rather than through the purse string, possibly related to an unrecognized intussusception. The closed purse string obliterates the rectal lumen before it is stapled closed by the PPH device [14, 15].

Further complications related to the PPH staple line range from asymptomatic pneumoretroperitoneum to gross pelvic sepsis requiring emergency resection. Rectal perforation is thought to result from ischemic dehiscence of a staple line that incorrectly includes the full thickness of the rectal wall and has been reported at a frequency of 0.1 % [16]. The integrity of the anastomosis should be checked in all cases and any defect repaired promptly. Pelvic sepsis after stapled procedures typically present with severe pain, fever, and urinary symptoms or frank septic shock within 7 days of surgery, although delayed presentation after 5 weeks has been reported. Cases associated with a recognized stapler malfunction are diagnosed earlier than those without, suggesting the need for a higher index of suspicion.

Rectovaginal fistula is a rare but devastating complication described only in association with stapled techniques. It is considered to be mediated by an ischemic injury rather than direct mechanical insult and consequently presents several days following surgery. The injection of saline into the anterior rectal submucosa or wall may reduce the possibility of including deeper structures in the purse string. Careful inspection and palpation of the posterior vaginal wall and rectovaginal septum while ascertaining the presence or absence of a prolapsed pouch of Douglas remain mandatory intraoperative precautions. Enterocele, which should be considered particularly in women who have undergone hysterectomy, contraindicates PPH due to the risk of intestinal perforation [17].

Tenesmus has not been included as a secondary outcome in meta-analyses but one prospective RCT reported a rate of 50 % at 1 year following PPH for fourth-degree hemorrhoids. Fecal soiling may be induced by a low staple line or internal sphincter fragmentation due to the insertion of the large caliber stapling device and should be carefully considered in multiparous women and perhaps men with elevated anal tone.

Reactive hemorrhage after PPH can be managed with submucosal injection of 1–2 ml of 1:100,000 adrenaline although it is often more effective to apply direct pressure with a finger or gauze and return the patient to theatre for suture ligation of the bleeding pedicle. Late bleeding from a granulomatous foreign body reaction to staples can occur between 6 weeks and 4 months and may resemble staple line polyps. Excision of the staples, "agrapphectomy," may be required.

Hemorrhoidal Arterial Ligation

Doppler-guided hemorrhoidal arterial ligation (HAL) or transanal hemorrhoidal dearterialization (THD) is a non-excisional technique which may be performed with a concomitant mucopexy. Systematic review (of observational studies and one prospective RCT), including patients with third- and in some cases fourth- degree hemorrhoids, has indicated that although early postoperative pain is not uncommon (18.5 %), there is otherwise minimal procedure-related morbidity [18]. Overall recurrence rates of prolapse and bleeding after a relatively short median follow-up period of 12 months were 9 and 8 %, respectively, while 5 % described defecatory pain and 2.3 % fissure. In patients with third- and fourth-degree hemorrhoids, a mucopexy was found to be associated with a nonsignificant reduction in the rate of relapse [18].

It has been demonstrated that neither PPH nor HAL completely interrupts the branches of the superior hemorrhoidal arteries as hypothesized. Bleeding from the staple line after PPH may be minimized by using the more hemostatic PPH3 device, tightening the stapling device fully, using an endoanal sponge, and underrunning of the anastomosis.

Conclusions

Contemporary meta-analysis has demonstrated that hemorrhoid recurrence is significantly less frequent after conventional than stapled hemorrhoidectomy, although the follow-up interval remains short. The main advantage therefore of stapled hemorrhoidectomy relates to reduced early postoperative pain and return to function, which remains an important concern. The use of LigaSure™ has a cost implication but has been demonstrated to offer comparable pain scores to the stapled technique. Acute postoperative pain resolves within 3 weeks after diathermy excision. There are no other significant differences in outcome on meta-analysis, though some rare complications particular to stapled hemorrhoidectomy are well documented.

The most appropriate technique can be selected with reference to the grade and symptoms which can be attributed to the patient's hemorrhoids. The presence of skin tags, which can be a significant concern to the patient, is included in modern classifications. Rubber band ligation, excisional hemorrhoidectomy, and stapled hemorrhoidectomy can be employed on a continuum. The choice between increased acute postoperative pain, common after excision, and rare but serious complications after stapled hemorrhoidectomy should be presented to the patient during preoperative counselling.

Fissure in Ano

Introduction

A recent Cochrane review has compared a number of techniques in the treatment of fissure in ano [19]. It was reaffirmed that the practice of anal stretch should be abandoned due to a higher rate of fissure persistence and flatus incontinence than other techniques. The review included botulinum toxin injection and variations of sphincterotomy as well as the relatively novel techniques of controlled balloon dilatation (a variant of anal stretch) and sphincterolysis which requires firm digital pressure to fragment the lateral fibers of the internal sphincter. Incontinence, which is usually minor, is the most serious complication with an incidence of less than 5 % in all but one series. Comparative RCTs would suggest that fissurectomy is less efficacious than unilateral partial lateral sphincterotomy or sphincterolysis which in turn may be less effective than bilateral partial lateral sphincterotomy. Comparison between trials was again hampered by differences in the definition of recurrence and length of follow-up.

The technique of lateral internal sphincterotomy may vary in relation to patient positioning (left lateral, lithotomy, or prone jackknife) and approach (open or closed and the direction of internal anal sphincter division).

A lateral rather than a posteriorly placed incision was favored by Eisenhammer, and this was supported by the work of Goligher and Bennett who recorded high rates of flatus (34 %) and fecal (15 %) incontinence following posterior sphincterotomy. However, the only RCT to compare these approaches ($n=41$) favored lateral sphincterotomy with respect to fissure healing time but did not demonstrate a difference in continence between posterior and lateral sphincterotomy in contrast to this well established principle [20].

Eisenhammer initially advocated division of four fifths the length of the internal sphincter although subsequently recommended only half be divided. Sphincterotomy to the dentate line reduces recurrence when compared with tailored sphincterotomy to the cephalad extent of the fissure with no difference in the rates of incontinence (Wexner scale).

A large nonrandomized series comparing the open and closed approaches with mean follow-up of 36 months reported persistent symptoms in 4 %, recurrence in 10 %, and a change in anal continence in 37 %. No significant difference in fissure resolution was detected; however, continence was impaired in a significantly higher proportion of patients after open sphincterotomy [21]. Lateral to medial closed division from the intersphincteric space minimizes inadvertent damage to the external sphincter in comparison to a medial to lateral division.

The advancement flap is an alternative treatment, typically used in the setting of a low-pressure fissure. In a small RCT in comparison with (DCR 1995 69) sphincterotomy, no difference in the rate of incontinence was noted although in 3 of 20 patients, the flap did not heal. A recent study supports the use of advancement flap in the treatment of high-pressure fissure, reporting an aggregate recurrence rate and wound failure rate of less than 6 % with no associated incontinence [22].

Recent study has demonstrated that patients with low-pressure fissure may have a different physiological response to botulinum toxin which paradoxically increases tone [23]. This treatment may be inappropriate for those with low anal tone therefore.

Chronic fissure may be associated with anal stenosis, particularly in those who have undergone hemorrhoidectomy. This may be treated with excision of the fissure, with posterior internal sphincterotomy, and if necessary with a broad based, tension-free VY advancement flap.

It is important to discriminate between fissure and ulcerative diseases of the anal canal which may be associated with HIV infection such as syphilis, chancroid, chlamydia, tuberculosis, herpes simplex, cytomegalovirus, squamous cell carcinoma, Kaposi's sarcoma, and B-cell lymphoma. All ulcers which are slow to heal should be biopsied and tested for acid fast bacilli. It may be difficult to distinguish between tuberculosis and Crohn's disease, and the identification of pulmonary disease may assist with the diagnosis. Formal investigation of the gastrointestinal tract may be appropriate in selected cases. Fissure may be the sole manifestation of Crohn's disease where the majority are situated in the anterior or posterior midline and are painful in approximately 50 % cases [24]. There is no role for internal sphincterotomy in these patients and medical treatment will treat the fissure in 70 % cases.

Prevention and Treatment of Complications

Flatus or fecal incontinence is the only major complication from sphincterotomy although several immediate complications are noted in the literature including ecchymoses or hematoma (2 %) and perianal abscess, fistula in ano, and hemorrhage (all 1 %). Hematoma usually results from inadequate manual pressure on the wound at the completion of the procedure. Hemorrhage may require suture ligation and is more common after the open technique. Perianal abscess is more common after closed sphincterotomy and is virtually always associated with a fistula initiated by inadvertent breach of the mucosa during closed sphincterotomy. If the correct plane has been developed during sphincterotomy, any subsequent fistula will be low and intersphincteric and therefore can be laid open.

Hemorrhoidal prolapse may also complicate internal sphincterotomy and since simultaneous hemorrhoidectomy has not been demonstrated to increase the rate of complications, it is reasonable to perform a prophylactic procedure for bulky hemorrhoids. However, hemorrhoidal tissue may make a substantial contribution to continence in the elderly.

The female sphincter is shorter and may be injured (structurally or functionally) during parturition. Perineal shortening should alert the clinician to the strong possibility of sphincteric injury. Obstetric injury is more common than once appreciated and may remain subclinical for a substantial period, and caution should be exercised when considering sphincterotomy. It is recommended that in those with a history of anal surgery or obstetric complication, anorectal physiology should be acquired to guide management. Nine out of ten women undergoing lateral sphincterotomy for fissure in ano were found to have unintentional complete division on postoperative ultrasound [25]. A retrospective analysis has demonstrated that the only predictor of postoperative incontinence after internal sphincterotomy was the length of the residual sphincter. Frank fecal incontinence is very rare, and if associated with inadvertent injury to the EAS, direct or overlapping repair may be performed with good results.

A randomized trial established that treatment under local anesthesia was associated with delayed healing in 50 % of cases, compared with only 3 % of those performed under general anesthesia [26].

Conclusions

Should conservative measures fail in the treatment of fissure, a trial of botulinum toxin can be performed. Where this also fails, a lateral sphincterotomy to the dentate line should be performed in men with normal tone and anorectal function. Current evidence suggests that advancement flap might be considered in all patients at risk of continence disturbance, for example, those with clinically abnormal anorectal function, previous anal surgery, and particularly in women with anterior fissure, a history of complicated labor, or multiparity. Should advancement flap fail, in any individual with such risk factors, anorectal physiology and endoanal ultrasound would be recommended prior to consideration of lateral sphincterotomy. Botulinum toxin may exacerbate symptoms in low-pressure fissure and further investigation might be considered to exclude alternative causes prior to consideration of primary surgical treatment with an advancement flap.

Fistula In Ano

Introduction

The complications of operative treatment for fistula in ano are (1) persistence of sepsis from inadequate drainage and (2) unacceptable fecal incontinence with reference to preoperative expectation. The treatment of complex disease (high transphincteric, suprasphincteric, or those with secondary extensions) may require a compromise between these two critical outcomes. Research into methods that can preserve sphincter integrity and reliably cure the fistula continues.

This section will not detail the possible reconstructive options following planned high division of the external sphincter but will outline a strategy to approach this problem. The treatment of recurrence utilizes the same principles as with primary disease albeit in a more complex anatomical context. Complex recurrences ought to be managed at a tertiary center. The best way to prevent such complications is to correctly treat the primary disease which itself demands a comprehensive appreciation of the fistula anatomy and the baseline anorectal function of the patient. Extrasphincteric fistulas arise from pelvic pathology and are not included in this chapter.

The published literature includes very few randomized trials which are generally underpowered. It is often not practicable to compare trials since follow-up is often short and populations under study are heterogeneous. It is difficult to define either complex fistula anatomy or outcomes. Recent Cochrane review reiterated the need for randomized trials and concluded from the 18 studies included that there was no significant difference in recurrence between the various techniques employed [27].

Park's classification of fistulae is based on the cryptoglandular hypothesis and is applicable in over 90 % of fistulae presenting in the United Kingdom. The remainder are secondary, associated with inflammatory bowel disease (predominantly but not exclusively Crohn's disease), pilonidal disease, hidradenitis suppurativa, malignancy, tuberculosis, and trauma (including iatrogenic) [28]. For this reason, routine histological evaluation of the fistula tract is recommended. In addition to the presence of a secondary cause, Miles defined the key attributes of a fistula to be the sites of the internal and external openings, the course of the primary tract, and the presence of any secondary tracts; indeed, the common reasons for surgical failure are inadequate treatment of the primary tract, secondary extensions, and, less commonly, an unrecognized secondary cause.

The goal of fistulotomy is to create an acute wound where the subsequent inflammatory process will result in wound healing. Infected niduses require drainage, the initiating diseased intersphincteric anal gland requires excision, and tracts must be completely de-epithelialized, requiring curettage and sharp dissection.

Patient Assessment

At the initial consultation, baseline continence including stool type must be established as well as risk factors for subclinical loss of function, such as previous anal surgery or childbirth, which may be unmasked following surgery. The impact of an equivalent loss of continence varies widely between individuals, and the importance of careful attention to the patient's attitudes and expectations cannot be overemphasized (Fig. 22.3).

Examination of the conscious patient allows assessment of global pelvic floor function through the surrogates of perineal position at rest and during straining and may also enable the accurate assessment of the sphincter cephalad to the primary tract. An accurate appreciation of this distance is essential for appropriate decision making. The internal opening may be palpated as a grain of sand or rice. A Graeme-Anderson oblique viewing proctoscope is ideal for visualizing this site in the clinic. Goodsall's rule generally applies though an important exception is the finding of

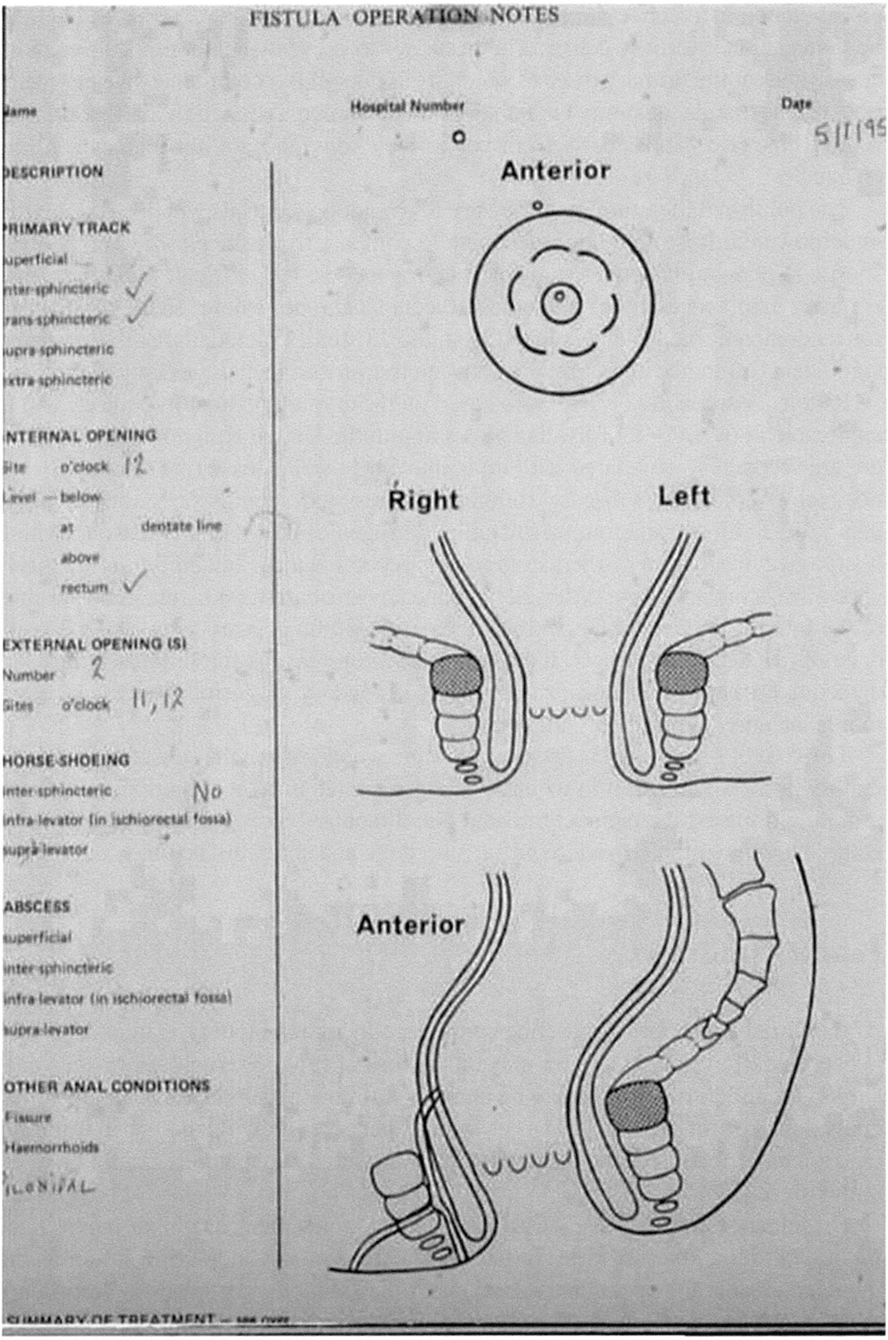

FISTULA OPERATION NOTES

Name | Hospital Number | Date 5/1/95

DESCRIPTION

PRIMARY TRACK
superficial
inter-sphincteric ✓
trans-sphincteric ✓
supra-sphincteric
extra-sphincteric

INTERNAL OPENING
Site o'clock 12
Level — below
at dentate line
above
rectum ✓

EXTERNAL OPENING (S)
Number 2
Sites o'clock 11, 12

HORSE-SHOEING
inter-sphincteric No
infra-levator (in ischiorectal fossa)
supra-levator

ABSCESS
superficial
inter-sphincteric
infra-levator (in ischiorectal fossa)
supra-levator

OTHER ANAL CONDITIONS
Fissure
Haemorrhoids
PILONIDAL

Anterior
Right
Left
Anterior

SUMMARY OF TREATMENT — see over

Fig. 22.3 The St. Mark's fistula proforma is used to clearly record the intra-operative findings.

unilateral or bilateral openings over 3 cm anterior to the anal verge which may represent anterior extensions of a posterior horseshoe. Induration of the levator plate may indicate a high primary tract in the roof of the ischiorectal fossa, a suprasphincteric fistula, or more commonly secondary extensions. The relationship between the tract and the anorectal ring – puborectalis posteriorly and the upper external sphincter anteriorly – can be assessed by asking the patient to contract the sphincters during digital examination. Sigmoidoscopy is obligatory to detect concomitant mucosal disease.

Preoperative imaging with gadolinium-enhanced STIR sequence magnetic resonance imaging is a valuable adjunct in surgical planning and is required in patients with recurrent fistula who are more likely to have associated deformity or a nonclassical tract orientation or in cases where examination has failed to convincingly clarify fistula anatomy. It is not possible to discriminate the mucosa, submucosa, or internal sphincter using MRI, and therefore, the internal opening may not be clearly seen.

Examination under anesthesia permits further characterization although with reduced muscle tone. The site of the external opening will often differentiate an intersphincteric (within the pigmented perianal skin) from a transphincteric or suprasphincteric fistula. If a cord is palpable immediately outside the external sphincter, a superficial transphincteric fistula is likely, which may be amenable to simple lay open. The internal opening is most commonly situated at the dentate line in the posterior midline where the decussating fibers of the EAS are weakest. It is this anatomical feature of the EAS which underlies Goodsall's rule. The internal opening may be palpable and inspected through gentle traction on the papillae which may be augmented through direct pressure on the tract to reveal a bead of pus at the internal opening. Instillation of hydrogen peroxide via the external opening may assist its identification. If the internal opening has epithelialized or scarred, a bulge may be seen at the dentate line. Hydrogen peroxide has the advantage of not staining the tissues, and bubbles formed at the internal opening assist in its localization. Alternatively, tethering or dimpling may be seen on opening an Eisenhammer retractor in the canal.

The fistula may run an eccentric course through the external and sometimes internal sphincters, and care must be taken when probing to avoid the creation of a false passage while leaving the true internal opening unrecognized. This will result in the creation of a more complex fistula. Where the course is not clear, the use of both the crypt hook and a suitable probe (via the internal and external openings, respectively) using a "fencing" movement may assist its identification. The placement of a loose-seton (Latin: bristle) suture can delineate the extent of sphincter involvement, may improve assessment in the conscious patient, and is used to eradicate sepsis prior to a definitive procedure.

In principle, intersphincteric and low transsphincteric (involving less than 30 % EAS) tracts may be laid open with reference to the baseline function of the patient.

If the internal opening is at the dentate and the tract is intersphincteric, then the anoderm and IAS are divided over the probe. If an intersphincteric dissection is required in order to drain extensions, for example, a curved incision reduces the chances of inadvertent damage to the sphincters. Great caution must be exercised in women with anterior transphincteric fistula where the canal is short and may have been injured during parturition. In this situation, division of 30 % of the EAS may result in unacceptably poor function. If a transphincteric tract is found to be high and doubt exists as to whether it can be opened safely, the IAS should be divided in order to excise the involved anal gland and the primary tract outside the EAS is laid open or excised. Effective lay open may require division of the anococcygeal ligaments to gain access to the deep postanal space in the case of high posterior tracts. Thereafter, a seton can be placed through the affected external sphincter and the implications of division discussed with the patient. Options thereafter include a long-term drainage seton, interval removal of the seton (after wound healing) with 40 % recurrence rate but preservation of sphincter function, and a snug or cutting seton to slowly divide the sphincter in an attempt to preserve function (minimal recurrence) or lay open (staged or otherwise) depending upon the amount of sphincter remaining [29] (Figs. 22.4a–e and 22.5).

High transphincteric and suprasphincteric tracts should not be laid open primarily due to the extent of external sphincter division. A high, apparently blind tract may represent an unrecognized extrasphincteric fistula arising from pelvic or abdominal sepsis or a presacral dermoid with a healed internal opening, though this scenario is now rare due to improved access to high-quality preoperative imaging.

When the primary tract cannot be defined using Lockhart-Mummery or lacrimal probes, dissection from the external opening may be undertaken in order to negotiate an acute bend in a horseshoe, for example, the tract may peter out before reaching the intersphincteric space. In this situation, the procedure should be abandoned to prevent iatrogenic injury which will render the situation more complex still. If dissection into the intersphincteric space is achieved but no internal opening can be found, it is likely to have healed and a one quadrant mucosectomy, to include this site, is effective.

Secondary tracts must also be identified and treated at this time. Persistence of granulation tissue despite curettage of the primary tract indicates a secondary tract or intersphincteric extension, which will require drainage. Removing granulation tissue with a curette (avoid the use of a probe in this situation) must be performed with great care under these circumstances in order to avoid iatrogenic breeches of unaffected anorectal mucosa. A finger should be placed within the anorectum to minimize this possibility, particularly when curetting supralevator extensions or within the intersphincteric space.

Wound care after lay open is an essential element of management, and the patient must digitate open wounds to prevent "bridging" of the granulation tissue which can predispose to recurrent localized sepsis which may initiate fistula recurrence. Marsupialization of the wound may contribute to successful outpatient management.

Division of the anorectal ring can result in total incontinence. Caudal to this level, the deficit in continence varies with the level of division and is reported to vary between 5 and 40 % [30]. The most important determinants of continence are the patient's preoperative function and the length of EAS cephalad to the fistula tract. The treatment of the cryptoglandular focus in the intersphincteric space is

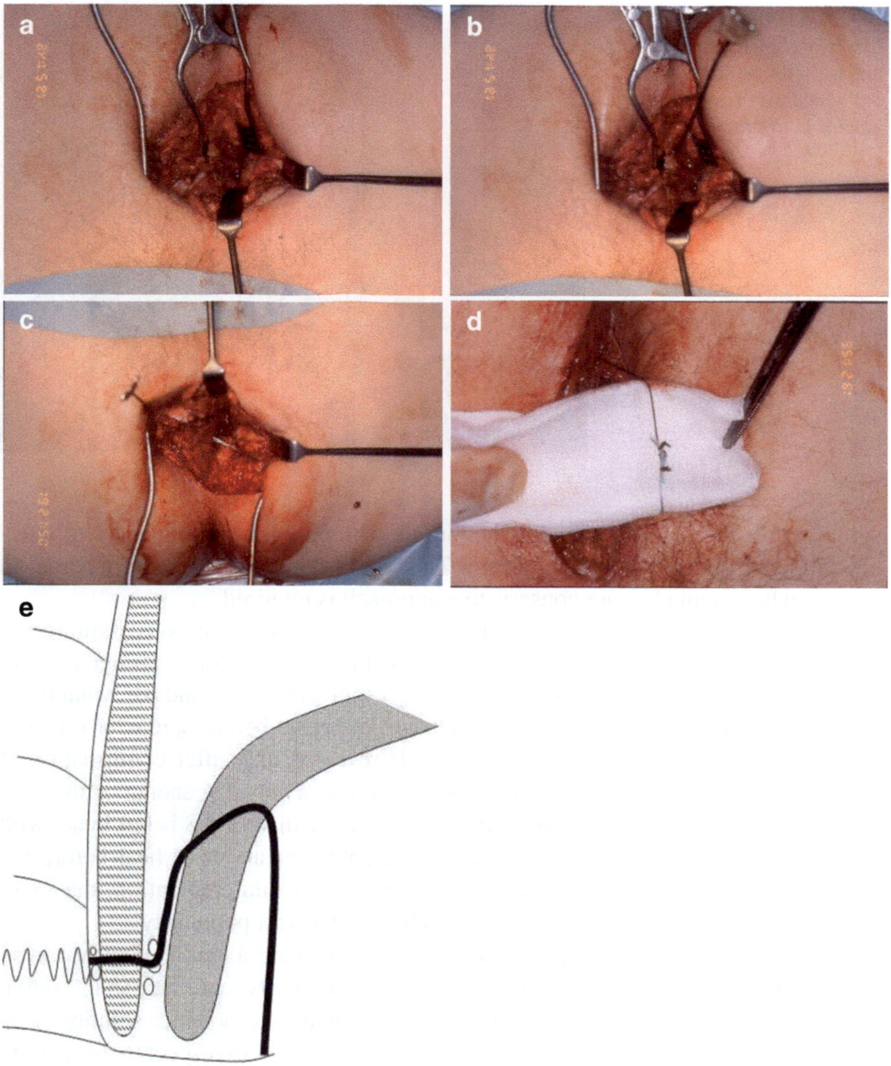

Fig. 22.4 (**a**) A fistula track in the 3'o'clock position has been dissected to the roof of the ischiorectal fossa and the anus has been obscured by a self-retaining retractor. (**b**) A probe is inserted into the external opening but cannot safely reach the internal opening. Thereafter, a second probe is inserted via the internal opening and guided through the physical contact or 'fencing' between the two probes. (**c**) The probe through the internal opening is thereby navigated safely into the wound superficial to the external sphincter and (**d**) a loose seton is placed to drain this track. (**e**) The configuration of the track is illustrated in the accompanying schematic.

achieved by laying open the internal sphincter to this level (typically at the dentate line) with a concomitant risk of 30 % mild mucus leak or loss of flatus control. The results of surgery are predicted better by clinical features than objective physiological measurements. In general, at least 2 cm of normal sphincter (or 1/3 entire sphincter length) above the fistula tract in a patient with normal continence and a solid

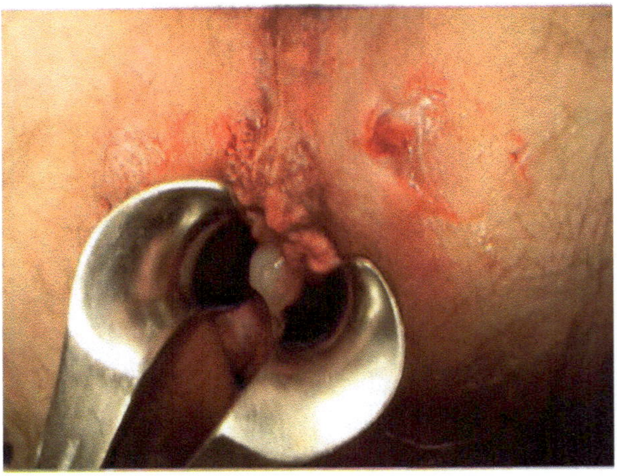

Fig. 22.5 Demonstrating a low transphincteric fistula in ano treated with fibrin glue but which may have been amenable to simple lay open.

stool permits the surgeon to divide the muscle with only the consequences of internal sphincter division described above. This is not the case in an anterior tract in women where a much more conservative approach is required.

Overlapping repair of the divided EAS has been reported to be successful (65 % grade I and II continence) and can be performed immediately or as a staged procedure where a stoma is raised at the time of high sphincterotomy and the wounds are allowed to heal with the consequent exclusion of sepsis before sphincter repair is undertaken [31]. Following this, the stoma is reversed only after confirmation of adequate function as indicated by the ability to retain a porridge enema or similar.

Staged fistulotomy is intuitively attractive since the distal EAS is left intact with the intention of allowing the partially divided sphincter above to heal before the sphincterotomy is completed. Despite high rates of fistula eradication, the functional results are highly variable and the technique has lost popularity.

The cutting seton is associated with high rates of fistula eradication; however, poor function and patient discomfort limit its acceptability, and the "snug" seton, which cuts more slowly and is more comfortable, may offer a better solution [32]. Patient selection for this technique is identical to lay open with respect to the amount of sphincter that can acceptably be divided. It has been recommended for patients with good preoperative function in whom less than two-thirds of the sphincter requires division (less than one-third anteriorly in women).

The use of advancement flaps is an attractive proposition since it avoids sphincter muscle division. Eltings's original principles remain pertinent; the tract must be separated from communication with the bowel, and adequate closure removal of all diseased tissue in the anorectal wall must be achieved [33]. Sphincter-preserving techniques are particularly prone to failure should sepsis not be completely eradicated from either the primary tract or secondary extensions. Further requirements are that the flap be well vascularized and tension-free and should be anastomosed to a site well distant to the excised internal opening. Mucosal flaps are associated with higher rates of recurrence, whereas deeper flaps are associated with unpredictable postoperative sphincter function which can be severe in the event of wound breakdown. Large internal openings (>2.5 cm) and the presence of infection are contraindications to advancement flap. The technique is impracticable in the densely inflamed "woody" perineum. Published results from selected series are variable, but overall success rates are in the region of 50–60 % with minimal functional morbidity. Preoperative antibiotics are indicted prior to advancement flap surgery.

The LIFT procedure (ligation of intersphincteric fistula tract) has been described and is based on an earlier technique developed at St. Mark's Hospital [34]. The operation involves excision of the intersphincteric component of the fistula alone, accompanied by ligation of the tract close to the internal opening and excision of granulation tissue in the remaining tract. The reported eradication rate varies between 40 and 94 % in reported series.

Fibrin glue has been used to avoid surgical dissection completely and early reports held promise. However, it does not facilitate host cell integration or revascularization and therefore does not function as a scaffold for repair. After degradation, fistula recurrence can manifest as "recurrent" sepsis despite healed internal and external openings. The fistula plug (porcine intestinal submucosa) was considered a superior biomaterial but results also demonstrate a recurrence rate of 50–60 %. These sphincter-sparing techniques have hitherto been examined only in the context of selected fistulae which may be treated without significant complication by more traditional methods. Sphincter-sparing techniques have not yet been demonstrated to compete with sphincter-dividing techniques in the treatment of more complex fistulae in ano.

Conclusions

The prevention of complications in surgery for fistula in ano depends upon a comprehensive appreciation of fistula anatomy which must be supplemented with high-quality imaging with contrast-enhanced magnetic resonance imaging when there is uncertainty on clinical assessment alone. This information enables appropriate surgical planning and patient counselling and must be correlated with clinical examination in the conscious and anesthetized patient.

Undrained sepsis propagates fistulation, increasing the complexity of future treatment, and must be controlled. Sphincter-sparing techniques have a substantial rate of failure but can be repeated if necessary in patients unwilling to entertain the implications of sphincter division. Fistulotomy and fistulectomy are the most effective techniques for fistula eradication though inevitably result in a degree of continence disturbance, related to the length of cephalad residual sphincter and preoperative anorectal function. Fistulectomy can be performed by different techniques (cutting seton, staged fistulotomy, lay open), but results are similar.

Recurrent, suprasphincteric, and extrasphincteric disease as well as sphincter reconstruction should be referred to a high-volume specialist center.

References

1. Favreau C, Siproudhis L, Eleouet M, Bouguen G, Bretagne JF. Underlying functional bowel disorder may explain patient dissatisfaction after haemorrhoidal surgery. Colorectal Dis. 2012; 14(3):356–61.
2. Nisar PJ, Acheson AG, Neal KR, Scholefield JH. Stapled hemorrhoidopexy compared with conventional hemorrhoidectomy: systematic review of randomized, controlled trials. Dis Colon Rectum. 2004;47(11):1837–45.
3. Jayaraman S, Colquhoun PH, Malthaner RA. Stapled versus conventional surgery for hemorrhoids. Cochrane Database Syst Rev (Online). 2006;(4): CD005393.
4. Nienhuijs S, de Hingh I. Conventional versus LigaSure hemorrhoidectomy for patients with symptomatic Hemorrhoids. Cochrane Database Syst Rev (Online). 2009;(1): CD006761.
5. Kraemer M, Parulava T, Roblick M, Duschka L, Muller-Lobeck H. Prospective, randomized study: proximate PPH stapler vs LigaSure for hemorrhoidal surgery. Dis Colon Rectum. 2005; 48(8):1517–22.
6. Sakr MF, Moussa MM. LigaSure hemorrhoidectomy versus stapled hemorrhoidopexy: a prospective, randomized clinical trial. Dis Colon Rectum. 2010;53(8):1161–7.
7. Shamliyan T, Wyman J, Bliss DZ, Kane RL, Wilt TJ. Prevention of urinary and fecal incontinence in adults. Evid Rep Technol Assess (Full Rep). 2007;161:1–379.
8. McCloud JM, Jameson JS, Scott AN. Life-threatening sepsis following treatment for haemorrhoids: a systematic review. Colorectal Dis. 2006;8(9):748–55.
9. Roe AM, Bartolo DC, Vellacott KD, Locke-Edmunds J, Mortensen NJ. Submucosal versus ligation excision haemorrhoidectomy: a comparison of anal sensation, anal sphincter manometry and postoperative pain and function. Br J Surg. 1987;74(10):948–51.
10. Correa-Rovelo JM, Tellez O, Obregon L, Duque-Lopez X, Miranda-Gomez A, Pichardo-Bahena R, Mendez M, Moran S. Prospective study of factors affecting postoperative pain and symptom persistence after stapled rectal mucosectomy for hemorrhoids: a need for preservation of squamous epithelium. Dis Colon Rectum. 2003;46(7):955–62.
11. Ohana G, Myslovaty B, Ariche A, Dreznik Z, Koren R, Rath-Wolfson L. Mid-term results of stapled hemorrhoidopexy for third- and fourth-degree hemorrhoids–correlation with the histological features of the resected tissue. World J Surg. 2007;31(6):1336–42.
12. Kakodkar R, Gupta S, Nundy S. Low anterior resection with total mesorectal excision for rectal cancer: functional assessment and factors affecting outcome. Colorectal Dis. 2006;8(8): 650–6.
13. Mauillon J, Thoumas D, Leroi AM, Freger P, Michot F, Denis P. Results of pudendal nerve neurolysis-transposition in twelve patients suffering from pudendal neuralgia. Dis Colon Rectum. 1999;42(2):186–92.
14. Giordano P, Bradley BM, Peiris L. Obliteration of the rectal lumen after stapled hemorrhoidopexy: report of a case. Dis Colon Rectum. 2008;51(10):1574–6.
15. Phillips R. Stapled obliteration of rectal lumen after PPH. Dis Colon Rectum. 2009;52(8):1525; author reply 1525-1526.
16. Ng KH, Ho KS, Ooi BS, Tang CL, Eu KW. Experience of 3711 stapled haemorrhoidectomy operations. Br J Surg. 2006;93(2):226–30.
17. Corman ML, Gravie JF, Hager T, Loudon MA, Mascagni D, Nystrom PO, Seow-Choen F, Abcarian H, Marcello P, Weiss E, Longo A. Stapled haemorrhoidopexy: a consensus position paper by an international working party – indications, contra-indications and technique. Colorectal Dis. 2003;5(4):304–10.
18. Giordano P, Overton J, Madeddu F, Zaman S, Gravante G. Transanal hemorrhoidal dearterialization: a systematic review. Dis Colon Rectum. 2009;52(9):1665–71.
19. Nelson RL. Operative procedures for fissure in ano. Cochrane Database Syst. Rev. 2010;(1).
20. Saad AM, Omer A. Surgical treatment of chronic fissure-in-ano: a prospective randomised study. East Afr Med J. 1992;69(11):613–5.

21. Garcia-Aguilar J, Belmonte C, Wong WD, Lowry AC, Madoff RD. Open vs. closed sphincterotomy for chronic anal fissure: long-term results. Dis Colon Rectum. 1996;39(4):440–3.
22. Giordano P, Gravante G, Grondona P, Ruggiero B, Porrett T, Lunniss PJ. Simple cutaneous advancement flap anoplasty for resistant chronic anal fissure: a prospective study. World J Surg. 2009;33(5):1058–63.
23. Lindsey I, Jones OM, Cunningham C. A contraction response of the internal anal sphincter to Botulinum toxin: does low-pressure chronic anal fissure have a different pathophysiology? Colorectal Dis. 2011;13(9):1014–8.
24. Sweeney JL, Ritchie JK, Nicholls RJ. Anal fissure in Crohn's disease. Br J Surg. 1988; 75(1):56–7.
25. Sultan AH, Kamm MA, Nicholls RJ, Bartram CI. Prospective study of the extent of internal anal sphincter division during lateral sphincterotomy. Dis Colon Rectum. 1994;37(10): 1031–3.
26. Keighley MR, Greca F, Nevah E, Hares M, Alexander-Williams J. Treatment of anal fissure by lateral subcutaneous sphincterotomy should be under general anaesthesia. Br J Surg. 1981; 68(6):400–1.
27. Jacob TJ, Perakath B, Keighley MR. Surgical intervention for anorectal fistula. Review update in Cochrane Database Syst. Rev. 2011;(11):CD002199.
28. Lunniss P, Phillips R. Anal fistula: evaluation and management. In: Phillips R, editor. Colorectal surgery. Edinburgh: Elsevier Saunders; 2009. p. 223–43.
29. Buchanan GN, Owen HA, Torkington J, Lunniss PJ, Nicholls RJ, Cohen CR. Long-term outcome following loose-seton technique for external sphincter preservation in complex anal fistula. Br J Surg. 2004;91(4):476–80.
30. Abcarian H. The 'lay open; technique. In: Phillips R, Lunniss PJ, editors. Anal fistula: surgical evaluation and management. London: Chapman & Hall Medical; 1996. p. 73–80.
31. Engel AF, Lunniss PJ, Kamm MA, Phillips RK. Sphincteroplasty for incontinence after surgery for idiopathic fistula in ano. Int J Colorectal Dis. 1997;12(6):323–5.
32. Hammond TM, Knowles CH, Porrett T, Lunniss PJ. The Snug Seton: short and medium term results of slow fistulotomy for idiopathic anal fistulae. Colorectal Dis. 2006;8(4):328–37.
33. Elting AW. The treatment of fistula in ano: with especial reference to the whitehead operation. Ann Surg. 1912;56(5):744–52.
34. Rojanasakul A, Pattanaarun J, Sahakitrungruang C, Tantiphlachiva K. Total anal sphincter saving technique for fistula-in-ano; the ligation of intersphincteric fistula tract. J Med Assoc Thai. 2007;90(3):581–6.

Chapter 23
Prevention and Treatment of Major Complications After Closure of Abdominal Wall and Repair of Abdominal Wall Hernias

Salvador Morales-Conde, María Socas, and Antonio Barranco

Keywords Postoperative • Complications • Abdominal wall hernias • Infection • Laparoscopic • Seroma • Mesh

Closure of Abdominal Wall

Early Postoperative Complications After Closure of Abdominal Wall

Wound complications that occur after closure of laparotomy remain challenging. Early wound complications included subcutaneous wound infection, deep wound infection, dehiscence, fistula, and suture sinus. Surgical site infections and wound and tissue dehiscence are the most frequent postoperative complications in gastrointestinal surgery that surgeons have to deal with, and usually both of them are related one to another. In fact, concurrent infection is a risk factor for abdominal wound dehiscence, and the prevention of wound infection would reduce substantially the incidence of dehiscence and herniation in abdominal wounds. Presence of bacteria in the healing tissue affects all processes of healing and promotes impairment of collagen synthesis and release of proteolytic enzymes, which promotes dehiscence by decreasing the suture-holding capacity of the tissue [1]. When present, infection and disruption of wounds and tissues are associated with a

S. Morales-Conde • M. Socas • A. Barranco (✉)
Department of Surgery,
Hospital Universitario Virgen del Rocio, Sevilla, Spain
e-mail: antoniobarrancomoreno@gmail.com

M.A. Cuesta, H.J. Bonjer (eds.), *Treatment of Postoperative Complications after Digestive Surgery*, DOI 10.1007/978-1-4471-4354-3_23,

higher risk of reoperation and a prolonged postoperative admission [2]. On the other hand, disruption of the local vascular supply, thrombosis of the vessels, and tissue hypoxia [3] bacterial contamination in the wound will affect the process involved in healing increasing the risk of wound infection, delayed healing, and dehiscence.

As it has been mentioned, traditionally, local factors such as the degree of contamination and the surgical technique have been regarded as strong predictors for surgical site infection, wound dehiscence, and hernias [4]. Literature supports, however, the concept that patient's factors are a major determinant of wound outcome following surgery, and systemic factors such as high age, gender, lifestyle, and coexisting morbidity play a significant role in the pathogenesis of these complications [5, 6]. In fact, lifestyle such as smoking and comorbidity such as diabetes, cardiovascular disease, and lung disease have been associated in different studies with surgical site infections and dehiscence of tissue and wounds [7, 8], which are being involved with several pathogenetic mechanisms. Smoking, microvascular disease, and severe lung disease are known to cause peripheral tissue hypoxia [9], which increases the risk of wound infection and dehiscence [10]. In addition, some studies suggest that hypoxia, smoking, and diabetes reduce collagen synthesis and oxidative killing mechanisms of neutrophils [11, 12]. On the other hand, following elective operations, perioperative blood loss was a predictor of postoperative tissue and wound complications in a dose-dependent manner when adjusting for other risk factors and confounders. This finding confirms previous reports [13] and suggests that hypovolemia and reduction of tissue oxygenation by loss of red blood cells are detrimental to healing and increase the risk of infection and tissue dehiscence [14, 15].

Different studies demonstrate also a significantly higher incidence of postoperative tissue and wound complications in emergency than elective surgery [16]. In emergency surgery, peritonitis in terms of localized pus or diffuse peritonitis was a strong predictor of wound and tissue complications. As shown by others, wound infection is likely to occur when peritonitis with a large intra-abdominal bacterial load and bacteremia is present, despite intravenous antibiotics administered perioperatively [17, 18].

It has been also described how optimal wound healing requires adequate nutrition. Nutrition deficiencies impede the normal processes that allow progression through stages of wound healing. Malnutrition has also been related to decrease wound tensile strength and increase infection rates. Malnourished patients can develop infections and delayed wound healing that result in chronic nonhealing wounds. Chronic wounds are a significant cause of morbidity and mortality for many patients and therefore constitute a serious clinical concern [19].

How to Prevent Early Wound Complications

There have been major advances in the management of patients undergoing surgery in order to prevent wound complications including aseptic techniques, prophylactic antibiotics, and advances in surgical approaches such us minimally invasive surgery. Prevention of wound infection requires standard principles of infection control after laparotomy, being essential sterile technique and conscientious efforts to avoid wound contamination. Perioperative systemic antibiotics, depending on the type of surgery, may reduce wound infection rates in the wounds that are closed primarily.

But, as it has been mentioned, wounds are exquisitely sensitive to hypoxia, which is common and preventable. Perioperative management can be adapted to promote postoperative wound healing and resistance to infection. Along with aseptic technique and prophylactic antibiotics, maintenance of perfusion and oxygenation of the wound is paramount. There is strong clinical evidence that once perfusion is assured, the addition of increased inspired oxygen substantially reduces site infection in at-risk patients.

There is enough data to establish that intraoperative care of patients has repercussions far into the postoperative period. The impact of anesthetic technique on wound healing and resistance to infection is becoming an important factor in order to avoid early wound complications. The most important factors include temperature management, increased arterial oxygen tension (PaO_2), pain control, fluid management, and, as it has been long recognized, appropriate sterile technique and administration of prophylactic antibiotics. All but the last relate particularly to maintaining perfusion and oxygenation of the wound.

All anesthetics tend to cause hypothermia by causing vasodilatation, which redistributes heat from core to periphery in previously vasoconstricted patients and increase heat loss, and by decreasing heat production. Vasoconstriction is uncommon intraoperatively, but it is often severe in the immediate postoperative period when thermoregulatory threshold returns to normal. The onset of pain with emergence from anesthesia adds to this vasoconstriction. Pain control should be addressed intraoperatively so that patients do not have severe pain upon emergence from anesthesia. Maintenance of normothermia intraoperatively has been shown to decrease the wound infection rate by two-thirds in patients undergoing colon surgery [20]. Rapid rewarming of hypothermic patients in the postanesthesia care unit also appears to be effective.

Surgical stress results in increased intravenous fluid requirements. Inflammatory mediators cause both vasodilatation and an increase in vascular permeability [21]. Optimizing the perioperative fluid administration remains a controversial challenge. Current best recommendations include replacing fluid losses based on standard recommendations for the type of surgery, replacing blood loss, and replacing other ongoing fluid loss.

All vasoconstrictive stimuli must be corrected simultaneously to allow optimal healing. Volume is the last to be corrected because vasoconstriction for other reasons induces diuresis and renders patients hypovolemic. Assessing perfusion is critical. Unfortunately, urine output is a poor and often misleading guide to peripheral perfusion. Markedly low output may indicate decreased renal perfusion, but normal or even high urine output has little correlation to wound and tissue PO_2. Physical examination of the patient is a better guide to dehydration and vasoconstriction.

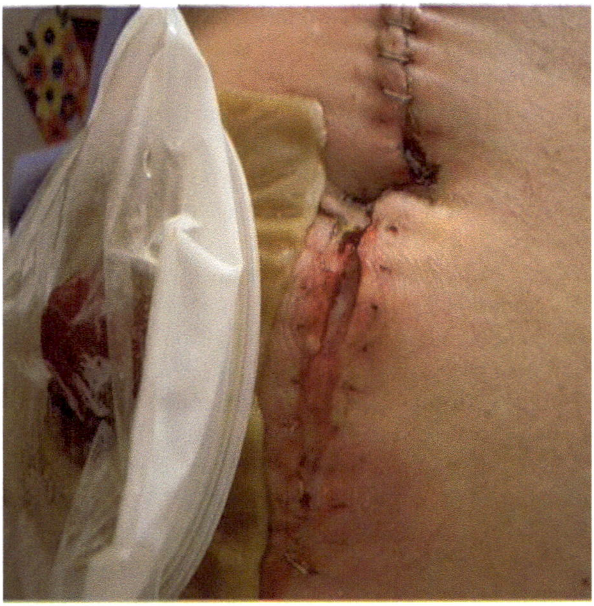

Fig. 23.1 Wound abscess

Regarding local management of the wounds, topical antibiotics and antiseptics are not of proven value and may interfere with wound healing or cause tissue injury. In grossly contaminated wounds, leaving the skin/subcutaneous tissue open is advisable. Systemic antibiotics do not reduce wound infection rates in wound that are managed by open methods. Necrotizing fasciitis is purportedly less frequent when contaminated wounds are left open.

Prevention of dehiscence/evisceration entails avoidance of infection, technical errors in closure, minimization of tension on the wound closure, and avoidance of wound ischemia. Edematous, distended intestine in the multiply operated abdomen results in the tense fascia closure which has a high rate of dehiscence. Severe edema and distention may preclude fascia closure even after attempts at intestinal decompression. Alternative strategies avoid dehiscence, damage to the fascial edges, bowel injury from evisceration, and abdominal compartment syndrome [22]. When an abdominal wall stoma is required, an important strategy is to place it remote from the reoperative open wound if possible to avoid secondary contamination. But when a fistula appears in an open abdomen, the situation becomes a problem difficult to deal with.

Early Diagnosis of Early Wound Complications

The diagnosis of wound infection is made from the identification of pus which is discharged from the closed wound, but classic signs of inflammation, such as induration or erythema, suggest infection (Fig. 23.1). Fever in the operated patient is a nonspecific finding of little value in the diagnosis. In the open wound, advancing cellulitis and progressive wound necrosis of the soft tissue margins confirm the diagnosis. Cultures are useful from the wound in the multiply operated patient and

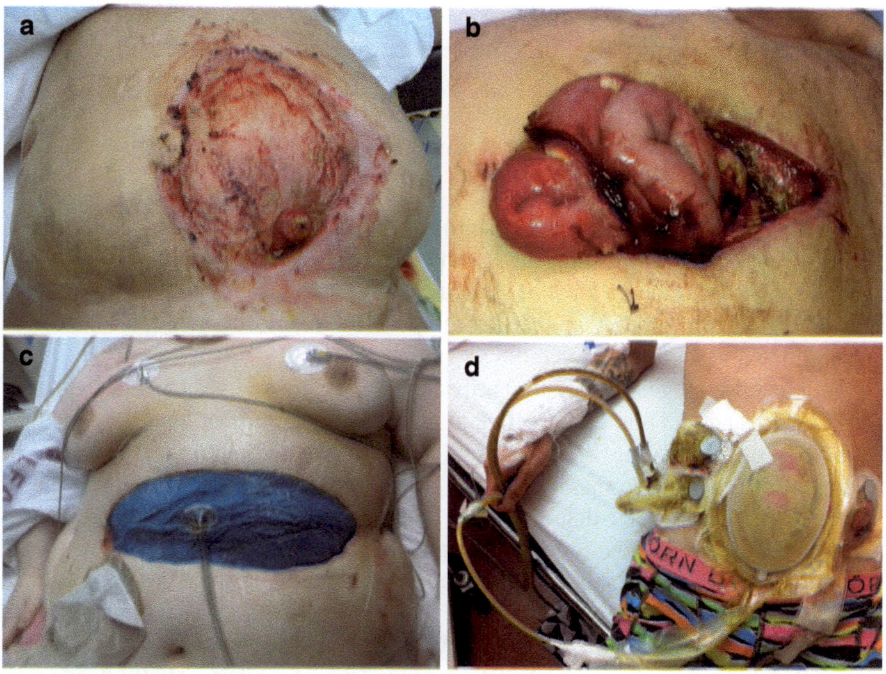

Fig. 23.2 (**a**) open abdomen with intestinal fistula; (**b**) Dehiscence of the wound; (**c**) VAC therapy; (**d**) Care of open abdomen with intestinal fistulas

will reflect the source of contamination responsible for the infection. Open surgical wounds that are culture positive or have superficial exudate but are without either necrosis or cellulitis should not be considered infected.

Necrotizing fasciitis is a clinical diagnosis from the identification of necrosis and suppuration of the wound fascia. The infection will be noted to invade laterally from the midline wound. Necrotic fat is commonly present from the subcutaneous space but skin or muscle may show minimal changes. Cultures are of value for the selection of antibiotics. Late necrotizing infection from multiply operated open wounds may reflect resistant nosocomial pathogens from the intensive care unit environment, and require cultures.

The diagnosis of dehiscence/evisceration is purely a clinical observation. Fascial separation is usually heralded by discharge of serous, bloody, or suppurative fluid from a closed wound. Opening the wound confirms the fascial separation (Fig. 23.2b). Fascial separation in the already open wound is readily seen.

How to Treat Early Wound Complications

Even with appropriate perioperative management, some wounds become infected or fail to heal. Management of wound infection from the closed abdominal wound is removal of skin sutures, opening and drainage of pus, and mechanical debridement of fibrin. Systemic antibiotics are not necessary unless necrotic soft tissue or a perimeter of cellulitis is present. If it is a simple case of infection, the wound will generally heal rapidly by secondary intention with just attention to basic care. If other complicating factors are involved, it may take more effort to achieve healing. In either case, basic proper wound care is crucial to ensure success. Basic care to avoid infection include:

- The first step to ensure a proper care of a wound includes reducing the bacterial load, especially by washing the wound gently. All open wounds are contaminated with bacteria and most of them are normally resident on the skin.
- Saline kept refrigerated or at room temperature should be avoided in order to avoid local vasoconstriction.
- Antibacterial agents, including antibacterial soaps, betadine, bleach, hydrogen peroxide, and alcohol, are effective at reducing bacterial load, but they do so at the cost of inactivating white cells and harming granulating tissue.
- It is also important to maintain moist wound environment, since moist wounds heal about 50 % faster than dry ones. The open wound is managed with moist gauze dressings without topical antiseptics or antibiotics.
- Invasive infection in open wounds requires debridement of necrosis. Localized debridement may spare elements of muscle or posterior fascia. Small areas of debridement may create fascial defects, and if no bowel is exposed, these small defects may be subsequently managed by secondary intention or small split-thickness skin grafts when culture is negative. In advanced stage, when necrotizing fasciitis exists, the dead tissues need to be debrided until only viable bleeding tissue remains.
- The vacuum-assisted closure (VAC) therapy has been also demonstrated to accelerate the healing process in open wounds (Fig. 23.2c).
- Regarding systemic antibiotics, we should take under consideration the fact that gram stain of exudate may guide antibiotic choice. Antibiotic choices are selected based on in-hospital protocols.
- While taking care of local wound it is important to pay attention to systemic factors. Nutrition and perfusion are essential to improve wound healing.

Open abdomen is another condition to deal with. There are some conditions in which closure of the fascial layer and skin may not be favorable in some surgical conditions, such us peritonitis, trauma, or mesenteric ischemia. The definitive closure of the abdominal wall is not possible, and a laparotomy is created to facilitate reexploration or to prevent abdominal compartment syndrome (Figs. 23.2a, d). Regarding the technique and material used for the temporary closure, no prospective randomized data exists, but mesh materials are commonly used. They provide drainage of infectious material, permit visual control of the underlying viscera, facilitate access to the abdominal wall, preserve the fascial margin, enable healing by secondary intention, and allow mobilization of the patient. In the case of decreasing intra-abdominal pressure, meshes can be trimmed to centralize the rectus muscle and to facilitate definitive closure. Nonabsorbable meshes have been frequently reported to cause enteric fistulae and persistent infection necessitating mesh explantation; for that reason the use of absorbable mesh material is common in these patients, but it should be determined in the near future the role of biological meshes in these types of wounds. While these infectious complications appear to occur less frequently with the use of absorbable materials, these meshes will finally lead to an incisional hernia, requiring repair with nonabsorbable mesh after a period of 6–12 months [23].

But new systems such as the vacuum-assisted fascial closure (VAFC) therapy can be used in open abdomen under a carefully applied protocol. The use of VAFC may result in significantly higher fascial closure rates, obviating the need for subsequent hernia repair in most patients [24]. The utility of this technique is not limited to the early postoperative period, but it can be successful as much as 3–4 weeks after initial operation. VAFC differs from these and other techniques in that it prevents both fascial retraction and visceral adherence, allowing for continuing attempts at abdominal closure several weeks after laparotomy. This is an extension of the standard vacuum pack technique and has two important components allowing for later closure. The first is the perforated polyethylene sheet placed over the bowel. This must be tucked under the fascial edges to prevent adherence. The second is the thick polyurethane sponge as opposed to the surgical towel used in the original technique. This provides suction to the cross section of the abdominal wall, preventing fascial retraction by creating constant medial tension on the fascia without injuring it as some similar techniques using suture might.

Late Postoperative Complications After Closure of Abdominal Wall

Incisional hernia is a late complication following abdominal surgery, occurring as a result of breakdown or loss of fascial closure and, as such, an iatrogenic disease. The incidence after laparotomy has been reported as ranging between 4 and 12 % in large series [25], but the true incidence is probably underestimated [26]. Many incisional hernias are asymptomatic, but if symptoms are present, an incisional hernia may be associated with major morbidity, loss of time from productive employment, and diminished quality of life. Given the financial cost of incisional hernia repair and the disappointing recurrence rates, incisional hernia remains a significant challenge for most surgeons.

A number of factors associated with incisional hernia have been identified, some of which are local, such as wound infection, surgical technique [27], and surgeon's experience, and some systemic, such as older age, male sex, and altered collagen metabolism [28]. In addition, a lifestyle factor such as obesity or smoking has been found to be associated with incisional hernias [29, 30].

Postoperative wound infection is a well-documented risk factor for early dehiscence of incisional wounds and fascia and for later development of incisional hernia [25]. The pathogenesis is related to proliferation of bacteria in a wound, which affects each process involved in healing leading to decreased collagen synthesis, decreased bursting strength of the abdominal wall, and an increased risk of dehiscence.

Re-laparotomy is the strongest predictor for incisional hernia. Reoperations have previously been found to increase the rate of abdominal wound dehiscence and may also be responsible for the development of incisional hernia [31], especially due to the need of re-suturing a relatively nonvascular scar tissue of the fascia. In addition, patients undergoing re-laparotomy are likely to have bacterial contamination of the wound and may in addition have peritonitis, which increase the risk of wound infection and delayed healing.

Regarding the systemic factors that may influence on the presence of incisional hernias, we observe how high age is associated with atrophy of the abdominal wall and changes in connective tissue. Inherent connective tissue disorders may result in a deterioration of abdominal wall connective tissue and the tensile strength of scar tissue may be decreased. Diabetics are prone to wound infection, which impairs wound healing. Moreover, atherosclerosis in diabetics may impair wound healing, as may obesity, which is often the cause of diabetes development. Corticosteroids have a deleterious effect on wound healing and are used by large groups of patients, especially those with pulmonary disease. In addition, malnutrition, radiotherapy, smoking, and cancer are known to cause impaired wound healing.

Smoking is another factor to be considered since several pathogenic mechanisms seem to be involved. Peripheral tissue hypoxia, which may be caused by smoking, increases the risk of wound infection and dehiscence, presumably through reduction of the oxidative killing mechanism of neutrophils, which constitute a critical defense against surgical pathogens. In addition, decreased collagen deposition in surgical test wounds has been found in smokers, a mechanism that may further attenuate the fascia in addition to the reduced collagen I–collagen III ratio present in incisional hernia. Degradation of connective tissue caused by an imbalance between proteases and their inhibitors may also be responsible. The latter mechanism, which is enhanced by smoking, is believed to cause tissue-destructive disorders like abdominal aorta aneurysm and pulmonary emphysema. Both diseases are associated with abdominal wall herniation. In fact, the incisional hernia rate has been reported as high as 31 % following midline laparotomy for abdominal aorta aneurysm repair.

Increased intra-abdominal pressure has been identified as another important factor that influences the development of incisional hernias after a laparotomy. Several conditions cause increased intra-abdominal pressure, such as chronic pulmonary disease with cough, obesity, ascites, prostatism, constipation, pregnancy, and ileus. During raised intra-abdominal pressure the strain put on the abdominal wall scar is increased, which could lead to wound failure and subsequent hernia development.

How to Prevent Late Postoperative Complications

The control of any of the aspects, previously mentioned, that influence hernia development will help to prevent incisional hernias, but surgical factors also play an important role. Some types of incisions, such as the lateral paramedian and transverse incisions have proven to cause less incisional hernias than, for example, the midline incisions. This is caused by several factors, including the anatomical structures that are cut by the incision, since richly vascularized structures heal better than avascular structures, while division of major arteries may result in impaired wound healing. Another important factor is the pulling force of the abdominal muscles, which is mainly transverse. This means that the wound edges in vertical incisions are likely to be separated by this force, while transverse wound edges are approximated.

Suture technique is also an important factor involved in incisional hernia development. The length of the suture used to close the abdomen should exceed the length of the wound by at least four times (suture length to wound length ratio 4:1) [32, 33]. The length of the stitch, or tissue bite, should at least be one centimeter, but not bigger than 5 cm. The suture should include aponeurotic tissues, may include muscle, but not peritoneum or subcutaneous tissue, and may be either interrupted or continuous. It is important to realize that the tensile strength of the wound increases to approximately 50 % at 4 weeks after operation. After 6–12 months, the wound reaches 80 % of its original strength. Suture materials should remain their tensile strength for at least 6 weeks to allow the wound to regain sufficient tensile strength. Rapidly absorbable suture materials, such as polyglyconate (Vicryl), should not be used, while slowly absorbable materials such as polydioxanone (PDS) perform equally well as nonabsorbable materials, such as nylon and polypropylene [34, 35]. Multifilament sutures result in an increased incidence of wound infection and should therefore not be used. In addition to type of incision and suture technique, prevention of wound infection by aseptic techniques will prevent wound infection, together with prophylactic antibiotics, atraumatic surgical technique, meticulous hemostasis, and removal of necrotic and breakdown tissues [36].

Early Diagnosis of Late Postoperative Complications

As we have seen, it has been suggested that early development of incisional hernias is caused by perioperative factors, such as surgical technique and wound infection, together with systemic factors, such as connective tissue disorders. Burger et al. [36] conducted a study in order to determine whether incisional hernias develop early after abdominal surgery might be predictive. Patients who underwent a midline laparotomy were submitted to a CT scan during the first postoperative month. The distance between the two rectus abdominis muscles was measured on these CT scans, after which several parameters were calculated to predict incisional hernia development, being hernia development established clinically. The average and maximum distances between the left and right rectus abdominis muscles were significantly larger in patients with subsequent incisional hernia development than in those without an incisional hernia. Altogether, 92 % of incisional hernia patients had a maximum distance of more than 25 mm compared to only 18 % of patients without an incisional hernia. This study concluded that incisional hernia occurrence can thus be predicted by measuring the distance between the rectus abdominis muscles on a postoperative CT scan, although its clinical manifestation may take years. On the other hand, this study shows the importance of perioperative factors in incisional hernia development and how prevention should focus on controlling this type of factors.

The diagnosis of incisional hernia is normally made based on clinical examination. However, small hernias, hernias in obese patients or patients with abdominal pain, distension, or various other factors can be difficult to diagnose. In cases in which there is clinical uncertainty of the diagnosis of an incisional hernia, ultrasound or CT scan, and even magnetic nuclear resonance, can be used to detect these clinically unsuspected incisional hernias. CT scan can show the exact size, location, and content of each incisional hernia. The evaluation of postsurgical abdomen by CT scan should include a careful assessment of previous laparotomy sites in search of occult incisional hernias that may be the source of the patient's abdominal symptoms.

How to Treat Late Postoperative Complications

The treatment of late postoperative complications, such as incisional hernias, must follow the basic principles of ventral hernia repair.

Abdominal Wall Hernia Repair

Open or laparoscopic mesh implantation for hernia repair of abdominal wall defects has been the gold standard treatment since it appears to reduce the rate of recurrence by an average of 30–50 % in comparison with nonmesh herniorrhaphy. However, the use of prosthetic materials is not without potential clinical problems and might lead to various complications such as seromas, adhesions, acute and chronic pain, migration of the mesh, rejection, and mesh-related infections [37, 38].

Mesh-related infection, along with seroma formation, is the most common complication following ventral hernia repair. Risk factors for surgical site infection after mesh implantation include gender, age over 70, comorbidities (diabetes, obesity), operating time, and the prophylactic use of drainages. Mesh-related infection rates are also associated [37] to the type of mesh, type of surgical technique used to place the mesh (laparoscopic or open), relationship of the mesh to the subcutaneous tissue, perioperative use of prophylactic antibiotics, sterile technique to apply the mesh, mesh placement in contaminated wounds, and systemic factors such as smoking and immunosuppression.

Elective primary mesh hernia repair is considered a clean surgery, with infection rates of up to 8 % being reported [37], being in most of the cases a problem related to open repair. On the other hand, one of the main advantages of laparoscopic ventral hernia repair is the lower mesh infection rate, especially when compared to open repair. But the main problems associated to the laparoscopic approach are adhesion and seroma formations.

The influence of the type of mesh on overall mesh-related complications is very important. The choice of the proper mesh to repair a ventral hernia, either by laparoscopic or open approach, may influence on the results and not only on the recurrence rate. Type of biomaterial, pore size, and weight are important factors that lead surgeons to select one or other mesh depending on the approach, the surgical field, the risk factors associated to the patient, and the risk of recurrence based on the size of the defect.

The development of polypropylene prosthetics revolutionized surgery for the repair of abdominal wall hernias. A tension-free mesh technique has drastically reduced recurrence rates for all hernias compared to tissue repairs and has made possible to reconstruct large ventral defects that were previously irreparable. The repair of abdominal wall defects is one of the most commonly performed general surgical procedures, and more research is needed to investigate the interaction of abdominal wall forces on a ventral hernia repair or the required amount or strength of the foreign-body material necessary for an adequate hernia repair.

The long-term consequences of implantable prosthesis are not without concern. The body generates an intense inflammatory response to the prosthetic that results in scar plate formation, increased stiffness of the abdominal wall, and shrinkage of the biomaterial. Reducing the density of the prosthetic material and creating a "lightweight" mesh theoretically induces less foreign-body response, results in improved abdominal wall compliance, causes less contraction or shrinkage of the mesh, and allows for better tissue incorporation, but the potential increase of recurrence should be still investigated. Different studies of the laboratory data and short-term clinical follow-up have been reviewed to provide a strong basis or argument for the use of "lightweight" prosthetics in hernia surgery.

Infection

How to Prevent Infection

New improved techniques and stricter aseptic protocols in the operating room have contributed to a decrease in wound infection rates after hernia repair. Principles to avoid wound infection must be followed after any laparotomy. Due to the special features of implant devices, the best way to treat an implant-related infection without destroying the implant is to take the appropriate measures to avoid initial exposure to infection agents.

Preoperative administration of antimicrobial agents in clean surgical procedures such as primary hernioplasty has been a matter of considerable debate for years, but a recent meta-analysis published by Sanabria et al. [39] of the accumulated evidence suggests that infection rates were decreased by almost 50 % in patients who received antimicrobial prophylaxis.

Considerable efforts are being made to develop techniques that will restrain the fundamental mechanism for implant-related infections, which are bacterial adhesion and colonization of artificial surfaces and biofilm formation. Various strategies such as the previously mentioned antimicrobial prophylaxis and mesh coatings of antimicrobial biomaterials are being developed, but so far there is a lack of data regarding the influence of this coated material in infection rate. Apart from antibiotic coating, silver, gold, titanium, carbonitride, polyglactin, gelatine, and other biomaterials have been used as coatings, with different mechanism of action.

Laparoscopic ventral hernia repair compared with open mesh techniques has been proven to induce a lower incidence of surgical wound infections, probably due to the lack or relatively limited physical contact of the mesh with the surgical wound during surgery.

The type of mesh is also of vital importance regarding the development or not of an infection. Monofilament polypropylene is the most frequently used biomaterial for open repair of an abdominal wall defect due to the low infection rates compared with other nonabsorbable types of meshes. The biocompatibility and the large pore size of this PP textile permit the relatively uncompromised inflammatory response of the immune system on the surface of this material. Surgical infection promoted by implantation of biomaterials is caused by infection and proliferation of bacteria into and within the pores and interstices of these synthetic materials. When pores are less than 10 μm, bacteria averaging 1 μm cannot be eliminated by macrophages and neutrophilic granulocytes, which are too large to enter a 10-μm three-dimensional pore. Totally macroporous prostheses, containing pores larger than 75 μm, deter housing and growth of bacteria by allowing macrophages, rapid fibroplasias, and angiogenesis, which also prevent infiltration and growth of bacteria. On the other hand, totally microporous prostheses (pores less than 10 μm) and macroporous prostheses with multifilamentous and microporous components are similar to braided suture materials, and by harboring bacteria, they can promote their growth, likewise resulting in biomaterial-related infection. Based on these principles, some authors have concluded that in cases of infection, the totally macroporous prostheses do not have to be removed, which leads us to select the proper mesh based on the risk factors of a wound to develop an infection.

Hernia repair is considered a clean operation, nevertheless, when bowel opening or abdominal wound infection has previously occurred, this procedure becomes contaminated; thus, the use of a prosthetic material was thought for years to be contraindicated. However, recent studies suggest that minor morbidity, minimal risk of infection, and minor wound-related mortality are observed after mesh placement in contaminated tissues.

Early Diagnosed Infection

Surgical wound infections are the most commonly encountered type of infection, presenting at an early postoperative stage, usually days or a few weeks after the mesh placement. The symptoms and signs are typical of local acute inflammation: pain, erythema, swelling with locally increased temperature, and confined tenderness.

Inappropriate treatment of surgical wound infections may be complicated by the formation of discharging fistula, intra-abdominal abscess, or, rarely, osteomyelitis. The emergence of systemic symptoms such as fever, chills, or rigor and malaise should urge prompt investigations and initiation of therapeutic actions before sepsis occurs.

Deep-seated mesh infections generally manifest in the early postoperative period, but infrequently they can also be observed as a late-onset phenomenon that is delayed for month or years (up to 4–5 years after the operation) [40]. Deep-seated infections may result from persistent fluid collection (seromas) leading to chronic sepsis. Symptoms can be chronic, recurrent, or totally absent until the progression to sepsis.

The combination of clinical presentation, physical examination, laboratory values, and previous medical history is usually adequate to establish a diagnosis. However, when there are doubts regarding differential diagnosis, two noninvasive imaging techniques could provide the diagnosis. Abdominal ultrasound and CT scan may reveal the inflammatory process in the adipose tissue around the implant as well as complications related to mesh infection such as the presence of a fistula or an intra-abdominal abscess. Diagnostic puncture of a mesh-related seroma when there is no sign of inflammation should be carefully considered and not performed routinely, since there is a high risk of transforming a potentially aseptic reaction to an infectious process through the introduction of bacteria into the previously aseptic seromas.

Treat Infection

The therapeutic options available following the development of mesh-related infection can be separated according to the type and severity of infection and the type of implanted mesh.

- Superficial wound infections after prosthetic material implantation may have better prognosis and may be treated conservatively using proper intravenous antimicrobial coverage and drainage when signs of accumulated exudates exist. However, the use of drainage is still controversial due to insufficient evidence.
- Deep-seated infections of the mesh required prolonged antibiotic treatment in combination with percutaneous or open drainage, since it has been demonstrated to be effective to restrain the infectious process. However, when extensive infections is present, due to biofilm formation and limited penetration of the drug in the area, mesh removal and surgical cleaning of the wound pose the best possible treatment to eradicate the infection. Hernia recurrence could be a postoperative complication if adequate fibrous tissue has not developed earlier.

The choice between conservative and surgical treatment could also be influenced by the type of implanted mesh. Structural (monofilament or multifilament) and biochemical (hydrophobic or hydrophilic) properties influence the potential response of the infection to the administered antibiotics. Clinical findings in combination with recent in vitro experiments suggest that infected hydrophobic meshes, such as PTFE and ePTFE, are most likely to be removed in order to achieve complete cure.

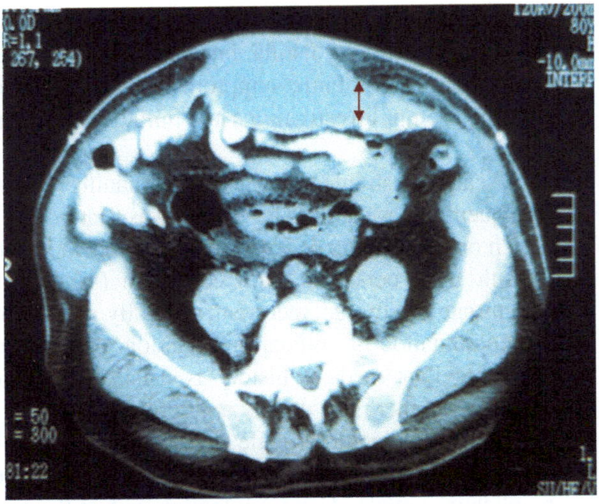

Fig. 23.3 Seroma could be related to recurrence, since it could disattach the tacks due to its weight (disattachment of the tackers of the inner crown is indicated by the *arrow*)

Seroma After Laparoscopic Ventral Hernia Repair

The potential complications related to seroma formation include pain, discomfort to the patient, and cellulitis, being the most important complication of them the possibility of getting infected. The infection of a seroma is considered one of the most challenging complications since it might lead to mesh removal and recurrence.

The rate of cellulitis and infection after laparoscopic ventral hernia repair varies from one series to another. Seroma-related cellulitis is considered by some authors to be a common problem that it is present in most of the patients in whom a seroma is detected [41]. This cellulitis can lead to mesh infection, postoperative morbidity, and further need for operative care. Some authors have proposed the administration of 7 days of postoperative prophylactic antibiotics to decrease the rate of patients with seroma developing cellulitis [41].

Seroma after laparoscopic ventral hernia repair could also be related to recurrence, since the weight of this serous fluid between the mesh and the anterior abdominal wall could increase the tensile strength on the fixation of the mesh and therefore disattach tackers (Fig. 23.3) from its original fixation to the anterior wall and be responsible of an improper anchoring of the mesh right after surgery, which may influence in the presence of recurrence in the future. In fact, some authors have observed at reoperation, due to recurrences, how they appeared to be due to mesh detachment, and this fact might be related to the presence of a seroma.

How to Prevent Seroma

The real importance of seroma formation and the influence of them in the quality of life in the postoperative period of the patient are also still to be determined. But it can be concluded that seroma is not really a key factor in the postoperative period after this surgery and its simple presence cannot be considered a complication. But it would be better to avoid it since, in some cases, it could be responsible for some sort of discomfort to the patient and because it could confuse both patients and surgeons about a possible recurrence.

Different methods are being proposed lately in order to decrease seroma formation, but since the method of describing the presence of seroma is not described in the same way by different authors, it is difficult to determine the effectiveness of one method compared to the other. Some authors have proposed that defect closure confers a strong advantage in laparoscopic ventral hernia repair, since there is a shift of the paradigm towards more physiologic abdominal wall reconstruction, and especially because defect closure essentially eliminated postoperative seroma. These authors advocate routine use of the closure of the defect technique during laparoscopic ventral hernia repair [42], but for other authors, such as Palanivelu et al. [43], this maneuver of closing the defect has no influence in the rate of seroma formation.

Other methods have been described to decrease the rate of this serous fluid between the mesh and the sac, such us cauterization of the hernia sac [44] and use of argon bean to treat the hernia sac or to excise it, and to decrease the seroma-related complications, such us the use of postoperative antibiotics to decrease the incidence of seroma-related cellulitis and decrease the possibility of mesh removal due to this cellulitis [41].

The studies conducted to reduce the presence of seromas, like the one described by Fernandez-Lobato et al. [45] and JP Chevrel, by using fibrin glue after conventional open ventral hernia repair, together with other publications of the reduction of seroma with the same substance in other pathologies like breast surgery or plastic and reconstructive surgery, made us develop a protocol looking for a solution to also decrease the presence of seroma. We have conducted a clinical study in which we have observed that the use of fibrin glue in the sac after laparoscopic ventral hernia repair seems to have an important value in the laparoscopic treatment of abdominal wall hernias in reducing seromas, while favoring, on the other hand, the ingrowth of meshes.

Early Diagnosed Seroma

Seroma, defined as serous fluid retention between the mesh and the anterior abdominal wall, is present in most of the cases after laparoscopic ventral hernia repair, as different series that analyzed its presence by radiological exams show. Its presence cannot be considered a complication since patients do not even detect them in most of the cases. For these reasons, it is important to define that seroma must be considered an incident after this surgery which may lead to complications.

The real incidence of seroma after this procedure is difficult to be determined and not being properly documented and analyzed since its presence varies from one series to another. Different studies have shown how seroma formation is very

Table 23.1 Clinical incidence of seroma after laparoscopic ventral hernia repair

Author	Clinical seroma (%)
3rd Parker et al. [77]	0.5
Morales-Conde et al. [78]	2.1
Heniford et al. [55]	2.6
Ferrari et al. [79]	2.6
Carbonell et al. [80]	2.7
Heniford et al. [55]	3
Bedi et al. [47] (systematic review)	5.4
Kaafarani et al. [57]	6.8
Uranues et al. [81]	7
Varnell et al. [58]	8.5
Tessier et al. [56]	9
Perrone et al. [50]	10.7
Farrakha et al. [82]	10.9
Sodergren et al. [83]	14.5
Sharma et al. [51]	25
Chowbey et al. [84]	32
Edwards et al. [41]	32.3
Edwards et al. [41]	33
Susmallian et al. [49]	35
Birch et al. [85]	78

Table 23.2 Radiological incidence of seroma after laparoscopic ventral hernia repair

Author	Radiological seroma (%)
Morales-Conde et al. [78]	95.2
Susmallian et al. [49]	100

variable, ranging the different series from 0.5 to 78 % [46] (Table 23.1), being the rate of the systematic review published by Bedi et al. of 5.4 % [47]. But this data is related to the presence of clinical seroma following different criteria, since one of our studies [48] and the study conducted by Susmallian et al. [49] show that seroma is present in radiological exams in almost all cases (Table 23.2).

One of the main problems related to the variety of these results is that seromas have been considered following different criteria by different authors. For some authors it is considered just a complication [43], for others it is considered one of the main complications of this technique [50] or even as the most common sequel of this surgery [51], but others just think it is a minor complication [52] or an incident [6].

On the other hand, an additional problem related to the description of seromas is observed in most of the series: authors have been using different parameters, difficult to be measured, to quantify the rate of seroma formation. Some authors have included the definition of "significant seroma" [42] or "prolonged seroma"; others described seroma as a fluid retention that requires surgical intervention [53] or the need to be punctured [54]; or based on the time lasting after surgery, lasting more than 4 weeks [55], more than 6 weeks [56], or even more than 8 weeks [57]; or they

Table 23.3 Clinical classification of seroma

Type 0		*No clinical seroma*	No clinical seroma
	0a	Neither clinical nor radiological seroma	
	0b	No clinical seroma, but it can be detected by radiological exams	
Type I		*Clinical seroma lasting less than 1 month*	Incident
Type II		*Clinical seroma lasting more than 1 month*	
	IIa	Between 1 and 3 months	
	IIb	Between 3 and 6 months	
Type III		*Minor seroma-related complications*	Complication
	IIIa	Clinical seroma lasting more than 6 months	
	IIIb	Important discomfort which does not allow normal activity	
	IIIc	Pain	
	IIId	Cellulitis	
Type IV		*Major seroma-related complications*	
	IVa	Need to puncture the seroma to decrease symptoms	
	IVb	Infection	
	IVc	Recurrence related to seroma	
	IVd	Mesh rejection related to seroma	

are just defined as "a symptomatic seroma" [58] or by the presence of a complication such as seroma-related cellulitis.

Based on these facts, in order to early diagnose a seroma, we have to determine first what we want to diagnose, since seroma is going to be present in almost all the case if its presence is determine by ultrasound or CT scan.

For that reason we propose a clinical classification of seroma after laparoscopic ventral hernia repair in order to unify different criteria so we can establish in the near future in the surgical literature the proper incidence of seroma and its clinical importance (Table 23.3).

Treat Postoperative Seroma

It is difficult to know, based on the literature, the best method to manage patients presenting seromas and theirs complications in the postoperative period. Different treatment options for postoperative seromas have been described including observation for spontaneous resolution, percutaneous aspiration [41], closed suction drainage, abdominal blinders, and sclerosant [59]. While some groups recommend puncturing the seroma just in case of pain or discomfort, other groups recommend not doing it in order to avoid contamination. Most of the authors considered that spontaneous resolution of seroma occurs in the vast majority of the cases, being not necessary to puncture any of them or the number of seromas that need to be aspirated is very low. But, it can also be observed in the literature review that the reasons that lead different authors to puncture seromas and the complications of this invasive approach are also not well defined. Based on this data, we have observed that the rate of seromas being punctured varies from one author to another, from 0 to 33.3 %.

Adhesions After Laparoscopic Ventral Hernia Repair

The formation of adhesions is an extremely complex process, which has not been well-determined so far. As a result, many of the studies on this phenomenon are still empirical, but the results published are so far promising and it is possible that we can control this process in the near future, whether stimulating or inhibiting it, depending on the circumstances. The consequence of these studies could lead in the future to use prosthetic materials for intra-abdominal placement in laparoscopic surgery of the abdominal wall, with no risk of creating adhesions and the subsequent consequences, such as fistulas or bowel occlusion.

In the meantime, while we try to determine the different factors involved in adhesion formation, the ideal material and substance to prevent them are still far from being found. Different studies performed so far have proved that it is possible to reduce the quantity and the quality of these adhesions, but not to prevent them completely. Full tissue integration without adhesion formation is still a challenge for intra-abdominal mesh materials.

Different factors have been related to the process of adhesion formation, but the need of the bowel and the intraperitoneal organs to isolate foreign agents, such us prosthetic materials, sutures, and bacteria, seems to have an important role in this issue. However, during laparoscopic repair of ventral hernia, the presence of intraperitoneal adhesions is not a result of only the material itself, since other experimental studies have related them to other factors: spiral tacks, improper placement and fixing of the mesh, or leaving the parietal side of these materials exposed to the intra-abdominal viscera [60] (Fig. 23.4).

On the other hand we also have a lack of information about the healing process involved on adhesion formation. It would be interesting for the future to determine

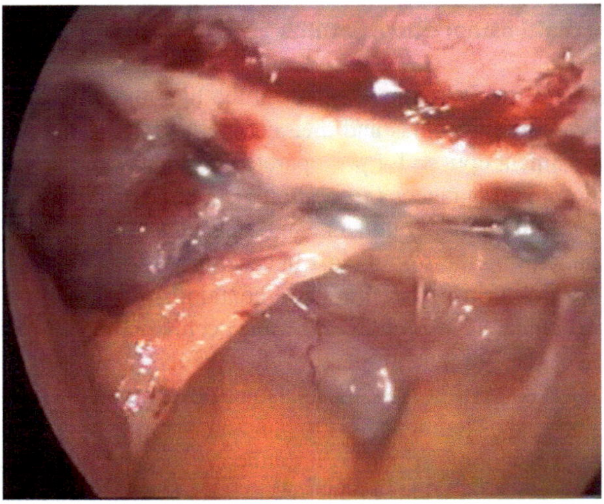

Fig. 23.4 Adhesions to the edge of the mesh after laparoscopic ventral hernia repair

the critical moment in which adhesions to the prosthetic materials are formed. For that reason some authors have designed different studies by using sequential laparoscopy to monitor the real-time adhesion formation process and the critical period when most adhesions form [61].

If we analyze the factors involved on adhesion formation when a mesh is placed intraperitoneally, we can determine the following:

- Material: Different studies published [62] have shown how porosity of the material is considered as one of the most important factors related to adhesion formation and ingrowth. Large porosity has been related to an increase amount of adhesions. Polypropylene meshes are considered a high porosity prosthetic material which creates an important scar tissue involved in adhesion formation. On the other hand, a low porosity material, such as ePTFE (expanded polytetrafluoroethylene) [62, 63], produces a capsule of tissue that covers the mesh, forming few or no adhesions. So, we can conclude that pore size of mesh is critical in the development and maintenance of abdominal adhesions and tissue ingrowth, but it has been demonstrated, however, that a reduction in the amount of material and an increase in pore size results in better mesh biocompatibility with a potential reduction of adhesion formations [64, 65], as it has been trying to demonstrate with the new "low weight" polypropylene. These large-pore polypropylene meshes in the intra-abdominal position showed a reduced inflammatory tissue reaction, so they could be considered an alternative for the future development of intraperitoneal onlay meshes [66]. In fact, new studies with reduced weight polypropylene mesh have demonstrated a smallest change in the adjacent tissue pliability/compliance and smallest amount of adhesion than conventional polypropylene [67]. On the other hand, these factors should be also analyzed in the future regarding the pore size of other materials such as PTFE. The large pore size, thinner meshes such as condensed PTFE (c-PTFE), led to better tissue integration compared to the other meshes with PTFE based or polypropylene. Through hydrophobic chemistry, low profile, and increased pore size, c-PTFE balances the rapid resolution of the inflammatory and wound healing response that resists adhesion formation, with efficient integration within the surrounding abdominal tissue [68].
- Surgical technique to place the mesh: An experimental study conducted by our group [60] has demonstrated the influence of the surgical technique during mesh placement during laparoscopic ventral hernia repair. In this study, most of the adhesions to the ePTFE meshes were observed at the edges compared to the central part of this prosthetic material. The potential reasons of these adhesions were analyzed, and it could be seen how adhesions were formed to the undesired exposition of the parietal face of the prosthesis or to tackers improperly introduced into the mesh. These issues demonstrate the need of a meticulous technique to avoid complications related to adhesions, such us bowel occlusion and/or perforation. The mesh must be properly extended so the parietal face do not end expose to the bowel and tackers should be introduced all the way into the mesh to avoid them hanging from the anterior abdominal wall.

- Role of fixation on adhesion formation: As it has been said previously adhesions to spiral tacks may occur and we have observed them in experimental study. Resent clinical papers have even reported cases of obstruction and/or perforation of the small bowel resulting from a band adhesion caused by a displaced spiral tacker [69, 70].
- Surgical trauma: Surgical trauma to the bowel or to the peritoneal surface of the anterior abdominal wall, during the process of adhesiolysis, has some influence in adhesion formation, even if the ideal mesh to be placed intra-abdominally is used. Adhesions result from the normal peritoneal wound healing response and develop in the first 5–7 days after injury. Adhesion formation and adhesion-free re-epithelialization are alternative pathways, both of which begin with coagulation which initiates a cascade of events resulting in the buildup of fibrin gel matrix. If not removed, the fibrin gel matrix serves as the progenitor to adhesions by forming a band or bridge when two peritoneal surfaces coated with it are apposed [71]. The band or bridge becomes the basis for the organization of an adhesion, especially if a foreign-body reaction is added to the process when a mesh is placed intra-abdominally, becoming of great importance the surgical trauma on the surface of the bowel [72].

How to Prevent Adhesions

Little clinical information based on preoperative findings is available about adhesions to biomaterials placed intra-abdominally. RH Koehler at al. [73] published a multi-institutional study of adhesions to implanted expanded polytetrafluoroethylene (ePTFE) mesh at reoperation in patients who had previously undergone laparoscopic incisional hernia repair done with the same mesh implantation technique. In this large series of reoperations after laparoscopic incisional hernia repair, no or minimal formation of adhesions to implanted ePTFE mesh was observed in 91 % of cases, and no severe cohesive adhesions were found. This study shows how the selection of the proper mesh may reduce the incidence of adhesion formation.

On the other hand, as it has been already mentioned, a meticulous technique is one of the most important factors involved in reducing adhesion formation: avoid unnecessary surgical trauma on the surface of the peritoneum and on the serosa of the bowel, avoid the parietal face of the mesh to be exposed to the abdominal cavity, and avoid the spiral tacks to be hanging from the mesh due to an improper introduction through the prosthetic material.

But, since these circumstances are not usually possible to avoid due to the process of adhesiolysis needed or to the location of the defect that makes difficult to place properly the mesh or the tackers, alternative method to avoid adhesion is under investigation. Moreover, efforts to prevent or reduce adhesions have been unsuccessful, hindered by their empirical basis, the lack of good predictive animal models, and the biochemical complexities of adhesiogenesis. The two major strategies for adhesion prevention or reduction are adjusting surgical technique, as it has been already proposed, and applying adjuvants.

Different studies have been published using a variety of substances to prevent adhesion formation to the prosthetic materials with different results: hyaluronic acid/carboxymethyl cellulose (HA/CMC) membrane has been used as an effective measure to prevent polypropylene-induced adhesions; taurolidine 2 % solution has been proposed as a cost-effective alternative to HA/CMC membranes when a polypropylene mesh is used in direct contact with the abdominal viscera; hyaluronate sodium in the form of a bioresorbant membrane has also been demonstrated to significantly reduce the development of intra-abdominal adhesions found after implantation of a polypropylene mesh in the context of surgical hernia repair; and a collagen foil (CF) has also been used to reduce adhesion formation.

Looking for a cost-effective alternative to reduce adhesion formation during laparoscopic ventral hernia repair to the mesh placed intra-abdominally, we have conducted different studies with two substances that can guarantee a good coverage of the complete surface of the mesh, even if we use a large prosthetic material [74, 75]. The two substances used are fibrin glue (Tissucol ®, Baxter Biosurgery, Vienna, Austria) and hyaluronidase cream. Both substances have been able to decrease, in an animal model, the number and the quantity of the adhesions to both polypropylene and ePTFE meshes. The reduction of adhesions with hyaluronidase cream is a consequence of an acceleration in the normal process of healing needed to create adhesions. This factor may also influence in the reduction of adhesion with fibrin glue, but may also be related to other facts: the mechanical barrier that the fibrin glue produces 3–5 min after its application, and the capsule of new tissue created by the fibrin glue with a different process of healing compared to the inflammatory process necessary to create an adhesion.

Early Diagnosed Adhesions

Laparoscopic ventral incisional hernia repair involves intra-abdominal placement of a synthetic mesh, and the possibility of formation of severe visceral adhesions to the prosthesis is a principal concern. Adhesions cause increased morbidity and mortality, with subsequent socioeconomic consequences. Zinther et al. [76] have recently published a structured literature search of medical databases based on English literature published until September 2009 in order to assess the presence of adhesions to implanted synthetic mesh after laparoscopic ventral hernia repair. The search identified transabdominal ultrasonography (TAU) and cine magnetic resonance imaging (cine MRI) as relevant tools matching the search criteria. In all, 12 publications concerning TAU and four publications concerning cine MRI were identified. Both TAU and cine MRI seem able to identify intra-abdominal adhesions using visceral slide with accuracy of 76–92 %. Unfortunately, the studies are biased by being nonblinded, which influenced the final sensitivity, specificity, and accuracy. Accordingly, a need exists for a systematic well-conducted double-blinded comparative study to validate these radiologic techniques.

Treat Postoperative Adhesions

Adhesions do not need to be treated unless complications, such as chronic pain, bowel occlusion, or fistulas, appear.

References

1. Ahrendt GM, Tantry US, Barbul A. Intra-abdominal sepsis impairs colonic reparative collagen synthesis. Am J Surg. 1996;171:102–7.
2. Longo WE, Virgo KS, Johnson FE, et al. Risk factors for morbidity and mortality after colectomy for colon cancer. Dis Colon Rectum. 2000;43:83–91.
3. Niinikoski J. Tissue oxygenation in hypovolaemic shock. Ann Clin Res. 1977;9:151–6.
4. Keill RH, Keitzer WF, Nichols WK, et al. Abdominal wound dehiscence. Arch Surg. 1973;106:573–7.
5. Burger JW, van't Riet M, Jeekel J. Abdominal incisions: techniques and postoperative complications. Scand J Surg. 2002;91:315–21.
6. Riou JP, Cohen JR, Johnson Jr H. Factors influencing wound dehiscence. Am J Surg. 1992;163:324–30.
7. Dunne JR, Malone DL, Tracy JK, et al. Abdominal wall hernias: risk factors for infection and resource utilization. J Surg Res. 2003;111:78–84.
8. Myles PS, Iacono GA, Hunt JO, et al. Risk of respiratory complications and wound infection in patients undergoing ambulatory surgery: smokers versus nonsmokers. Anesthesiology. 2002;97:842–7.
9. Hopf HW, Hunt TK, West JM, et al. Wound tissue oxygen tension predicts the risk of wound infection in surgical patients. Arch Surg. 1997;132:997–1004.
10. Sorgensen LN, Kallehave F, Christensen E, et al. Less collagen production in smokers. Surgery. 1998;123:450–5.
11. Black E, Vibe-Petersen J, Jorgensen LN, Madsen SM, Agren MS, Holstein PE, Perrild H, Gottrup F. Decrease of collagen deposition in wound repair in type 1 diabetes independent of glycemic control. Arch Surg. 2003;138:34–40.
12. Sørensen LT, Nielsen HB, Kharazmi A, Gottrup F. Effect of smoking and abstention on oxidative burst and reactivity of neutrophils and monocytes. Surgery. 2004;136:1047–53.
13. Yasuda K, Shiraishi N, Adachi Y, Inomata M, Sato K, Kitano S. Risk factors for complications following resection of large gastric cancer. Br J Surg. 2001;88:873–7.
14. Hartmann M, Jonsson K, Zederfeldt B. Effect of tissue perfusion and oxygenation on accumulation of collagen in healing wounds: randomized study in patients after major abdominal operations. Eur J Surg. 1992;158:521–6.
15. Esrig BC, Frazee L, Stephenson SF, Polk Jr HC, Fulton RL, Jones CE. The predisposition to infection following hemorrhagic shock. Surg Gynecol Obstet. 1977;144:915–7.
16. Makela JT, Kiviniemi H, Juvonen T, Laitinen S. Factors influencing wound dehiscence after midline laparotomy. Am J Surg. 1995;170:387–90.
17. Alves A, Panis Y, Trancart D, Regimbeau JM, Pocard M, Valleur P. Factors associated with clinically significant anastomotic leakage after large bowel resection: multivariate analysis of 707 patients. World J Surg. 2002;26:499–502.
18. Schmit PJ, Hiyama DT, Swisher SG, Bennion RS, Thompson Jr JE. Analysis of risk factors of postappendectomy intra-abdominal abscess. J Am Coll Surg. 1994;179:721–6.
19. Stechmiller JK. Understanding the role of nutrition and wound healing. Nutr Clin Pract. 2010;25:61–8.
20. Kurz A, Sessler DI, Lenhardt R. Perioperative normothermia to reduce the incidence of surgical-wound infection and shorten hospitalization. N Engl J Med. 1996;334:1209–15.

21. Holte K, Sharrock NE, Kehlet H. Pathophysiology and clinical implications of perioperative fluid excess. Br J Anaesth. 2002;89:622–32.
22. Schein M, Wittmann DH, Aprahamian C, Condon RE. The abdominal compartment syndrome. The physiological and clinical consequences of elevated intra-abdominal pressure. J Am Coll Surg. 1995;180:745–53.
23. Schachtrupp A, Fackeldey V, Klinge U, Hoer J, Tittel A, Toens C, Schumpelick V. Temporary closure of the abdominal wall (laparostomy). Hernia. 2002;6(4):155–62.
24. Miller PR, Meredith JW, Johnson JC, Chang MC. Prospective evaluation of vacuum-assisted fascial closure after open abdomen. Planned ventral hernia rate is substantially reduced. Ann Surg. 2004;239(5):608–14.
25. Carlson MA, Ludwig KA, Condon RE. Ventral hernia and other complications of 1,000 midline incisions. South Med J. 1995;88:450–3.
26. Yahchouchy-Chouillard E, Aura T, Picone O, Etienne JC, Fingerhut A. Incisional hernias, I: related risk factors. Dig Surg. 2003;20:3–9.
27. Hodgson NC, Malthaner RA, Ostbye T. The search for an ideal method of abdominal fascial closure: a meta-analysis. Ann Surg. 2000;2(31):436–42.
28. Klinge U, Si ZY, Zheng H, Schumpelick V, Bhardwaj RS, Klosterhalfen B. Abnormal collagen I to III distribution in the skin of patients with incisional hernia. Eur Surg Res. 2000;32:43–8.
29. Israelsson LA, Jonsson T. Overweight and healing of midline incisions: the importance of suture technique. Eur J Surg. 1997;163:175–80.
30. Sugerman HJ, Kellum Jr JM, Reines HD, DeMaria EJ, Newsome HH, Lowry JW. Greater risk of incisional hernia with morbidly obese than steroid-dependent patients and low recurrence with prefascial polypropylene mesh. Am J Surg. 1996;171:80–4.
31. Adye B, Luna G. Incidence of abdominal wall hernia in aortic surgery. Am J Surg. 1998;175(5):400–2.
32. Israelsson LA, Jonsson T. Incisional hernia after midline laparotomy: a prospective study. Eur J Surg. 1996;162(2):125–9.
33. Israelsson LA, Jonsson T. Suture length to wound length ratio and healing of midline laparotomy incisions. Br J Surg. 1993;80(10):1284–6.
34. Hodgson NC, Malthaner RA, Ostbye T. The search for an ideal method of abdominal fascial closure: a meta-analysis. Ann Surg. 2000;231(3):436–42.
35. Van't Riet M, Steyerberg EW, Nellensteyn J, et al. Meta-analysis of techniques for closure of midline abdominal incisions. Br J Surg. 2002;89(11):1350–6.
36. Burger JW, Lange JF, Halm JA, Kleinrensink GJ, Jeekel H. Incisional hernia: early complication of abdominal surgery. World J Surg. 2005;29(12):1608–13.
37. Falagas ME, Kasiakou SK. Mesh-related infections after hernia surgery. Clin Microbiol Infect. 2005;1:3–8.
38. Bliziotis IA, Kasiakou SK, Kapaskelis AM, Falagas ME. Mesh-related infection after hernia surgery: case report of an emerging type of foreign-body related infection. Infection. 2006;1:46–8.
39. Sanabria A, Domínguez LC, Valdivieso E, Gómez G. Prophylactic antibiotics for mesh inguinal hernioplasty: a meta-analysis. Ann Surg. 2007;3:392–6.
40. Delikoukos S, Tzovaras G, Liakou P, Mantzos F, Hatzitheofilou C. Late-onset deep mesh infection after inguinal hernia repair. Hernia. 2007;1:15–7.
41. Edwards C, Angstadt J, Whipple O, Grau R. Laparoscopic ventral hernia repair: postoperative antibiotics decrease incidence of seroma related cellulitis. Am Surg. 2005;71(11):931–5.
42. Orenstein SB, Dumeer JL, Monteagudo J, Poi MJ, Novitsky YW. Outcomes of laparoscopic ventral hernia repair with routine defect closure using "shoelacing" technique. Surg Endosc. 2011;25(5):1452–7.
43. Palanivelu C, Jani KV, Senthilnathan P, Parthasarathi R, Madhankumar MV, Malladi VK. Laparoscopic sutured closure with mesh reinforcement of incisional hernias. Hernia. 2007;11(3):223–8.
44. Tsimoyiannis EC, Siakas P, Glantzounis G, Koulas S, Mavridou P, Gossios KI. Seroma in laparoscopic ventral hernioplasty. Surg Laparosc Endosc Percutan Tech. 2001;11(5):317–21.

45. Fernández Lobato R, García Septiem J, Ortega Deballon P, Martín Lucas FJ, Ruíz de Adana JC, Limones Esteban M. Tissucol application in dermolipectomy and incisional hernia repair. Int Surg. 2001;86(4):240–5.
46. Birch DW. Characterizing laparoscopic incisional hernia repair. Can J Surg. 2007; 50(3):195–201.
47. Bedi AP, Bhatti T, Amin A, Zuberi J. Laparoscopic incisional and ventral hernia repair. J Minim Access Surg. 2007;3(3):83–90.
48. Morales-Conde S. Laparoscopic ventral hernia repair: advances and limitations. Semin Laparosc Surg. 2004;11(3):191–200.
49. Susmallian S, Gewurtz G, Ezri T, Charuzi I. Seroma after laparoscopic repair of hernia with PTFE patch: is it really a complication? Hernia. 2001;5(3):139–41.
50. Perrone JM, Soper NJ, Eagon JC, Klingensmith ME, Aft RL, Frisella MM, Brunt LM. Perioperative outcomes and complications of laparoscopic ventral hernia repair. Surgery. 2005;138(4):708–15.
51. Sharma A, Mehrotra M, Khullar R, Soni V, Baijal M, Chowbey PK. Laparoscopic ventral/ incisional hernia repair: a single centre experience of 1,242 patients over a period of 13 years. Hernia. 2011;15(2):131–9.
52. Barbaros U, Asoglu O, Seven R, Erbil Y, Dinccag A, Deveci U, Ozarmagan S, Mercan S. The comparison of laparoscopic and open ventral hernia repairs: a prospective randomized study. Hernia. 2007;11(1):51–6.
53. Rosenberg J, Burcharth J. Feasibility and outcome after laparoscopic ventral hernia repair using proceed mesh. Hernia. 2008;12(5):453–6.
54. Morales-Conde S, Cadet H, Cano A, Bustos M, Martin J, Morales-Mendez S. Laparoscopic ventral hernia repair without sutures–double crown technique: our experience after 140 cases with a mean follow-up of 40 months. Int Surg. 2005;90(3 Suppl):S56–62.
55. Heniford BT, Park A, Ramshaw BJ, Voeller G. Laparoscopic repair of ventral hernias: nine years'experience with 850 consecutive hernias. Ann Surg. 2003;238(3):391–9.
56. Tessier DJ, Swain JM, Harold KL. Safety of laparoscopic ventral hernia repair in older adults. Hernia. 2006;10(1):53–7.
57. Kaafarani HM, Hur K, Hirter A, Kim LT, Thomas A, Berger DH, Reda D, Itani KM. Seroma in ventral incisional herniorrhaphy: incidence, predictors and outcome. Am J Surg. 2009; 198(5):639–44.
58. Varnell B, Bachman S, Quick J, Vitamvas M, Ramshaw B, Oleynikov D. Morbidity associated with laparoscopic repair of suprapubic hernias. Am J Surg. 2008;196(6):983–7. discussion 987-8.
59. Schoenmaeckers EJ, Raymakers JF, Rakic S. Complications of laparoscopic correction of abdominal wall and incisional hernias. Ned Tijdschr Geneeskd. 2010;154(45):A2390.
60. Morales-Conde S, Cadet I, Tutosaus JD, Carrasco P, Palma F, Morales-Méndez S. Macroscopic evaluation of mesh incorporation placed intraperitoneally for laparoscopic ventral hernia repair. Experimental model. Proceedings of the 7th World Congress of Endoscopic Surgery (Singapore June 1-4, 2000). Monduzzi Editore. Bologna, Italy. 2000:455–460.
61. Bellón JM, Rodríguez M, García-Honduvilla N, Pascual G, Gómez Gil V, Buján J. Peritoneal effects of prosthetic meshes used to repair abdominal wall defects: monitoring adhesions by sequential laparoscopy. J Laparoendosc Adv Surg Tech A. 2007;17(2):160–6.
62. Bellón JM, Contreras LA, Buján J, Carrera-San Martín A, Gimeno MJ, Jurado F. Influence of the porosity of prosthetic biomaterials implanted in the abdominal wall on the healing process. Cir Esp. 1996;57:296–302.
63. Matthews BD, Pratt BL, Pollinger HS, Backus CL, Kercher KW, Sing RF, Heniford BT. Assessment of adhesion formation to intra-abdominal polypropylene mesh and polytetrafluoroethylene mesh. J Surg Res. 2003;114(2):126–32.
64. Schug-Pass C, Tamme C, Tannapfel A, Köckerling F. A lightweight polypropylene mesh (TiMesh) for laparoscopic intraperitoneal repair of abdominal wall hernias: comparison of biocompatibility with the DualMesh in an experimental study using the porcine model. Surg Endosc. 2006;20(3):402–9.

65. Conze J, Rosch R, Klinge U, Weiss C, Anurov M, Titkowa S, Oettinger A, Schumpelick V. Polypropylene in the intra-abdominal position: influence of pore size and surface area. Hernia. 2004;8(4):365–72.
66. Conze J, Junge K, Weiss C, Anurov M, Oettinger A, Klinge U, Schumpelick V. New polymer for intra-abdominal meshes-PVDF copolymer. J Biomed Mater Res B Appl Biomater. 2008;87(2):321–8.
67. Novitsky YW, Harrell AG, Cristiano JA, Paton BL, Norton HJ, Peindl RD, Kercher KW, Heniford BT. Comparative evaluation of adhesion formation, strength of ingrowth, and textile properties of prosthetic meshes after long-term intra-abdominal implantation in a rabbit. J Surg Res. 2007;140(1):6–11.
68. Voskerician G, Rodriguez A, Gingras PH. Macroporous condensed poly(tetra fluoro-ethylene). II. In vivo effect on adhesion formation and tissue integration. J Biomed Mater Res A. 2007;82(2):426–35.
69. Peach G, Tan LC. Small bowel obstruction and perforation due to a displaced spiral tacker: a rare complication of laparoscopic inguinal hernia repair. Hernia. 2008;12(3):303–5.
70. Ladurner R, Mussack T. Small bowel perforation due to protruding spiral tackers: a rare complication in laparoscopic incisional hernia repair. Surg Endosc. 2004;18(6):1001.
71. Holmdahl L, Risberg B, Beck DE, Burns JW, Chegini N, diZerega GS, Ellis H. Adhesions: pathogenesis and prevention-panel discussion and summary. Eur J Surg Suppl. 1997;577:56–62.
72. Dinsmore RC, Calton Jr WC, Harvey SB, Blaney MW. Prevention of adhesions to polypropylene mesh in a traumatized bowel model. J Am Coll Surg. 2000;191(2):131–6.
73. Koehler RH, Begos D, Berger D, Carey S, LeBlanc K, Park A, Ramshaw B, Smoot R, Voeller G. Minimal adhesions to ePTFE mesh after laparoscopic ventral incisional hernia repair: reoperative findings in 65 cases. JSLS. 2003;7(4):335–40.
74. Martín-Cartes J, Morales-Conde S, Suárez-Grau J, López-Bernal F, Bustos-Jiménez M, Cadet-Dussort H, Socas-Macías M, Alamo-Martínez J, Tutosaus-Gómez JD, Morales-Mendez S. Use of hyaluronidase cream to prevent peritoneal adhesions in laparoscopic ventral hernia repair by means of intraperitoneal mesh fixation using spiral tacks. Surg Endosc. 2008;22(3):631–4.
75. Martín-Cartes JA, Morales-Conde S, Suárez-Grau JM, Bustos-Jiménez M, Cadet-Dussort JM, López-Bernal F, Morcillo-Azcárate J, Tutosaus-Gómez JD, Morales-Méndez S. Role of fibrin glue in the prevention of peritoneal adhesions in ventral hernia repair. Surg Today. 2008; 38(2):135–40.
76. Zinther NB, Zeuten A, Marinovskij E, Haislund M, Friis-Andersen H. Functional cine MRI and transabdominal ultrasonography for the assessment of adhesions to implanted synthetic mesh 5–7 years after laparoscopic ventral hernia repair. Hernia. 2010;14(5):499–504.
77. Parker III HH, Nottingham JM, Bynoe RP, Yost MJ. Laparoscopic repair of large incisional hernias. Am Surg. 2002;68:530–3.
78. Morales-Conde S. A new classification for seroma after laparoscopic ventral hernia repair. Hernia 2012;16:261–7.
79. Ferrari GC, Miranda A, Sansonna F, et al. Laparoscopic repair of incisional hernias located on the abdominal borders: a retrospective critical review. Surg Laparosc Endosc Percutan Tech. 2009;19:348–52.
80. Carbonell AM, Kercher KW, Matthews BD et al. The laparoscopic repair of suprapubic ventral hernias. Surg Endosc. 2005;19:174–7.
81. Uranues S, Salehi B, Bergamaschi R. Adverse events, quality of life, and recurrence rates after laparoscopic adhesyiolisis and recurrent incisional hernia mesh repair in patients with previous failed repair. J Am Coll Surg. 2008;207:663–9.
82. Farrakha M. Laparoscopic ventral hernia repair using expanded polytetrafluorethylene-polyester mesh compound. Surg Endosc. 2006;20:820–3.
83. Sodergren MH, Swift I. Seroma formation and method of mesh fixation in laparoscopic ventral hernia-repair-highlights of a case series. Scand J Surg. 2010;99:24–7.
84. Chowbey PK, Sharma A, Khullar R, et al. Laparoscopic ventral hernia repair. J laparoendosc Adv Surg Tech A. 2000;10:79–84.
85. Birch DW. Characterizing laparoscopic incisional hernia repair. Can J Surg. 2007;50:195–201.

Chapter 24
Treatment of Open Abdomen Approach

Miguel A. Cuesta and Jurriaan B. Tuynman

Keywords MOF • Sepsis • Fistulas • Stomas • Abdominal wall • Open abdomen

The treatment by open abdomen approach is very difficult to prevent. Performing surgery with a good indication and applying good surgical judgment and skills can in most cases prevent this problem. But given severe complications—mostly leakages of anastomosis or repeated surgical reoperations in the abdomen—surgeons may encounter the double problem of the sepsis of the abdominal cavity not being solved and also the closure of the abdominal wall not being possible. The best attitude in this sick patient, mostly cared in the intensive care unit, is to leave the abdomen open for adequate drainage of fistulas, care of stomas maintaining the possibility to inspect, and treat new problems. Practical problems are:

1. Respiratory insufficiency and insufficiency of other organs (MOF). This is a very important part of the treatment of these patients on the ICU. In general, MOF of more than double organ insufficiency is related to a progressive mortality rate.
2. General treatment of ongoing sepsis. Treatment with antibiotics will be selective and based on cultures. Long treatment with antibiotics will include antifungal therapy.
3. Feeding the patient. This is a very important part of the treatment. A feeding team will decide together with the surgeon what the best strategy for the patient can be. The best is the enteral feeding option, but sometimes in the case of fistulas, this is very difficult or even impossible. Alternative option will be the TPN and, if possible, the collection of the leaked fluids being returned through a more distal fistula with good passage to the stomas or the rectum. Whatever the course

M.A. Cuesta, MD (✉) • J.B. Tuynman
Department of Surgery, VU University Medical Center,
Amsterdam, The Netherlands
e-mail: ma.cuesta@vumc.nl

M.A. Cuesta, H.J. Bonjer (eds.), *Treatment of Postoperative Complications after Digestive Surgery*, DOI 10.1007/978-1-4471-4354-3_24,

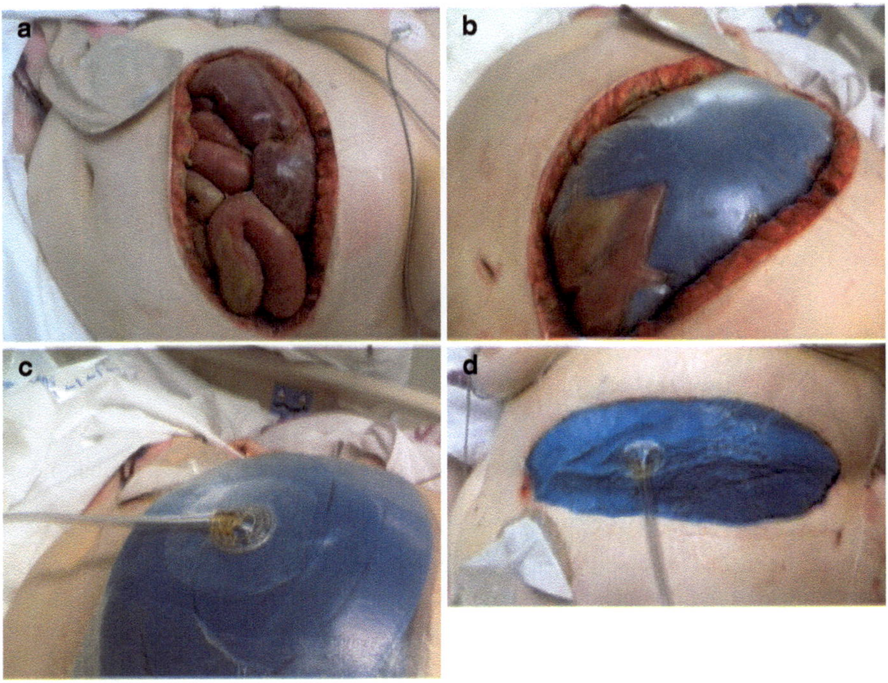

Fig. 24.1 (a–d) Vacuum-assisted closure device (VAC)® (KCI Medical, San Antonio, TX)

chosen, the total amount of calories and nutrients will have to be determined and administered well in order to get the patient in an optimal anabolic situation.

4. Care of the wound. It is essential to obtain an adequate drainage of all leakages coming out of the abdomen. If possible, a vacuum system or a most simple wound manager with suction drains will keep the abdomen constantly well drained and keep at the same time the wound clean. The vacuum system will provide a stimulus of the granulating tissue and closure of the wound (Fig. 24.1a–d). Care of the stomas is important too, avoiding leakages and permitting adequate care of the skin. In the end an adequate drainage along with the abovementioned measures will best contribute to the recovery of the patient. The treatment involved is clearly multidisciplinary.

How to close the wound, fistulas (and stomas) after an open abdomen treatment? There are two possibilities:

1. If the wound is granulating and patient is recovering and no intestinal fistulas are present, definitive closure of the wound may be postponed until a better recovery of the patient, e.g., 6 months later, may have occurred. In the latter case, a temporary closure can permit an easier care of the wound. Temporary closure of it can be achieved by means of a splits skin graft.
2. In the presence of intestinal fistulas (and stoma's) and if the patient is recovering, closure can be attempted 6 weeks later. This is the minimum period of time needed to permit the loosening of the adhesions between intestinal

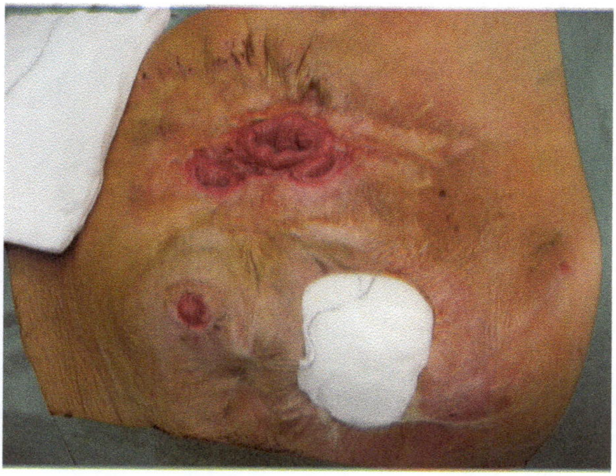

Fig. 24.2 Scar and intestinal fistulas

loops so that the operation becomes possible. There are different possibilities involved:

(a) Complete closure of everything, being fistulas, stomas, and definitive abdominal wall closure.
(b) Closure of intestinal fistulas and temporary closure of abdominal wall, e.g., Vicryl mesh® in order to facilitate an optimal oral feeding and a good intestinal transit, thereby avoiding the risks of taking down stomas.

Whatever the course taken, it will depend on the condition of the patient and the experience of the surgeon on what to do.

Steps to do are:

1. Resect the whole scar of the open abdomen; with this approach the skin will be never the problem. A tangential excision of the granulating surface will be done with the knife without damage to the underlying intestinal loops. In this way and by maintaining as much as possible fascia, we enter the abdomen (Figs. 24.2, 24.3 and, 24.4).
2. In the abdomen, complete inspection of the loops has to be carried out. This work can be done by digital dissection and with scissors. One must take care to minimize the serosa and intestinal loop perforations. Most of the time this is impossible to avoid.
3. Dissect adequately the intestinal fistulas and stomas and make a plan. Do not perform sequential anastomosis in the small bowel within a short distance; the principle is to conserve the maximum of bowel with a minimum of anastomosis. Anastomosis will have a good perfusion, no tension, and an adequate patency. Close all the serosa defects and bowel perforation in horizontal direction thereby not compromising the patency of the bowel.
4. Inspect the bowels again, now controlling the closure of the stomas, if distal in the left colon by using methylene blue.

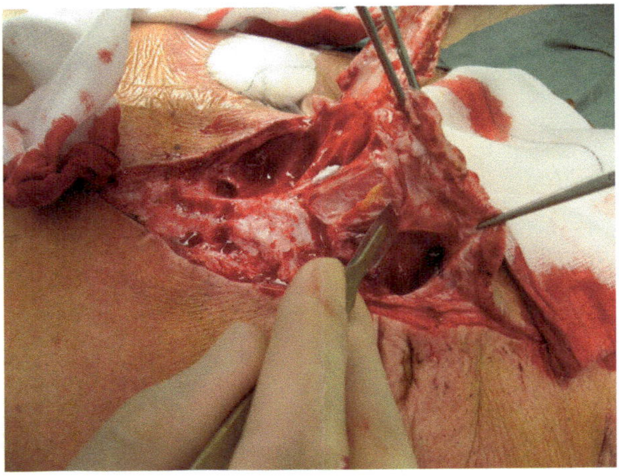

Fig. 24.3 Tangential excision of the scar

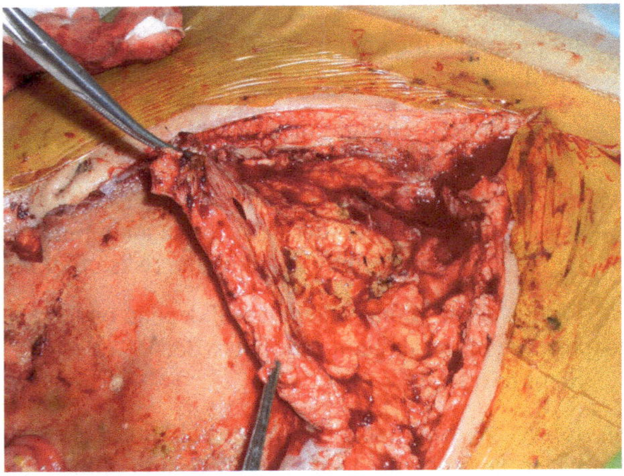

Fig. 24.4 Abdomen after excision of the scar

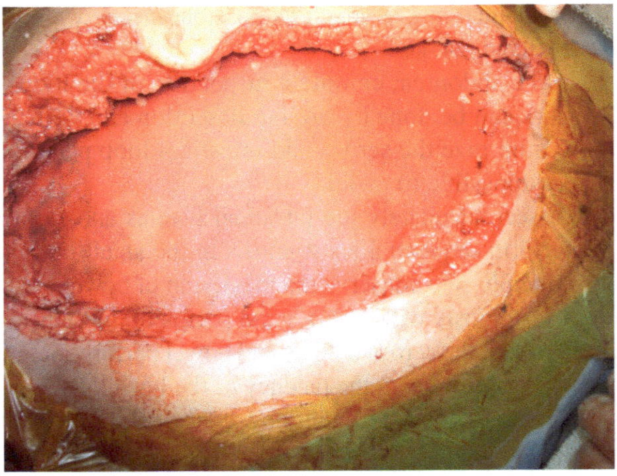

Fig. 24.5 Mesh fixed to fascia in order to close the abdomen

5. Close all the defects (fistulas and stomas) in the abdominal wall. Do this from the inside using a thick thread.
6. Finally, after leaving some drainage intra-abdominally, now follow the procedure of closure of abdominal wound (Fig. 24.5). The most perfect way is using some combination of muscular plasty, e.g., component separation technique (Ramirez plasty) with a mesh. This would be an ideal situation but impossible at this stage. We prefer to cover the bowels with omentum and over this to put a mesh, mostly double, e.g., Parietex® or in the case of present residual sepsis, a double Vicryl mesh® attached to the fascia with a continuous reabsorbable running suture. Between the fascia mesh and the subcutaneous tissues, two drains are left to keep this space clean and dry.
7. After drainage, subcutaneous tissues and skin have to be closed

Discussion

Bjorck et al. and De Waele et al. stressed the indications, causes, risks, and management of the open abdomen, describing different treatment strategies [1, 2]. Interesting is the use of the topical negative pressure by means of the vacuum-assisted closure to the management of open abdomen with and without enteric fistulae. D'Hondt et al. reported the experience with topical negative-pressure (TNP) therapy in the management of enteric fistulae using the vacuum-assisted closure (VAC) device (KCI Medical, San Antonio, TX). They described that nine patients with 17 enteric fistulae in an open abdomen were treated with topical TNP therapy [3]. Surgery with take down of the fistulae and abdominal closure was planned 6–10 weeks later. Three fistulae closed spontaneously. The median time from the onset of fistulization to elective surgical management was 51 days. No additional fistulae occurred during VAC therapy. They concluded that although previously considered a contraindication to TNP therapy, enteric fistulae can be managed successfully with TNP therapy. Surgical closure of fistulae is possible after several weeks

References

1. Bjorck M, D'Amours SK, Hamilton AE. Closure of the open abdomen. Am Surg. 2011;77 Suppl 1:S58–61.
2. De Waele JJ, Leppaniemi AK. Temporary abdominal closure techniques. Am Surg. 2011;77 Suppl 1:S46–50.
3. D'Hondt M, Devriendt D, Van Rooy F, et al. Treatment of small-bowel fistulae in the open abdomen with topical negative-pressure therapy. Am J Surg. 2011;202:20–4.

Chapter 25
Establishing the Pneumoperitoneum and Closing the Trocar Sites During Laparoscopic Surgery

Miguel A. Cuesta and H. Jaap Bonjer

Keywords Pneumoperitoneum • Trocar sites • Laparoscopic surgery • Veress needle • Closed entry • Open entry • Hernia

The way to establish the pneumoperitoneum forms the initial part of any laparoscopic intervention. There are two ascertained ways for undertaking this important part of the operation, the first by means of the Veress needle and the second by the open method. Taking into account all variations introduced, four ways can be delineated: (a) Veress needle, (b) the open Hasson technique, (c) direct trocar placement without prior pneumoperitoneum, and (d) the optical view technique. A review of each method is now provided.

Regarding the Veress needle, the potential danger of using it is the occurrence of visceral or vascular injury. We note that Bonjer et al. have performed a retrospective study of the literature to compare the closed laparoscopy and open laparoscopy in terms of safety [1]. Data on closed laparoscopy in 489,335 patients and in open laparoscopy in 12,444 patients were culled. The rates of visceral and vascular injury were respectively 0.083 and 0.070 after closed laparoscopy and 0.048 and zero after open laparoscopy. Mortality rates after closed and open laparoscopy were respectively 0.003 and zero. In this study, Pearson Chi^2 analysis demonstrated a statistically significant difference in terms of visceral and vascular injury between closed and open laparoscopy, there was no such difference for mortality rates. The conclusion by Bonjer et al. was that in laparoscopic surgery the open establishment of pneumoperitoneum is advocated because it is safer than the closed method.

In 2003, Merlin et al. did a systematic review of the safety and effectiveness of methods used to establish pneumoperitoneum in laparoscopic surgery [2]. Their meta-analysis was carried out on prospective, nonrandomized studies of open

M.A. Cuesta, MD (✉) • H.J. Bonjer PhD, FRCSC
Department of Surgery, VU University Medical Center, Amsterdam, The Netherlands
e-mail: ma.cuesta@vumc.nl; j.bonjer@vumc.nl

M.A. Cuesta, H.J. Bonjer (eds.), *Treatment of Postoperative Complications after Digestive Surgery*, DOI 10.1007/978-1-4471-4354-3_25,

versus closed access. Their findings regarding open access indicated a trend towards a reduced risk of major complications, with a 95 % confidence interval (ci) of 0.09–1.03. Open access was also associated with a trend towards a reduced risk of access site herniation, ci 0.04–1.03, and concerning nonobese patients, a 57 % reduced risk of having minor complications. Additionally, they located a trend of fewer conversions to laparotomy. Data on major complications gained from studies of direct trocar versus needle/trocar access were inconclusive. Yet, minor complications were fewer when engaging direct trocar access, a phenomenon predominantly owing to a reduction in extraperitoneal insufflation.

In 2004, Jansen et al. did an extensive inquiry regarding closed versus open-entry technique [3]. A questionnaire was submitted to the members of the Dutch Society of Gynaecological Endoscopy and Minimal Invasive Surgery, and the results were combined with a Medline literature search. They recorded complications from January 1997 to December 2001 and divided the data on methods in two groups: group 1 cases of Veress needle or first trocar and group 2 cases of open-entry technique. Procedures were performed by 187 gynecologists in 74 hospitals. The majority of the specialists (57 %) performed the closed-entry laparoscopy and had recorded 31 complications (0.1 %) of the 31.532 interventions. In cases of previous laparotomy or obesity, most of the gynecologists used an alternative insufflation, namely, the Palmer's point. The rest of the specialists used both entry techniques.

In those cases of expected adhesions, or of previous laparotomy, or of obese or else very thin patients, an open entry was used. The specialists reported 20.027 closed procedures and 579 open procedures, having complication rates of 0.12 and 1.38 %, respectively. Significantly, more visceral lesions were found at open entry in group 2. Moreover, their literature search showed a calculated average of the entry complication rates holding for the closed-entry technique regarding visceral and vascular lesions of 0.44 per 1,000 procedures and 0.31 per 1,000 procedures, respectively. They found no evidence of abandoning the closed-entry technique in laparoscopy. However, selection of patients for open or alternative entry procedures is still recommended in this study.

Varma and Gupta published in 2008 a national survey in the United Kingdom by questionnaire and a systematic literature search. They described the national guidelines and survey as well as the medicolegal ramifications concerning the different entry techniques [4]. Their conclusions were "despite widespread awareness of laparoscopic entry guidelines, there remains considerable variation in the techniques adopted in clinical practice. Unless practice concurs with recommendation guidance, women undergoing laparoscopy will be exposed to increased and unnecessary operative risks. Laparoscopic entry-related injury in an uncomplicated woman is according to UK legal case law considered to be a negligent practice."

In 2012, Ahmad et al. reviewed the laparoscopic entry techniques using the Cochrane's search strategies [5]. They reviewed 28 randomized controlled trials with 4,860 individuals undergoing laparoscopy and evaluated 14 comparisons.

They concluded that an open-entry technique is associated with a significant reduction in failed entry when compared to a closed-entry technique, with no difference in the incidence of visceral or vascular injury. Significant benefits were noted with the use of a direct-entry technique when compared to the Veress needle.

The use of the Veress needle was associated with an increased incidence of failed entry, extraperitoneal insufflation, and omental injury; direct trocar entry is therefore a safer closed-entry technique.

Moreover, the SAGES guidelines [6] concluded that "there are no demonstrable differences in the safety of open versus closed techniques for establishing access; decisions regarding choice of technique are left to the surgeon and should be based on individual training, skills, and case assessment" (Level I, grade A).

Closure of the Trocar Sites

Trocar sites of 10 mm and gigger should be closed. There are available different closure techniques [7].

The incidence of port-site hernia is between 1 and 2 % for the sites >10 mm.

In order to prevent this complication, consensus has been established to close the ports that are 10 mm or larger. In a review of 647 patients who underwent a laparoscopic operation during a period of 3 years, Moran et al. found a port-site hernia incidence of 1.23 %, all being symptomatic and all requiring surgical correction [8]. The moment when herniation occurs is interesting; an early postoperative herniation is associated with significant morbidity. This complication should be considered in those patients presenting with postoperative bowel obstruction. Engaging in a meticulous closure of port sites of 10 mm and wider could reduce the incidence of hernia. It is obvious that at the moment of diagnosis, the fascia defect is larger than the original 10 mm that then the best way to repair it will be by means of a laparoscopic correction with a mesh, thereby also paying attention to have closed all the new trocar sites.

References

1. Bonjer HJ, Hazebroek EJ, Kazemier G, et al. Open versus closed establishment of pneumoperitoneum in laparoscopic surgery. Br J Surg. 1997;84:599–602.
2. Merlin TL, Hiller JE, Maddern GJ, et al. Systematic review of the safety and effectiveness of methods used to establish pneumoperitoneum in laparoscopic surgery. Br J Surg. 2003;90:668–79.
3. Jansen FW, Kolkman W, Bakkum EA, et al. Complications of laparoscopy: an inquiry about closed- versus open-entry technique. Am J Obstet Gynecol. 2004;190:634–8.
4. Varma R, Gupta JK. Laparoscopic entry techniques: clinical guideline, national survey, and medicolegal ramifications. Surg Endosc. 2008;12:2686–97.
5. Ahmad G, O'Flynn H, Duffy JM, et al. Laparoscopic entry techniques. Cochrane Database Syst Rev. 2012;2, CD006583.
6. Closure of trocar sites guidelines for the clinical application of laparoscopic biliary tract surgery. Practice/clinical guidelines published on: 01/2010 by the Society of American Gastrointestinal and Endoscopic Surgeons (SAGES).
7. Shaler Z. Port closure techniques. Surg Endosc. 2007;21:1264–74.
8. Moran DC, Kavanagh DO, Sahebally S, Neary PC. Incidence of early symptomatic port-site hernia: a case series from a department where laparoscopy is the preferred surgical approach. Ir J Med Sci. 2012;181:463–6.

Chapter 26
Final Considerations

Miguel A. Cuesta and H. Jaap Bonjer

Keywords Prevention of complications • Evidence base medicine • Postoperative complications • Operative technique • Training • Developments • Surgery

The objective of this book has been to stress how important it is to prevent postoperative complications by a proper indication for engaging surgery and having a good operative technique. Especially the indication for surgery must be discussed multidisciplinary; it is no longer acceptable that such a determination would only be the work of a solitary surgeon. Having a good surgical technique may imply a lot of things, such as proper standard training based on evidence-based surgery; using techniques demonstratively better than others; and having knowledge of the type of anastomosis and dissection as, for instance, when to mobilize or not the splenic flexure in rectum cancer surgery.

More evidence on preventing postoperative complications will be required to accomplish these objectives, thereby stimulating an optimal training and continuous and permanent learning to adopt new developments. We note that the introduction of laparoscopic surgery and currently the fast track have changed many aspects of daily practice, reducing hospital stay and complication rates. And thereby not forgetting that surgical times are becoming more complicated with the introduction of neoadjuvant protocols, for each patient is unique, and individualization of surgery has become a reality.

All authors and contributors to this book have succeeded to address these points, thereby stimulating us to go further. It also prompts some considerations I would like to share.

M.A. Cuesta, MD (✉) • H.J. Bonjer, PhD, FRCSC
Department of Surgery, VU University Medical Center, Amsterdam, The Netherlands
e-mail: ma.cuesta@vumc.nl; j.bonjer@vumc.nl

M.A. Cuesta, H.J. Bonjer (eds.), *Treatment of Postoperative Complications after Digestive Surgery*, DOI 10.1007/978-1-4471-4354-3_26,

Complications are inherent in surgical work! We have the audacity to treat a surgical disease by means of the knife! Surgical treatment as such means trauma, as it will create an inflammatory response—local as well as general—and an immune response. Patients undergo in surgery profound physiological alterations. The issue now becomes: How to define surgical complications in this context? We can define a complication as an alteration of a smooth and prompt recovery of the patient after an operation. Examples are a wound infection or venous thrombosis but also a urinary infection. Observing and documenting carefully, we realize that almost all patients will have some sort of complication, mostly minor, but also major. Dr. Dindo has defined the principles of an optimal classification for gastrointestinal complications. For young surgeons and residents, it is very important not only to learn about proper indications for surgery and corresponding operative techniques but certainly also to detect postoperative complications early and to treat these adequately. An essential learning point I want to stress is that detection and treatment of complications are very much multidisciplinary practices, as the different authors appointed out so well in their respective chapters about complications. In modern surgery, the internist, gastroenterologists, and radiologist need to work together to accomplish the objective to detect early and to treat adequately the postoperative complications occurring. Early detection means proper and careful clinical observation. If the patient is doing well and recovers quickly, then he/she can go home, but when certain factors appear, such as abdominal pain and fever, because a patient does not progress properly or even is getting sick, laboratory studies and eventually CT-scan diagnosis must become a standard performance. Doing this promptly relates positively to better outcomes, less complications, and less mortality. All authors have stressed these important basic points in their respective chapters. Lack of progress in being timely means having complications!

A much more difficult topic and more subjective to value is how to treat major complications. At the same time, we recognize an abundance of evidence in this volume on how to treat major complications and when to do so.

All authors have stressed such points and we can be grateful for their candor. A golden standard implied in each chapter is the maxim that in case of a major complication, the surgeon first must save the life, second must save the organ, and third must save the cosmetics. At the same time, it is unavoidable that adequate treatment of the sepsis will imply radical measures. This affirms again that multidisciplinary cooperation is of paramount importance for gaining excellence.

Remarkably, all authors expressed their willingness to engage in permanent learning regarding surgery. In particular, I laud the work of many residents and young surgeons, who by writing clearly about the complicated cases have been able to portray their own performance of professional practice understandably for a broad audience. Finally, we must recognize with distinction the essential role of the anesthesia and intensive care personnel on whom all of us rely day in and day out for performing the challenges of major surgery.

Index

A

Abdominal wall closure
  early postoperative complications
    degree of contamination, 288
    diagnosis, 290–291
    patient's factors, 288
    prevention, 288–290
    treatment, 291–293
  late postoperative complications
    diagnosis, 295–296
    patient's factors, 293–294
    prevention, 294–295
    treatment, 296
Abdominal wall hernia repair
  adhesions
    diagnosis, 307
    fixation role, 306
    materials, 305
    prevention, 306–307
    surgical technique, 305
    surgical trauma, 306
    treatment, 308
  infection
    diagnosis, 298–299
    prevention, 297–298
    treatment, 299
  "lightweight" prosthetics, 297
  mesh-related infection, 296
  seroma
    clinical classification of seroma, 303
    clinical incidence, 302
    prevention, 300–301
    radiological incidence, 302
    symptomatic seroma, 302–303
    tacker disattachment, 300
    treatment, 303
Achalasia, 38, 68
Acute appendicitis, 211–213
Acute pancreatitis
  complication
    enterocutaneous fistula, 195
    infected necrosis, 195
    intra-abdominal bleeding, 196
    mortality, 196
    new-onset organ failure, 195
    pancreatic fistula, 196
    PANTER trial, 196
    rate of complication, reduce, 197
    treatment strategy, 195–196
  health care utilization and costs, 196–197
  intervention, 194
  liquefaction process, 191–192
  necrotizing acute pancreatitis, 191–192
  obstructive jaundice/mechanical ileus, 193
  organ failure, 191
  perioperative care, 194
  peripancreatic necrosis infection, 193
  postoperative management, 195
  sterile pancreatic necrosis and
      peripancreatic collection, 191
  systemic inflammatory response
      syndrome, 191
Adjustable gastric band (AGB), 102, 104
Adrenal glands
  adrenal incidentalomas, 203
  adrenocortical cancer, 204
  alpha/beta blockers, 203
  anesthesiology, 203
  fine-needle aspiration biopsy, 202–203
  hyperaldosteronism, 203
  hypercortisolism, 203
  MIBG, 203

M.A. Cuesta, H.J. Bonjer (eds.), *Treatment of Postoperative Complications after Digestive Surgery*, DOI 10.1007/978-1-4471-4354-3,

Adrenal glands (*cont.*)
minimally invasive approach, 204
retroperitoneal adrenalectomy, 205
transperitoneal approach, 204–205
AGB. *See* Adjustable gastric band (AGB)
Anal fissure, proctology
advancement flap, 274–275
complications, 275–276
lateral internal sphincterotomy, 274
Anal fistula, proctology
complications, 276–277
fistulotomy, 277
Park's classification, 277
patient assessment
advancement flaps, 282
anesthesia, 279
cryptoglandular treatment, 281
cutting seton, 282
examination, 277
fibrin glue, 283
Goodsall's rule, 277, 279
hydrogen peroxide, 279
initial consultation, 277
internal and external opening, 279–280
intersphincteric and low transsphincteric, 279–280
LIFT procedure, 283
preoperative imaging, 279
removing granulation tissue, 280
Sphincter-preserving techniques, 282–283
wound care, 280
Anastomotic healing, 9, 229
Appendicectomy. *See* Small bowel surgery

B

Bariatric surgery
AGB, 102, 104
bacterial overgrowth, 102
biliopancreatic diversion, 102, 107, 120–121
complications, 121
duodenal switch, 102, 106, 120–121
early postoperative complications, 110–111
LAGB
band erosion, 115–116
band slip and pouch dilatation, 114–115
normal situation, 113
port-site infections, 116
tube breakage, 116–117
LSG, 117–119
mortality risk, 101
operative complications
internal hernia, 108–109
Roux-en-"O," 109
splenic injury, 108
trocar injuries, 107–108
operative times, 101
preoperative considerations
chronic disease and super obesity, 104–105
low-volume surgeons and hospitals, 105
male gender, 104
older age, 103
OS-MRS, 106
risk factors, 103, 107
type of surgery, 105
reeking diarrhea, 102
RYGB bypass, 102, 103, 111–112
sleeve gastrectomy, 102, 105
surgery timing, 121
VBG, 119–120
Bile duct injury (BDI)
cholecystectomy, 147
classification of
type A injury, 149–150
type B injury, 149, 151
type C injury, 149, 152
type D injury, 149, 153
CVS, 145–146
diagnosis, 148–150
fundus-first technique, 147
incidence of, 144
infundibular technique, 147
IOC, 148
litigation claims, 155–156
peroperatively diagnosed injury, 153–154
postoperatively diagnosed injury, 154–155
prevention, 144
psychological factors, 147
quality of life, 155–156
risk factors, 144–145
stopping rule, 147
Terblanche method, 148
treatment, 152
vasculo-biliary injury
accessory duct, 151
cause of, 149
infundibular technique, 149
ischemia, 152
RHA injury isolation, 152
vascular reconstruction/partial hepatectomy, 152
visceral and vascular injury, 143

Biliary anastomosis
diagnosis and grading, 177
incidence and definition, 176–177
management and outcome, 177, 178
prevention and risk factors, 177–178
Biliopancreatic diversion (BPD), 102, 107, 120–121
Bismuth-Corlette classification, 164–165
BPD. *See* Biliopancreatic diversion (BPD)

C
Classical injury. *See* Vasculo-biliary injury (VBI)
Clavien–Dindo classification, 14–16
Cochrane's search strategy, 320
Colorectal surgery, stress response
consort algorithm randomization, 2, 3
C-reactive protein outcome, 1–2, 4
fast-track postoperative care, 2
HLA-DR outcome, 1–3
interleukin-6 outcome, 2, 4
LAFA trial, 2
laparoscopy and fast-track perioperative care, 2
thoracic epidural anesthesia, 2
TME procedure, 2
Conventional hemorrhoidectomy, 268–271
C-reactive protein (CRP), 1–2, 4, 29, 249
Critical view of safety (CVS), 21, 145–146
Crohn's disease
reoperation, 220
surgical therapy, 219
technique, 220–221

D
Digestive tract surgery
case study, 30–31
clinical principles, 28
early diagnosis and repair, 28
early recognition and intervention, 27–28
infectious complications, 27
laboratory principles, CRP, 29
leakage rates, 27
patient condition assessment, 28
postoperative mortality, 27
quality control, 31–32
radiology principles, CT scanning, 29–30
wait-and- see policy, 31
Distal pancreatectomy, 205–206
Duodenal switch (DS), 102, 106, 120–121
Duodeno-pancreatic head surgery
anastomotic leakage
biliary anastomosis (*see* Biliary anastomosis)
enteric anastomosis (*see* Enteric anastomosis)
pancreatic anastomosis (*see* Pancreatic anastomosis)
chylous leakage
diagnosis and grading, 186
incidence and definition, 185–186
management and outcome, 186
prevention and risk factors, 187
delayed gastric emptying
diagnosis and grading, 184
incidence and definition, 183–184
management and outcome, 184–185
prevention and risk factors, 185
postpancreatectomy hemorrhage (PPH)
diagnosis and grading, 180
incidence and definition, 179–180
management and outcome, 180–183
prevention and risk factors, 183
PPPD, 171

E
Early recovery after surgery (ERAS) protocols, 10
End ileostomy, 255, 260, 261, 263
Endoscopic retrograde cholangiopancreatography (ERCP), 149–152, 162
Enteric anastomosis
diagnosis and grading, 178, 179
incidence and definition, 178
management and outcome, 179
prevention and risk factors, 179
Enterostomy, 109, 259, 260, 262
ERAS protocols. *See* Early recovery after surgery (ERAS) protocols
ERCP. *See* Endoscopic retrograde cholangiopancreatography (ERCP)
Esophageal surgery for benign disease
esophagomyotomy, 70
GERD, 67
Nissen fundoplication, 68–70
paraesophageal/hiatal hernia repair, 70–71
Esophageal surgery for cancer
anastomotic leakage
definition, 58
diagnosis, 58–59
incidence, 58
treatment, 59–60

Esophageal surgery for cancer (*cont.*)
- chylous leakage
  - definition, 60
  - diagnosis, 61
  - incidence, 60
  - treatment, 61–62
- classification, 54
- esophagectomy, 53
- late complications
  - fistula, 63–65
  - strictures, 65–66
- minimally invasive esophageal surgery, 56, 66–67
- nonsurgical complications
  - cardiac complications, 57
  - pulmonary complications, 56
- prognostication, 54
- RLN paralysis
  - definition, 62
  - diagnosis, 62
  - incidence, 62
  - treatment, 62–63
- severity of complications, 54, 55

Esophagojejunostomy leakage
- diagnosis, 89–90
- nutritional status optimization, 88
- surgical technique, 88–89
- treatment, 90–91

Esophagomyotomy, 70

F

Fast-track surgery
- complex elective open surgery, 48
- GI surgery, 21
- LAFA trial, 50–51
- laparoscopic *vs.* open surgery, 48–50

Fecal peritonitis
- abdominal CT, 229
- anastomotic leakage, 230
- inflamed/thickened bowel, 230
- intra-abdominal abscess, 231
- intraoperative flexible sigmoidoscopy, 230
- randomized controlled trials, 230
- tension-free anastomosis, 230

Finsterer-Bancroft-Plenk procedure, 85, 86

G

Gastric surgery
- bleeding ulcer repair, 94–98
- duodenal perforation closure, leakage, 93–94
- esophagojejunostomy leakage, 88–91
- intraluminal and intra-abdominal postoperative bleeding
  - abdominal angiography CT scan, 80, 81
  - anastomoses, 79–80
  - clinical manifestations, 80
  - endoscopic treatment, 82
  - initial resuscitation, 82
  - intra-abdominal bleeding, 82
  - jejunojejunostomy, 79
  - laboratory, 80
  - treatment, 81
- laparoscopic gastrectomy, 78–79
- morbidity and mortality rates, 76, 77
- MRC gastric cancer trial, 76
- neoadjuvant therapy, 75
- nonfatal complications, 78
- pancreatectomy, 77
- peritonitis
  - acute pancreatitis, 87
  - causes, 83
  - clinical manifestations, 85–86
  - closure techniques, 84–86
  - CT scan, 86
  - duodenal stump leakage, 84
  - local duodenal conditions, 84
  - postoperative diagnosis, 83
  - postoperative jaundice, 88
  - prevention, 83
  - relaparotomy, 83
  - treatment, 83–84, 86–87
- risks factors, 76, 77
- splenectomy, 77, 78
- stenosis-obstruction, 91–92

Gastroesophageal reflux disease (GERD), 38, 67

Gastrointestinal (GI) surgery
- hospital resources, 20–21
- hospital volume/surgeons volume, 20
- important factors, 19
- monitoring system, 22–24
- process of care
  - clinical observation, 22
  - early recognition and intervention, 21–22
  - fast-track surgery, 21
  - laboratory tests, 22
  - organizatorial aspects, 21
  - pain management, 21
  - patient selection, 21
  - perioperative care and surgical procedure standards, 21
  - structure and surgical outcome, 22, 23
- superficial wound infection, 19

GERD. *See* Gastroesophageal reflux disease (GERD)
GI surgery. *See* Gastrointestinal (GI) surgery

H
Hartmann's procedure, 242–244
Hemorrhoids, proctology
conventional hemorrhoidectomy, 268–271
hemorrhoidal arterial ligation, 273
LigaSure hemorrhoidectomy, 268
pelvic sepsis, 268
stapled hemorrhoidectomy, 271–272

I
Ileal pouch-anal anastomosis (IPAA), 237–239
International Study Group of Pancreatic Surgery (ISGPS), 172, 179–181, 184
Intra-abdominal abscess, 212, 213, 231
Intraductal papillary mucinous neoplasm (IPMN), 205
Intraoperative cholangiography (IOC), 128, 145, 148

J
Jejunojejunostomy, 79, 82

K
Klatskin tumors
Bismuth-Corlette classification, 164–165
complications and mortality, 167–168
diagnostic tools, 162
postoperative complications prevention, 162–164
preoperative approach, 162–164
surgery
hepaticojejunostomy, 166, 167
intraoperative ultrasonography, 166
liver resection surface, 166
prognostic factor, 166
PTC drains, 166
symptoms and differential diagnosis, 161–162

L
Laparoscopic adjustable gastric banding (LAGB)
band erosion, 115–116
band slip and pouch dilatation, 114–115
normal situation, 113
port-site infections, 116
tube breakage, 116–117
Laparoscopic colorectal resections
anastomotic leakage, 254–256
bowel ischemia and bleeding
fenestrated grasper, 251
left-sided resection, 249–251
right-sided dissection, 249, 250
splenic vein, 250, 251
vessel sealing equipment, 249
C-reactive protein, 249
diagnosis, 249
internal herniation, 252–253
laparoscopic approach, 247, 248
"late" conversion, 247–249
learning curve, 248
stool-loaded bowel, 248
treatment, 249
trocar site hernia, 247, 253–255
ureter damage, 251–252
Laparoscopic gastrectomy, 78–79
Laparoscopic Heller myotomy (LHM), 38–39
Laparoscopic ileocecal surgery
Crohn's disease
reoperation, 220
surgical therapy, 219
technique, 220–221
preoperative preparations, 217
proper plane, 218–219
Laparoscopic sleeve gastrectomy (LSG), 117–119
Laparoscopic surgery
closure techniques, 321
colon cancer surgery
Barcelona trial, 40, 41
COLOR I study, 41
cosmetic long-term effect, 43
COST study, 41
"intention to treat" principle, 42
MRC CLASICC study, 41
opaque wound dressing, 41
operating time, 44
postoperative quality of life, 44
postoperative recovery, 43
stage III colon cancer, 40
Transatlantic study, 41
esophageal surgery, 36–39
evidence-based surgery, 35
gastric surgery, 39–40
minimally invasive surgery procedure, 35
pneumoperitoneum
closed *vs.* open technique, 320
Cochrane's search strategy, 320

Laparoscopic surgery (*cont.*)
direct trocar placement, 319, 320
open Hasson technique, 319
optical view technique, 319
Palmer's point, 320
Pearson Chi² analysis, 319
safety and effective method, 319
SAGES guidelines, 319, 321
Veress needle, 319, 321
rectal cancer surgery, 44
Left colon, sigmoid, and rectal surgery
anastomosis
asymptomatic, 232–233
dramatic early leak, 231–232
fecal diversion, 234
ileoanal pouch, 237–238
LAR, 235
pelvic drains, 234
sigmoid, 235–237
subtle insidious, 232
fecal peritonitis
abdominal CT, 229
anastomotic leakage, 230
inflamed/thickened bowel, 230
intra-abdominal abscess, 231
intraoperative flexible sigmoidoscopy, 230
randomized controlled trials, 230
tension-free anastomosis, 230
Hartmann's procedure, 242–244
ileoanal pouch fistulas, 238–240
infection perineal, 241–242
perineal hernia, 242
presacral abscess, 234–235
rectovaginal fistulas, 240–241
LHM. *See* Laparoscopic Heller myotomy (LHM)
LigaSure hemorrhoidectomy, 268
Liver surgery
air embolism, 126–127
biliary complications, 128–129
indications, surgical technique, and morbidity, 123–125
infected collections, 129
intraoperative and postoperative bleeding
inferior vena cava, 124–125
origin of, 124
prevention, 125–126
treatment, 126
liver transplantation (*see* Liver transplantation (LT))
postoperative liver failure, 127–128
Liver transplantation (LT)
arterial complications
clinical features, 132
etiology, 131–132
prevention, 133
treatment, 133
biliary complications
arterial thrombosis, 138–139
bile duct, 137–138
biliary fistula, 135, 136
permeable hepatic artery, 136–137
reconstruction techniques, 135–136
T tube removal, 137
postoperative bleeding
diagnosis, 130
etiology, 130
predisposing factors, 129–130
prevention, 131
treatment, 131
venous complications
portal vein thrombosis, 134–135
vena cava thrombosis, 133–134
Loop enterostomy, 260
Low anterior resection (LAR), 235
LSG. *See* Laparoscopic sleeve gastrectomy (LSG)

M

Magnetic resonance cholangiopancreatography (MRCP), 88, 138, 150, 151, 153, 162, 177, 205
Medical quality, 13
Medical Research Council (MRC) gastric cancer trial, 76
Minimally invasive esophageal surgery (MIE), 56, 66–67
Minimally invasive esophagectomy (MIO), 36–37
Minimally invasive step-up approach, 8
Mono-iodo-benzyl-guanidine (MIBG), 203
Morbidity rates, 7–8

N

National Surgical Quality Improvement Program (NSQIP), 24
Nissen fundoplication, 68–69

O

Obesity surgery. *See* Bariatric surgery
Obesity surgery mortality risk score (OS-MRS), 106

Open abdomen approach treatment
abdomen excision, 315, 316
MOF, 313
ongoing sepsis, 313
Parietex®, 317
patient feeding, 313
tangential excision, 315, 316
vacuum-assisted closure device, 314
Vicryl mesh®, 315
Open Hasson technique, 319

P
Pancreatic anastomosis
diagnosis and grading, 172–174
incidence and definition, 172
management and outcome, 173–175
risk factors and prevention, 175–176
Paraesophageal/hiatal hernia repair, 70–71
Parietex®, 317
Pearson Chi2 analysis, 319
Percutaneous transhepatic cholangiography (PTC), 88, 149, 150, 153, 162, 166, 168
Perineal hernia, 242, 243
Peristomal sepsis, 262, 263
Peritonitis
acute pancreatitis, 87
causes, 83
clinical manifestations, 85–86
closure techniques, 84–86
CT scan, 86
duodenal stump leakage, 84
local duodenal conditions, 84
postoperative diagnosis, 83
postoperative jaundice, 88
prevention, 83
relaparotomy, 83
treatment, 83–84, 86–87
Postoperative pancreatic fistula (POPF), 172–176, 182
PPPD. *See* Pylorus-preserving pancreatoduodenectomy (PPPD)
Preoperative mechanical bowel preparation, 9
Preoperative setting, 8–9
Presacral abscess, 234–235
Proctological disorders
fissure
advancement flap, 274–275
complications, 275–276
lateral internal sphincterotomy, 274
fistula
complications, 276–277
fistulotomy, 277
Park's classification, 277
patient assessment, 277–283
hemorrhoids
conventional hemorrhoidectomy, 268–271
hemorrhoidal arterial ligation, 273
LigaSure hemorrhoidectomy, 268
pelvic sepsis, 268
stapled hemorrhoidectomy, 271–272
PTC. *See* Percutaneous transhepatic cholangiography (PTC)
Pylorus-preserving pancreatoduodenectomy (PPPD), 171, 178, 184–185

R
Rectovaginal fistulas (RVFs), 240–241
Recurrent laryngeal nerve (RLN) paralysis
definition, 62
diagnosis, 62
incidence, 62
treatment, 62–63
Right colectomy
duodenum, 221–222
ileocolic artery and ileocolic veins, 221
intracorporeal *vs.* extracorporeal anastomosis, 222–223
mediocaudal access, 222
peroperative complications
duodenum and small bowel injuries, 224–225
ileocolic and mesenteric artery, 224
structures, 223–224
postoperative complications
anastomotic leakage, 225–226
intra-abdominal abscess, 226
prolonged postoperative ileus, 226–227
RLN paralysis. *See* Recurrent laryngeal nerve (RLN) paralysis
Routine preoperative biliary stenting, 8
Roux-Y gastric bypass (RYGB) bypass, 102, 103, 111–112
RVFs. *See* Rectovaginal fistulas (RVFs)

S
SIRS. *See* Systemic inflammatory response syndrome (SIRS)
Sleeve gastrectomy, 102, 105
Small bowel surgery
acute appendicitis, 211–213
anastomosis, 209–210
Cochrane systematic review, 210
Crohn's disease., 209

Small bowel surgery (*cont.*)
intervention, 210–211
intestinal obstruction, 210–211
laparoscopic surgery, pregnancy, 214
types of, 210
Solid pseudopapillary neoplasm (SPPN), 205
Spleen
angiography, 200
complication, 202
gastric leakage, 202
laparoscopic splenectomy, 201
pancreatic fistula, 201–202
risk factors, 202
size assessment, 201
thrombocytopenia, 200
types, 199
Stapled hemorrhoidectomy, 271–272
Stenosis, 91–92, 111, 132–134, 137–139, 152, 164, 235–237, 264
Stoma surgery
bowel, 263
cecostomy, 263
complications, 263–264
end-ileostomy, 261
eversion colostomy, 260, 261
fistula, 265
fixation, 261
intestinal obstruction, 265
intestinal stomas/enterostomy, 259
loop ileostomy, 262
necrosis, 263, 265
stomal sepsis, 265
trephine, 260
visual inspection, 261–262
Surgical complications
Clavien–Dindo classification, 14–16
definition, 13
grades, 14
sequelae, 14
Systemic inflammatory response syndrome (SIRS), 85, 87, 94, 191, 193

T
Total mesorectal excision (TME) procedure, 2, 234
Trocar site hernia (TSH), 253–255

V
Vacuum-assisted closure (VAC) therapy, 291–292, 314
Vacuum-assisted fascial closure (VAFC) therapy, 293
Vasculo-biliary injury (VBI)
accessory duct, 151
cause of, 149
infundibular technique, 149
ischemia, 152
RHA injury isolation, 152
vascular reconstruction/partial hepatectomy, 152
Vertical banded gastroplasty (VBG), 119–120
Vicryl mesh®, 315

MIX
Papier aus verantwortungsvollen Quellen
Paper from responsible sources
FSC® C105338

If you have any concerns about our products,
you can contact us on
ProductSafety@springernature.com

In case Publisher is established outside the EU,
the EU authorized representative is:
Springer Nature Customer Service Center GmbH
Europaplatz 3, 69115 Heidelberg, Germany

Printed by Libri Plureos GmbH
in Hamburg, Germany